AIDS, Politics, and Music in South Africa

This book offers an original anthropological approach to the AIDS epidemic in South Africa. Based on more than 15 years' association with the region, it demonstrates why AIDS interventions in the former homeland of Venda have failed – and possibly even been counterproductive. It does so through a series of ethnographic encounters, from kings to condoms, which expose the ways in which biomedical understanding of the virus have been rejected by – and incorporated into – local understandings of health, illness, sex, and death. Through the songs of female initiation, AIDS education, and wandering minstrels, the book argues that music is central to understanding how AIDS interventions operate. It elucidates a hidden world of meaning in which people sing about what they cannot talk about, where educators are blamed for spreading the virus, and in which condoms are often thought to cause AIDS. The policy implications are clear: African worldviews must be taken seriously if AIDS interventions in Africa are to become successful.

Fraser G. McNeill is a Senior Lecturer in the Department of Anthropology and Archaeology at the University of Pretoria, South Africa. He was awarded a PhD by the Department of Anthropology at the London School of Economics in 2007 and received the Audrey Richards Prize from the African Studies Association, UK, in 2008 for his thesis. He is a co-author of the 2009 *AIDS Review* for the Centre for the Study of AIDS at the University of Pretoria, and he has published articles in *African Affairs* and *South African Music Studies*, as well as chapters in several edited volumes.

THE INTERNATIONAL AFRICAN LIBRARY

General Editors

J. D. Y. PEEL, *School of Oriental and African Studies, University of London*
SUZETTE HEALD, *London School of Economics and Political Science*
DEBORAH JAMES, *London School of Economics and Political Science*

The International African Library is a major monograph series from the International African Institute and complements its quarterly periodical *Africa*, the premier journal in the field of African studies. Theoretically informed and culturally sensitive ethnographies and studies of social relations 'on the ground' have long been central to the Institute's publications programme. The IAL includes works focused on development, especially on the linkages between the local and national levels of society; studies in the social and environmental sciences; and historical studies with social, cultural, and interdisciplinary dimensions.

For a list of titles published in the series, please see the end of the book.

AIDS, Politics, and Music in South Africa

Fraser G. McNeill
University of Pretoria, South Africa

International African Institute, London
and

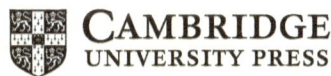

CAMBRIDGE
UNIVERSITY PRESS

32 Avenue of the Americas, New York NY 10013-2473, USA

Cambridge University Press is part of the University of Cambridge.

It furthers the University's mission by disseminating knowledge in the pursuit of education, learning and research at the highest international levels of excellence.

www.cambridge.org
Information on this title: www.cambridge.org/9781107417564

© Fraser G. McNeill 2011

This publication is in copyright. Subject to statutory exception and to the provisions of relevant collective licensing agreements, no reproduction of any part may take place without the written permission of Cambridge University Press.

First published 2011
First paperback edition 2014

A catalogue record for this publication is available from the British Library

Library of Congress Cataloguing in Publication data

McNeill, Fraser G., 1977–
AIDS, politics, and music in South Africa / Fraser G. McNeill.
  p. ; cm. – (International African library ; no. 42)
Includes bibliographical references and index.
ISBN 978-1-107-00991-2 (hardback)
1. HIV infections – Prevention – South Africa. 2. HIV infections – Social aspects – South Africa. 3. Music – South Africa. I. Title. II. Series: International African library ; no. 42.
[DNLM: 1. HIV Infections – prevention & control – South Africa. 2. Anthropology, Cultural – South Africa. 3. Health Knowledge, Attitudes, Practice – South Africa. 4. Music – South Africa. WC 503.6]
RA643.86.S6M386 2011
362.196'97920096–dc22   2011001950

ISBN 978-1-107-00991-2 Hardback
ISBN 978-1-107-41756-4 Paperback

Additional resources for this publication at
www.cambridge.org/9781107009912

Cambridge University Press has no responsibility for the persistence or accuracy of URLs for external or third-party internet websites referred to in this publication, and does not guarantee that any content on such websites is, or will remain, accurate or appropriate.

For other publications of the International African Institute, please visit its Web site at www.internationalafricaninstitute.org.

*For my mum, dad, and sister
and*
*in loving memory of
Humbulani Nekhavhambe:
1974–2007*

Soon we shall experience the death of birth itself if we go on at this rate.
Zakes Mda, *Ways of Dying* (1995)

Contents

Maps		*page* xi
Preface		xiii
Acknowledgements		xv
Abbreviations		xvii
Select Glossary of Tshivenda Terms in the Text		xix
1	Introduction: AIDS, Politics, and Music	1
2	The Battle for Venda Kingship	26
3	A Rite to AIDS Education? Venda Girls' Initiation, HIV Prevention, and the Politics of Knowledge	74
4	'We Want a Job in the Government': Motivation and Mobility in HIV/AIDS Peer Education	114
5	'We Sing about What We Cannot Talk About': Biomedical Knowledge in Stanza	154
6	Guitar Songs and Sexy Women: A Folk Cosmology of AIDS	180
7	'Condoms Cause AIDS': Poison, Prevention, and Degrees of Separation	203
8	Conclusion	232
	Appendix A: Songs on Accompanying Web Site	243
	Appendix B: 'Zwidzumbe' (Secrets)	244
	Appendix C: AIDS, AIDS, AIDS	250
	References	251
	Index	273

Maps

1. Limpopo Province (incorporating the former homeland of Venda) in South Africa. *page* xxii
2. Boundaries between the main kingdoms in the former homeland of Venda. xxiii
3. The Mphephu/Tshivhase border within Limpopo Province. xxiv
4. Selected villages referred to in the text. xxv

Preface

After leaving school in 1995, I decided to take a 'year out' – that quintessentially Western rite of passage – and ended up teaching English to adults in the Venda region of South Africa. Returning to Venda every year as the guitarist in a popular local reggae band, I found it impossible to escape the deeply held collective sentiment that all was not as it ought to be. South Africa's newly established democracy was under serious threat from something that most people knew as AIDS, but which no one wanted to talk about. By 2002, the football team for which I played in 1995 had lost almost half of its original squad to AIDS, all young men my age who succumbed to slow, painful, and humiliating deaths shrouded in public secrets and private suspicions.

Returning to Venda as a social anthropologist, I sought to make sense of this situation. Why, despite widespread prevention campaigns, does sexual behaviour remain largely unchanged? Why is there a stigma around condom use? Why is AIDS constructed as a public secret and how does this affect intervention projects? I established as the focus of my study the only people who were willing to talk openly about HIV, and who subsequently became amongst the main protagonists of this book: AIDS peer group educators.

Peer group education is a global phenomenon in the fight against HIV, and it takes various forms in different settings. In Venda, the groups are composed exclusively of young women who sing and dance at weekly public meetings, give out free condoms, and generally promote safer sexual behaviour. But it does not work, and in this book I explain why. In doing so, I take you on a journey from the lofty politics of kingship to the lowly places of gossip and rumour, demonstrating along the way that AIDS peer group education in this remote corner of South Africa is not part of the solution, but rather is part of the problem.

This book is an ethnographic account of AIDS told indirectly through my personal and ongoing sojourn in Venda, and the people that I have met along the way. Contrary to anthropological convention, I have not changed all the names of those whose knowledge I have plundered. My friends in Venda have been subject to my continual interrogations for more than fifteen years now, and most of them have asked to be identified by name in the text. However, when I do use pseudonyms, I let you know.

Many of the arguments I make in the following pages are either rooted in – or illustrated by – the analysis of songs. If you want to listen to the music you are reading about, songs referred to in the text can be downloaded free of charge from the Cambridge University Press Web site at www.cambridge.org/9781107009912.

Acknowledgements

I owe a massive thanks to Fiona Nicholson, Fliss Ingham, and Suzi Cook for their friendship, support, hot meals, and accommodation in Thathe Vondo over the last 15 years. Their house has often served as my second home, and I hope one day to repay their kindness. So many people have helped my research in Venda that it is impossible to acknowledge them all, and I apologise to anyone I have missed here. King Kennedy Tshivhase gave my research his blessing, oiling the wheels from the outset. Special thanks are also due to my research assistant and friend, Colbert Mushaisano Tshivhase. We did not always agree on the interpretation of events, but Colbert had a deep understanding of my anthropological aims and helped take my research in directions I had not considered. Much of what made its way into this book emerged from our late-night debates at Mapita's Tavern. Regular contributors to this often raucous forum were Mashamba Ligulube Mukwevho, Humbulani Nekhavhambe, Arinao Netshilema, Mulingoni Congo Mungoni, Pfene Nemugadi, David Davhidana, and Denga Tshivhase. Also, I have had the privilege of performing, recording, and writing music with Colbert Mukwevho and his brothers Mulalo, Sammy, Buddha, Clement, and Gift. Their creativity and musicianship will always inspire me. Jammin' in the Burnin' Shak with Harley, Cornerstone, and Percy was an absolute honour. Solomon Mathase taught me to play guitar Venda style and helped me translate the meaning of his songs. The peer educators allowed me to record and write about their songs, and Noriah Ralinala taught me the music and magic of female initiation. Thanks also to Traugott, Zilke, and Jeannie Fobbe; Zwiakonda Rathogwa; Justice Matshakatini; Rendani Tshautshau Nzhinga; Norman Sebe; Abel Neluvhalani; Betty Tshivhase; Mashudu Madache; Florence, Brenda and Mr Chauke; Vho Joe; Godfrey Dederen; Melville Jacobz; Musanda Shandukani Mudzunga; Vendula Rezacova; and Khosi T. N. Makhuya. In Thathe Vondo, my dog Simba proved a trusty and brave companion during the slow process of converting a thesis into a book.

Deborah James often went beyond the call of duty to assist me during my days at the London School of Economics (LSE), and I am very grateful for all the support she has given me. Jean Comaroff and Harry West examined my PhD thesis and provided me with insightful suggestions on how to develop the ideas. I have also benefited from the intellectual rigour imposed by participation in the weekly LSE anthropology seminars. Earlier versions of the arguments made in this book were rehearsed in conversations with Matthew Engelke, Jean La Fontaine, Isak Niehaus, Maurice Bloch, Charles Stafford, Olivia Harris, Michael Scott, Catherine Allerton, Fenella Cannell, Rita Astuti, Laura Bear, Mathijs Pelkmans, Michael Lambek, Girish Daswani, Emily Hitch, Jason Sumich, Maxim Bolt, George St Clair, Hans Steinmuller, Irene Calis, Giovanni Bochi, Casey High, Rory de Wilde, Nicolas Martin, Will Hammonds, Detlev Krige, Ilana van Wyk, Vicky Boydell, Elizabeth A. Hull, and Gwyn Prins. Also, Dave Turkon, Robert Thornton, and Alex Rodlach in the AIDS and Anthropology Research Group read and commented on earlier versions of Chapter 7. Mary Crewe, Jimmy Pieterse, and Johan Maritz at the Centre for the Study of AIDS and John Sharp in the Department of Anthropology and Archaeology at the University of Pretoria have helped me think of new directions for the future. In London, Chenjeri Shire ensured that I never forgot Tshivenda. Alistair Fraser compiled the maps. The editorial staff at Cambridge University Press and Stephanie Kitchen at the International African Institute have given me invaluable advice in the politics of publishing a monograph. Later, Mike Kirkwood turned the otherwise forbidding task of working through copyedits into a pleasure.

I gratefully acknowledge financial assistance from the Economic and Social Research Council (UK) and the Barcapel Foundation.

Abbreviations

Agriven	Venda Agricultural Corporation Ltd.
AIC(s)	African Independent Church(es): used in singular (AIC) as adjective
ANC	African National Congress
ARDC	Agric Rural Development Corporation
ARV	Antiretroviral
AusAID	Australian Agency for International Development
AZT	azidothymidine (ARV drug)
BEE	Black economic empowerment
BMF–STF	Bristol-Myers Squibb Foundation–Secure the Future
BONGO	Bank-organised NGO
CBI	Community-based initiative
CONTRALESA	Council of Traditional Leaders of South Africa
COPE	Congress of the People
COSATU	Congress of South African Trade Unions
DfID	Department for International Development
ELCSA	Evangelical Lutheran Church of South Africa
GEAR	Growth, Employment, and Redistribution Strategy
GONGO	Government-organised NGO
FAP	Forum for AIDS Prevention
FHI	Family Health International
HBC	Home-based care
HIV/AIDS	Human Immunodeficiency Virus/Acquired Immune Deficiency Syndrome
IKS	Indigenous knowledge systems
JOHAP	Joint HIV/AIDS programme
KAP	Knowledge, Attitudes and Practice
LHR	Lawyers for Human Rights
MDM	Movement for Democracy
MSF	Médecins San Frontières
NAPWA	National Association for People Living with AIDS
NDA	National Development Agency
NEPAD	New Partnership for Africa's Development

NGO	Non-governmental organisation
NMCF	Nelson Mandela Children's Fund
NPO	Non-profit organisation
NUM	National Union of Mineworkers
OVC	Orphans and vulnerable children
PEPFAR	President's Emergency Plan for AIDS Relief
PLWH	People Living with HIV and AIDS
PMTCT	Prevention of mother-to-child transmission
PPASA	Planned Parenthood Association of South Africa
PSG	Project Support Group
RDP	Reconstruction and Development Programme
SABC	South African Broadcasting Corporation
SACSIS	South African Civil Society Information Service
SAIRR	South African Institute of Race Relations
SANAC	South African National AIDS Council
SBP	Soutpansberg Petroleum
TAC	Treatment Action Campaign
TVBC (states)	Transkei, Venda, Bophuthatswana, and Ciskei (apartheid 'independent homeland states')
TDT	Tshivhase Development Trust
TTA	Tshivhase Territorial Authority
TTC	Tshivhase Tribal Council
UDF	United Democratic Front
USAID	United States Agency for International Development
VCT	Voluntary counselling and testing
VDC	Venda Development Corporation
VIPP	Venda Independence People's Party
VNP	Venda National Party
VSO	Voluntary Services Overseas (UK)
ZCC	Zion Christian Church

Select Glossary of Tshivenda Terms in the Text

Domba: The final rites of female initiation, performed after *vhusha*.
Domba la tshifularo: *Domba* of the first count.
Doroboni: In town.
Dzekiso: Name given to the senior wife of a king who will bear the heir to the throne.
Gota: Headman, in charge of a specific area under a *khosi*.
Hogo: Colloquialism for *murundu*, the male circumcision lodge, in which *hogo* is the main song.
Inyanga: Traditional healer (from isiZulu, but used widely in Tshivenda).
Khondomu: Condom.
Khoro: Weekly public meeting at a chief's kraal.
Khosi (plural, *mahosi*): Chief, 'senior traditional leader'.
Khosikhulu: Paramount king.
Khotsi: Father.
Losha: To greet humbly by putting palms of hands together, either seated or kneeling on the ground.
Mabundu: Non-alcoholic traditional maize drink.
Mahafhe: Alcoholic drink made from fermented maize meal.
Makhadzi: Paternal aunt. The king's *makhadzi* plays a special advisory and ritual role.
Malende: Songs and dances sung to accompany beer drinking or general festivities.
Malofha: Blood.
Malombo: Possession dance, rites of affliction.
Malwadze: Sickness.
Malwadze dza vhafumakadzi: The illnesses of women.
Mudabe (plural, *midabe*): Graduates of *vhusha* who instruct younger initiates.
Muduhulu: Sister's daughter.
Mudzimu (alternatively *Murena*): The Christian God.
Mufarakano (plural, *mafarakano*): Secret lover.
Mufhufha: Venda version of solitaire.
Mufumakadzi (plural, *vhafumakadzi*): Woman.

Mukololo (plural, *vhakololo*): Royal person.

Mukoma: Petty headman. The plural, *Vhakoma*, can be used as an honorific greeting for a *Mukoma*, but *Vhakoma* also refers to the chief's mother.

Mulayo (plural, *milayo*): Laws/rules, usually in reference to that which is associated with initiation schools.

Mulimo: Evil poison, as used by a witch.

Murundu: Male circumcision lodge.

Musanda: The name of the chief or king's royal courtyard.

Musevheto: Early initiation rites for very young girls.

Mushonga: Medicine.

Musiwana (plural, *vhasiwana*): Commoner.

Muti: Colloquialism for *mushonga*.

Mutupo (plural, *mitupo*): Clan.

Mvelele: Culture.

Ndumi: Male adviser to a traditional leader.

Ngoma: Drum.

Ngoma dza vhadzimu: Alternative term for the *malombo* possession ritual.

Nwenda (plural, *minwenda*): Traditional cloth worn by Venda women, originally made from salempore.

Shedo (plural, *mashedo*): Ritual apron worn by female initiates at the *vhusha* and *domba* ceremonies.

Sialala: Traditions, of former generations.

Singo: Name of the clan who crossed the Limpopo in the late 1600s, conquering *Vhangona* to form 'the Venda'. *Musingo* means 'elephant's trunk'.

Thabeloni: Prayer meetings held at sunset every night during the week before a funeral.

Thevhula: Rites of ancestral sacrifice.

Thivela: To prevent.

Thovhela: King.

Tshefu: Evil drug, as used by a witch.

Tshidzumbe (plural, *zwidzumbe*): Secret.

Tshifhase: Adolescent dance.

Tshigombela: A dance for women.

Tshikona: The Venda national reed dance, performed by men.

Tshilombe (plural, *zwilombe*): A male-dominated guitar genre.

Tshivhambo: Name given to the ritual hut in which female initiation rites take place.

Tshivhidzo: Emergency meeting held by a chief in times of crisis.

Venda: Used to refer to the physical locality where Venda people (singular, *Muvenda*; plural, *Vhavenda*) live. The language can be called Tshivenda or Luvenda, but is also referred to as Venda.

Vhadzimu (alternatively *Midzimu*): Ancestral spirits, no singular.
Vhamusanda (singular and plural): Headman.
Vhatei: Initiates in *vhusha* or *domba*.
Vhudsekani: Sexual intercourse.
Vhuhosi: Installation ceremony for a new headman, chief, or king.
Vhusha: Female initiation school attended after the first menses.
Vhutali wa midzimu: Ancestral wisdom.
Vhutungu: Poison from the natural world.
Zwilonda: Pimples/sores.
Zwirendo: Praises.

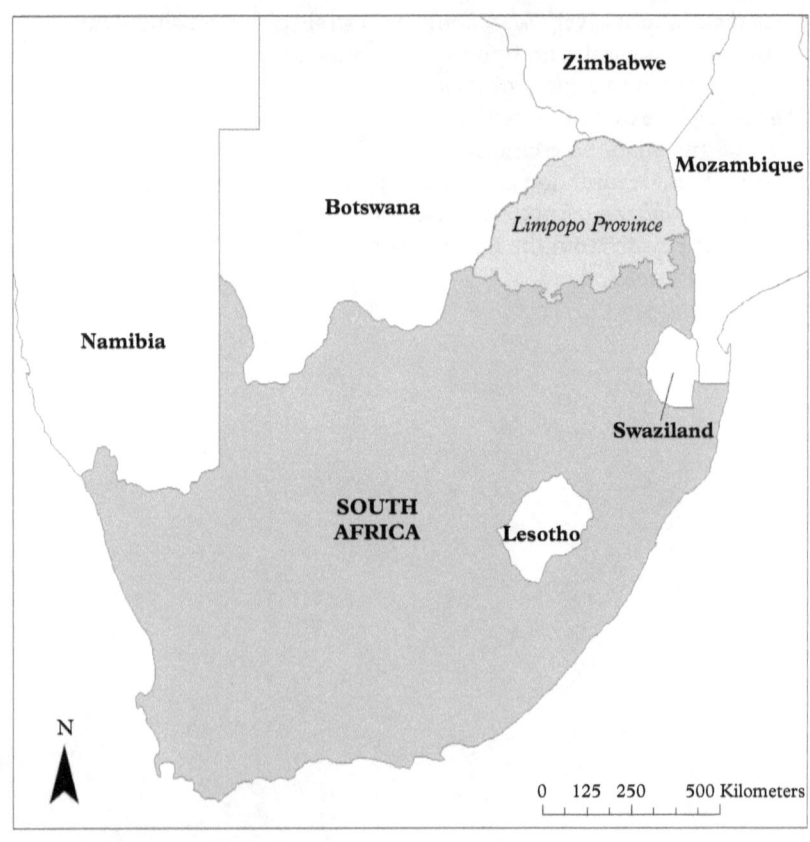

Map 1. Limpopo Province (incorporating the former homeland of Venda) in South Africa.

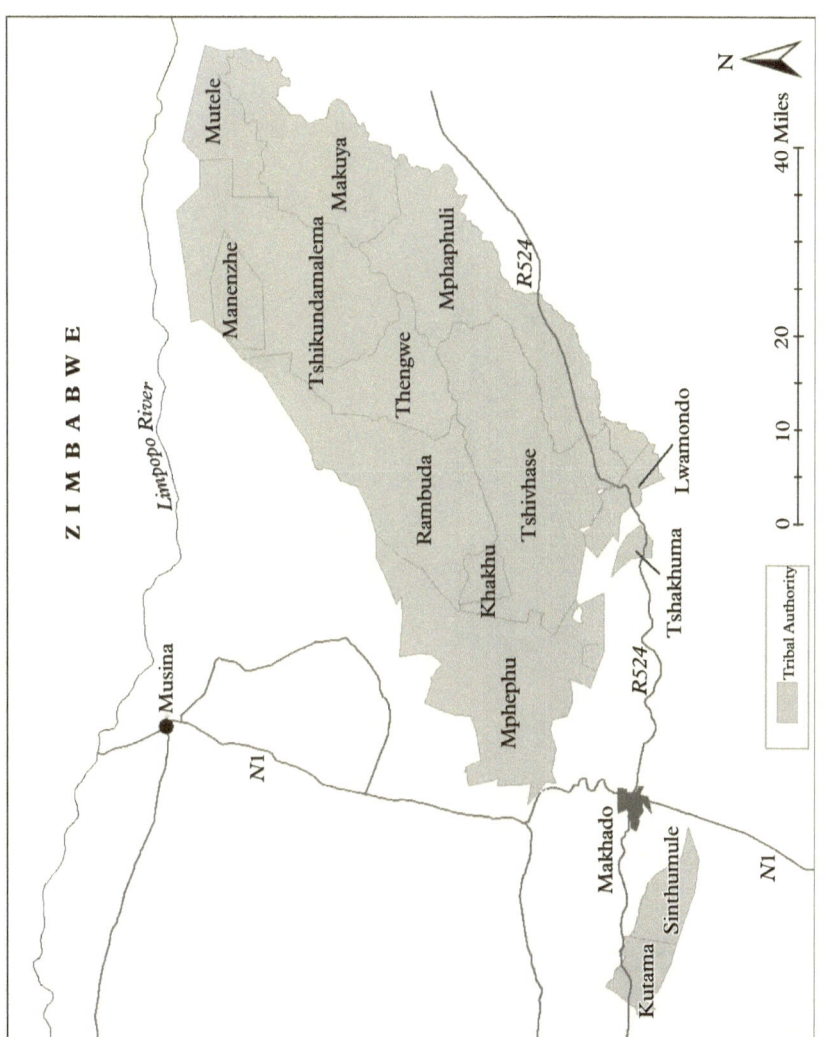

Map 2. Boundaries between the main kingdoms in the former homeland of Venda.

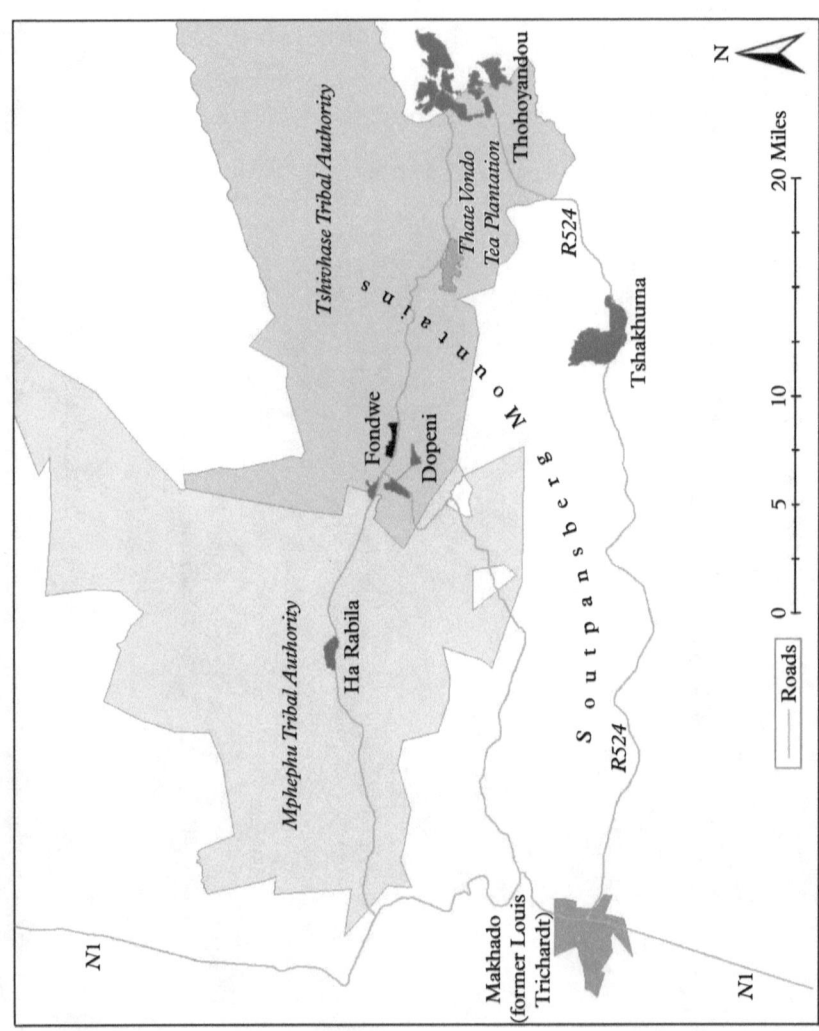

Map 3. The Mphephu/Tshivhase border within Limpopo Province.

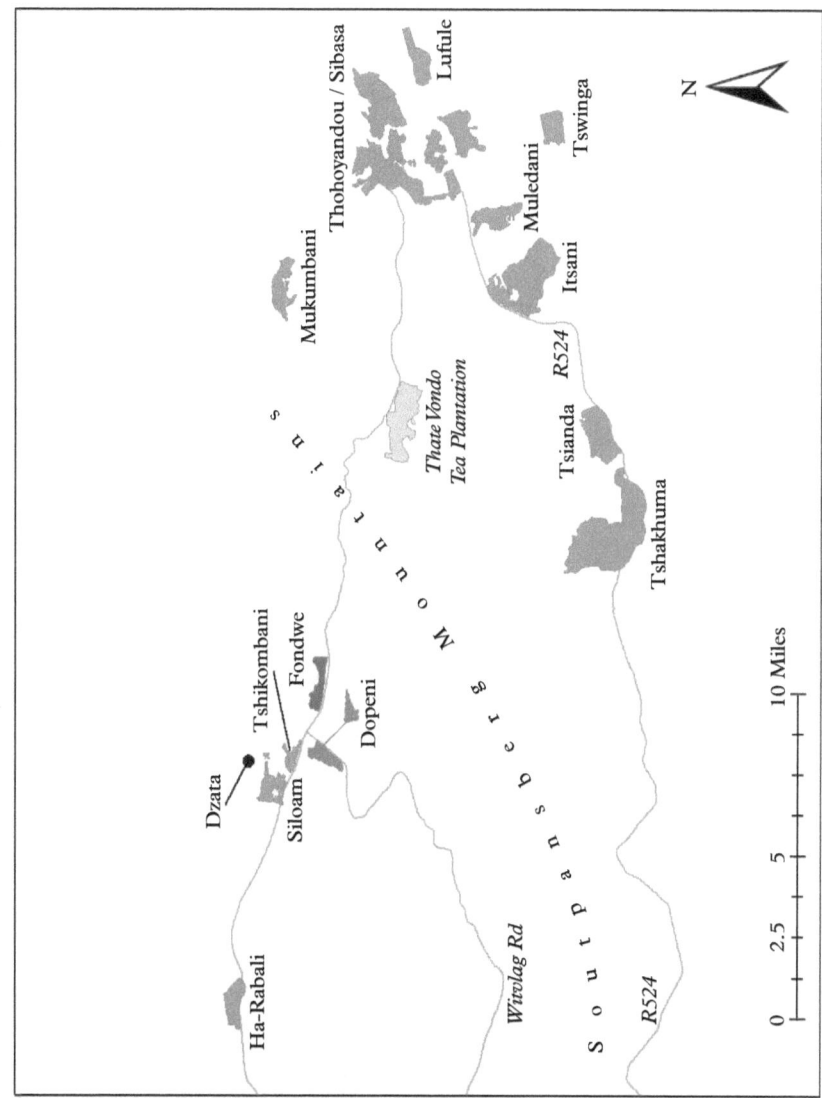

Map 4. Selected villages referred to in the text.

1 Introduction

AIDS, Politics, and Music

AIDS and Music in Venda

The peer educators had already gathered outside the Midway Bottle Store as I climbed out of the mini-bus taxi and headed through the barbed wire gates into the crowd. It was March 2005, late afternoon on a month-end Friday, and the usual mix of recently paid drinkers and thirsty beggars had taken up residence for the evening ahead. Slowly, a group of young women dressed in bright red skirts and smart polo shirts with 'Prevention is Better than Cure' on their backs formed a long line. In single file, each holding onto the performer in front of her in symbolic re-enactment of the famous Venda girls' initiation python dance (*domba*), they forced their way through the crowd towards the main seating area next to the bar. The song that accompanied their intrusion into the men's drinking session had a familiar melody, but it was not from the *domba* repertoire. Instead, it was based on a well-known song from the anti-apartheid days in praise of ANC stalwart Joe '*Ntate*' Modise.[1] The echo of peer educators singing in the sparse drinking arena prompted sporadic tenor and bass accompaniment from groups of men perched on empty beer crates, but the male and female vocal parts struggled to find harmony: the educators had changed the lyrics. Shuffle-stepping towards the bar, they were met with a combination of laughter, feigned shock, anger, and indifference as the audience made out the new words:

Khondomu ndi bosso!	Condom is the boss!
I thivhela malwadze!	It prevents sickness!
Khondomu nga i shume.	Use condoms!
Khondomu ndi bosso!	Condom is the boss!

---

[1] Joe Modise (1929–2001) played an important role in establishing the military wing of the ANC (*Umkhonto we Sizwe*) and was the South African Minister of Defence from 1994 to 1999.

The term Venda is used throughout in reference to the formerly 'independent' homeland under the apartheid regime. Whilst Venda remains in common usage, the area is now formally known as the Vhembe District of the Thulamela Municipality. Along with the previous homelands of Lebowa and Gazankulu, Venda currently forms part of South Africa's Limpopo Province (see maps).

I took a seat next to some elderly men who seemed bewildered by the scene unfolding before them. Within minutes they made excuses to leave, making their way to the shaded area outside. Several others followed suit, leaving a handful hunched over bottles of beer and cracking jokes under their breath as the peer educators' performance got into full swing. An introductory drama about a drunk man sleeping with an HIV-positive girl before returning home to beat his wife and children proved controversial with the remaining audience: 'You should know, you are the prostitutes!' someone yelled. 'Don't come here with your AIDS story!' shouted another.

Thriving on the hostility, and with almost military precision, the educators assembled into a choir formation. They began to sing more songs and more loudly, encouraging each other to drown out any dissenting voices among the half-drunk hecklers. Turning to shock tactics, thrusting clenched fists filled with packets of condoms into the air, they performed a well-known gospel tune and 'Jesus is number one!' became 'Condom is number one!' Their raised fists imitated the defiant symbol of anti-apartheid activists, and, as the chorus continued, the leader of the song broke ranks to patrol the hall. Now she bellowed from above, directing her attention towards the remaining groups of drinkers: 'AIDS is killing us like the *Boer*[2] used to! You fought apartheid, now fight with us against AIDS!'

This had the desired effect. Faces from outside reappeared to stare through open windows at the educators who, at least briefly, were the centre of attention. A large wooden penis was produced, and they demonstrated to the audience how to safely fit and remove a condom. Unexpectedly, the fake phallus was snatched by a young man who used it as a prop in his own improvised drama – in which, to the hilarious delight of the crowd, he selected a group of educators for an imaginary orgy. One of the elderly men returned from outside to collect his pouch of tobacco. Amid the laughter, I offered him a seat. Refusing politely, he whispered into my ear: 'These things that you see here, they are the illnesses of women (*malwadze dza vhafumakadzi*), they are not our concern.'

The old man's passing comments are a useful place to begin this book. They encapsulate the fault lines along which knowledge of HIV/AIDS has entered the politics of everyday life in the far north-eastern corner of South Africa. In doing so, they allude to the unintended consequences of implementing peer education projects among young women, identified by policy makers as a group at high risk of HIV infection.

---

[2] *Boer* (literally, farmer) is a Dutch word that is widely used in South Africa to refer to Afrikaans-speaking groups who migrated north from the Cape, away from British colonial control, in the early 1800s. During the anti-apartheid struggle, *Boer* became synonymous with conservative supporters of the Nationalist government.

As a loose demographic cluster, young women in South Africa are indeed more likely to test HIV-positive than any other group.[3] The thrust of the arguments presented in this book, however, challenges the conventional wisdom of 'participatory development' through which such women have assumed the role of AIDS educators. I show in the pages to come the ways in which educators have been framed as vectors of the virus, reinforcing a patriarchal aetiology through which men and older women explain sexually transmitted disease in terms of blood-related taboos and the build-up of pollution in the bodies of certain young women. This has resulted in a paradoxical situation whereby many men are more concerned about *whom* they sleep with, rather than how 'safe' the encounter may be. In this sense, the evidence from Venda presents considerable obstacles to the effectiveness of current approaches to AIDS awareness in the region.

Perhaps surprisingly, this is not necessarily a negative attribute: at least not for the educators. As experts in the bioscientific discourse of the pandemic, they are engaged in attempts to achieve upward social mobility by securing employment in various aspects of public health care. Indeed, a significant proportion of them have obtained some form of employment in government clinics, hospitals, and non-governmental organisations (NGOs). One such organisation is the Forum for AIDS Prevention (FAP),[4] an NGO that acts as an umbrella and central administrative body for the 600 or so peer educators in the Venda region. The FAP has a history of securing large government contracts for AIDS-related initiatives such as voluntary counselling and testing, and peer educators, with their well-honed knowledge and experience, stand a strong chance of being employed in these new projects.

Peer education itself, however, is barely remunerated. Volunteers receive a small monthly stipend and only those promoted to the rank of project coordinator collect a more substantial allowance. Nonetheless, in the current context of rising unemployment, where neoliberal restructuring has brought an abrupt decline in migrant remittances and sharp rises in the cost of living, volunteering has become an attractive proposition. In rural post-apartheid South Africa, where much of the population is heavily dependent on government benefits, volunteering is a potential harbinger of sustenance and self-advancement. The educators' desire to change the social and sexual health environment in this part of rural South Africa is thus matched by their aspirations to transcend and move away from the site of their volunteering.

---

[3] See <http://www.unaids.org/en/Regions_Countries/Regions/SubSaharanAfrica.asp> (accessed 6 February 2007).
[4] A pseudonym.

Singing songs of AIDS thus serves a dual purpose (cf. McNeill and James 2009). It exposes the general public to the safe sex message, fulfilling the obligations of the NGO, whilst touting a fluency in biomedical knowledge of the kind which is valued in the public health sector. Their songs and dances are designed and rehearsed in the settings of 'ongoing training' and 'workshops', organised in collaboration with various donor agencies with the specific aim of refashioning pre-existing songs into contemporary pedagogic aids. The intention is to form a kind of musical 'trap' (Gell 1999). They make simple lyrical and stylistic adjustments with the intention of drawing in the audience, having them sing along, and inducing them to notice the new lyrics. This, in turn, is intended to encourage open discussion about their meaning. The educators, as biomedical experts, are trained to step in at this stage of the performance and furnish the audience with authoritative information about HIV/AIDS, before distributing free condoms.

As part of their daily routine, then, peer educators mine the depths of Venda's rich musical traditions. The prolific musicality of this region was first made famous by John Blacking, whose ethnomusicological account began in the late 1950s and spanned three decades. Blacking emphasised the extent to which musical performance is a marker of life-cycle events. For example, a young woman can only perform the songs and dances of the *vhusha* initiation ceremony, where she is taught how to manage bodily pollution, after her first menses. After a few years, she can 'graduate' into the *domba*, where song lyrics and actions demonstrate the skills required to run a household and satisfy a husband. In a similar fashion, boys pass into manhood through *murundu*, the initiation lodge at which they learn to perform *hogo*. *Hogo* is also part of the male public repertoire, and is often invoked to complete a *tshikona* reed dance or spontaneously at beer drinks by groups of men who were initiated together.[5] Periods of sickness and healing are also marked musically. Rites of affliction (*ngoma dza vhadzimu*) are performed through a ceremony known as *malombo*, during which ancestors are invited to possess those who are sick, and expose the reason for their illness. Various forms of Zionist/Pentecostal musical expressions serve similar, and similarly specific, purposes: to expel demons, perform miracles, and heal the sick.

---

[5] *Tshikona* is the national Venda reed dance performed by males of all ages. They are grouped by age and social status (royal/commoner) into cohorts, one for each note of the heptatonic scale upon which the genre is based. I learned to play *veve*, one of the smaller pipes towards the end of the phrase. The six reed pipes, *thakula, phala, dangwe, kholomo, veve,* and *nzhingi*, are blown continuously in descending order, punctuated by the leading Kudu horn – *phala* – which starts and ends the phrase, followed directly again by *thakula* ('the lifter') that introduces a new melody. This is accompanied by an anti-clockwise progression of the dancers, who follow the steps of the leader (who can take the *tshikona* in any direction). See Stayt (1931: 320–3) and listen to *tshikona* on the website at http://www.cambridge.org/us/9781107009912.

In Blacking's schema, music is thus an audible and visible sign of social and political groupings, and each genre is symbolically situated in relation to the centre of traditional authority (Blacking 1965: 36–7). The girls' *domba* initiation dance (Blacking 1969a–1969e) and the men's *tshikona*, for example, are both controlled by and performed for chiefs. They display loyalty to specific royal lineages, and as such have taken centre stage in the vibrant political economy of post-apartheid Venda. Following national trends and in response to localised internecine disputes, a revitalisation of chieftainship within the context of the new democratic dispensation has had far-reaching consequences for the performers of these genres and the bodies of knowledge they represent.

The boys' circumcision lodge (*murundu*), on the other hand, is privately owned and subject to a minimal degree of control by rulers. Although a nominal fee is paid to the traditional leaders of the area, and the first night after *murundu* is spent by initiates at the royal kraal, it is substantially less subject to chiefly influence than female initiation. This is evident in terms of spatial location: female initiation takes place at royal homesteads; its successive levels, progressing from marginal outposts of political power to its centre, mirror the chiefly hierarchy of the polity itself. *Murundu*, in comparison, is conducted in a specially made secluded clearing deep in the bush (*thavhani*, literally 'on the mountain' or *hogoni*, after the famous circumcision song, *hogo*). This relative autonomy has been eroded by state institutions but not by those of the chiefship. Since the mid-1930s, government licences have been necessary to hold *murundu*, and representatives from the Department of Health and Welfare regularly inspect proceedings. This has limited the extent to which lodges are conducted in seclusion, and the state has become increasingly concerned about surgical hygiene during circumcision.

Male circumcision was introduced to the region in the early 1800s by Lemba or Sotho groups, whereas female initiation is earlier in origin, dating back to Vhangona occupancy of the Soutpansberg Mountains (see Chapter 2; Stayt 1931: 125–9; van Warmelo 1932: 125). During the Singo migration from north of the Limpopo River into Venda in the late seventeenth century, the invaders incorporated female initiation rites into their structures of government. As *murundu* came much later, possibly from the south, it remained at the periphery of political power. To this day, *murundu* is conducted mostly by Lemba men (Vhashavi): an endogamous clan who – albeit on somewhat dubious grounds – claim ancient Jewish ancestry (cf. Parfitt 2002). As a result of this particular historical development, men who are potentially in line to the succession of royal power in Venda are never circumcised, forging a physical manifestation of distinction between royalty (*Vhakololo*) and commoners (*Vhasiwana*).

Like the peer educators' songs, Blacking's Venda work exposes a duality. He sought to conceptualise the apparent contradiction between music as a signifier of fixed social positions and equally a source of, and force for, social change. Different genres therefore served disparate functions. He considered some music, such as that from girls' initiation schools and the various musical expressions of Christian hymnody, as conservative in influence, the former reinforcing pre-existing positions in a rigid patriarchal hierarchy and the latter being rooted in the strictures and structures of a missionary past. On the other hand, he saw a potentially transformative quality in the Zionist-style independent African church music (Blacking 1995b), in *tshikona* (Blacking 1973: 51), and in the now extinct *bepha* musical expeditions involving competitive displays by youngsters of rival royal homesteads (Blacking 1962). For Blacking, then, musical performance could cement the hierarchies established through generational, gendered, and royal ties, whilst also being 'an expression of alternative visions of social order . . . [with] . . . an almost heroic capacity to alter the world' (James 2006: 72–4).

Blacking argued that, through these latter musical traditions, and *tshikona* in particular, performers engage in symbolic reconstructions of the social order by establishing harmonious relationships through complex intertwined yet integrated performances. In this way potential and actual enemies may be brought together through a state of being he called 'virtual time', bringing 'peace to the countryside' (Blacking 1973: 51) in the vested interests of chiefs and their subjects. This belief in the capacity of music to alter the world advantageously led Blacking to draw an analogy between 'humanly organised sound' and the realisation of 'soundly organised humanity' (Blacking 1973: 95): an insight which has proved productive for subsequent studies of musical traditions in Southern Africa (James 2006).[6]

This tension between music's ambiguous qualities is apparent in peer educators' songs. They reaffirm the volunteers' status as young women in an unyielding patriarchal structure, whilst simultaneously incorporating the revolutionary spirit of the anti-apartheid movement, via musical form, into AIDS education. In more practical terms, their performances create the possibility of material benefits, of earning a fixed income and achieving upward social mobility. Thus, the analysis of peer education music points to the shortcomings of categorising specific genres as having an 'either/or' effect. AIDS educators in Venda, like countless other performers throughout the world, weave local elements into songs and dances that hold more national and international significance. They blur the boundaries between, and perhaps even create new genres, through the syncretic and strategic blending of various musical traditions to harness the particular zeitgeist of their post-apartheid experience.

---

[6] See, for example, Coplan (1994), Erlmann (1991; 1996), James (1999), and Muller (1999).

Their songs represent a creative rearrangement of existing repertoires. As young women, however, the composers/performers of these songs have limited options. Again this points to their position in a gendered stratification of social status. Their alternatives include *malende* (beer drinking/celebratory songs), certain public aspects of female initiation (from the three consecutive stages of *musivheto*, *vhusha*, and *domba*), *tshigombela* (a widely performed but exclusively female genre with a particular form and technique), missionary and Zionist/Pentecostal-style church music, and a variety of non-gender-specific popular music such as songs of the struggle or singles from local and national charts. Music performed exclusively by men, such as that from the *tshikona* reed dance, songs from *murundu*, and *tshilombe* guitar music, fall outside of their potential repertoire. A *domba* girls' initiation dance can thus be fused with a popular anti-apartheid melody, and that melody can be laced with lyrics declaring AIDS as the new apartheid, or condoms as the second coming of Jesus Christ. Through this *bricolage*, peer educators seek to present 'the illnesses of women' as the illnesses of the nation, and the performers are at once fixed into the social structure, and potentially liberated from it, through performance.

However, the biomedical knowledge dispensed by peer educators is in play with competing – but not necessarily incommensurable – ideas about what AIDS is, where it came from, and how to prevent it. In these, scientific explanations have had to contend with a robust, but flexible, body of ritual knowledge. This knowledge, like the biomedicine touted by the peer educators, is explicitly concerned with the maintenance of healthy sexual and social reproduction. However the modes of transferring the two bodies of knowledge rely on very different social settings. Ancestral knowledge is transferred from ritual elders to initiates through the songs and dances of initiation ceremonies in ritual contexts that have flourished under recent processes of 'retraditionalisation'. In seeking to transfer this knowledge, ritual elders and traditional leaders act not only to gain a sense of control over the initiates, but to quell the consequences of a widely perceived 'crisis' through which they blame the erosion of generational/ancestral respect for the unprecedented recent increase in deaths (cf. Comaroff and Comaroff 2004). This book explores the relationship between these two bodies of scientific and ancestral knowledge against the backdrop of socio-cultural divisions of gender and generation through which people in Venda make sense of AIDS in their everyday lives.

Post-Apartheid Venda: Africa's Eden?

Depending on the time of year, the landscape within which this medley of song and dance takes place varies dramatically. After the variable summer rain from December to February, the countryside near the Soutpansberg mountain range, around which much of Venda is clustered, transforms into a vibrant hilly collage of deep greens and rich, reddish browns. If the rain has been favourable, rivers cut through the countryside, filling the lakes and dams. Villages of varying size and stature pepper the mountainsides, each falling under the control of a particular chief (*Khosi*, plural *Mahosi*) who, in turn, answers to the superior structures of regional traditional authorities – who answer, ultimately, to their employers in the provincial government's Office of the Premier.

To the far north and east, smaller and more sporadic villages mark the edges of the Soutpansberg. On this periphery, the deep greens fade into a dryer, dusty brown savannah that drops down towards the Indian Ocean via the former homeland of Gazankulu, the Kruger National Park, and on to Mozambique. To the north, Venda stretches towards the border towns of Musina and Beitbridge, across the Limpopo River, and into Zimbabwe (see maps).

A driver approaching Venda from the south along the highway from Johannesburg is greeted by large roadside billboards that entice him with promises of what lies ahead. From the outskirts of Pretoria they read: 'Limpopo: a Different World, Only Hours Away!', 'Venda, Experience the Land of Legend', 'The Road to the REAL Africa' until, eventually, on arrival, a sign proclaims 'Welcome to Africa's Eden!' On the huge posters, pictures of a *domba* initiation dance fade into picturesque snapshots of village life with earthenware pottery. Sparkling waterfalls feed the ancient, sacred Lake Fundudzi. Superimposed on this idyllic scene, artistic impressions of wildlife allude to a border with the Kruger National Park, another untouched corner of Africa. The driver might imagine himself as journeying into the past, to a forgotten, mystical land where humans live in harmony with nature and time stands still.

By marketing the Limpopo Province, and specifically the Venda region, as 'Africa's Eden', post-apartheid tourism bosses have drawn on a widely held stereotype. Tshivenda-speaking people (Vhavenda; singular, Muvenda) have long been portrayed as mysterious, insular, and culturally unique among South African ethnic groups. Several overlapping factors have contributed to this portrayal of a Venda ethnic identity. Geographically, the region is remote, nestling – as we have heard – at the foot of the Soutpansberg in the extreme north-east of the country. This peripheral location has led to a 'myth of Venda isolation' (Ralushai 1977) and of Venda resistance to outside influence. A well-known anecdote seems to prove this. During the so-called *Mfecane* in the nineteenth century, Shaka's regiments are said to have been unable to penetrate the inhospitable terrain or conquer the cunning Venda warriors, who hid in high mountain gullies and crushed the approaching Zulu aggressors by rolling large boulders down into their path.

The stereotypical representation of Venda as a remote and mystical hinterland is exacerbated by demographic and linguistic factors. Constituting just over one million people, only 2.3 per cent of the total South African population (Statistics South Africa 2003), Vhavenda are second only to amaNdebele as the country's smallest ethnic group. Unlike the siNdebele, isiZulu or isiXhosa languages, however, Tshivenda is not of Nguni origin, but is from 'the north' (*vhukaranga*) and has more affinity with the vast Niger-Congo linguistic cluster that includes Shona in Zimbabwe and Lozi in Zambia. For this reason, Tshivenda is not easily understood by Zulu or Xhosa speakers, and Vhavenda people in Johannesburg are often mistakenly referred to as *Makwerekwere* (foreigners).[7] Moreover, although many Vhavenda were recruited to become migrant labourers in the gold mines on the Rand and diamond mines near Pretoria, they often disguised their true ethnicity, for fear of minority victimisation, by speaking only in isiZulu at the workplace and in labour compounds. For this reason, they were largely excluded from studies of the South African migrant work force of the time (cf. Moodie 1994 or McNamara 1980).

The small group that originated in a place of distant mountains and who seemed to speak in a foreign tongue yet could blend into the cityscape were, and still are, treated with suspicion and renowned for their supposedly secretive character. This gave rise, inter alia, to the notion that Vhavenda are mythical masters of the occult who possess an extraordinary ability to invoke witchcraft: a conviction that has been reinforced by the perceived proliferation of witch killings and perpetual allegations of medicine murder (colloquially, '*muti* murder') in the area. Between 1985 and 1995, an estimated 389 alleged witches were murdered in the (then) Northern Province (Niehaus 2001a: 188; Ralushai et al. 1996). Sociological explanation of this episode has presented it partly in terms of young, male ANC Youth League 'comrades' reacting against the political authorities and traditional leaders who supported and often became office holders in the Bantustan governments.

Framing Venda as a part of Africa's Eden seems inappropriate in this macabre context. And yet in another sense the government's advertising strategy is an accurate depiction of bountiful fruitfulness: the omnipresent agricultural industry that is the cornerstone of Limpopo's economic contribution to the country.[8] Whilst most commercial-scale farming is to be

---

[7] This is a relatively recent derogatory term for non-South African black people, particularly those from the Niger-Congo area. Whilst Nguni and Niger-Congo languages share a certain amount of grammatical structure, the vocabularies and tonal qualities of the languages differ significantly.

[8] The most recent statistics available are from Statistics South Africa (2001). In early 2009, data from the 2006 census for Limpopo Province were as yet unavailable. In 2001, 'Agricultural related work' was second only to 'Community services' as the most common form of employment in Vhembe District.

found on farms that were part of the old 'white South Africa', there is also remarkably fertile land to be found within the borders of the previous homeland. This takes the form of bright red soil that nurtures in virtually every Venda homestead a selection of avocado, maize, mango, banana, orange, cherry, lemon, and pawpaw trees, the fruits of which are either consumed by the family or sold at roadside markets. However, private or community-run orchards in which the main subsistence crop of maize could be cultivated for the production of surplus have become less common in recent years. Through a combination of atypical drought, flash floods, and inadequate access to microfinance, and despite state-sponsored initiatives to reverse the trend, most communal farming projects in Venda have collapsed. This has left families reliant on commercially produced maize which, like all foodstuffs in recent years, has been subject to significant increases in retail price.

Despite Venda's potential for natural abundance, then, daily life in the region is characterised by socio-economic hardship and political trends broadly similar to those found in other parts of rural South Africa (cf., for example, Oomen 2005 in Sekhukhuneland; Ngwane 2004 in Transkei; White 2004 in KwaZulu-Natal). Recent government attempts to provide basic services such as water and electricity have been implemented very slowly, and supplies remain infrequent and unreliable. According to the most recently available government statistics, over 70 per cent of households in the Venda region still cook on wood fires, and fewer than 3 per cent have a water tap in the house (Statistics South Africa 2001). The burden of providing fuel and water is borne by women and children, who have little option but to make daily trips to collect them. With few exceptions, roads and the mini-bus taxis that traverse them are in various stages of disrepair. Opportunities for employment are scarce, with both personal and household incomes suffering as a result.

School leavers generally aspire to work 'in town' (*doroboni*), with destinations such as Polokwane, Pretoria, or Johannesburg in mind, while some even seek work abroad (*seli ha lwange* ['across the sea']). This small minority, mostly children of wealthy families, have achieved employment in Europe (mostly the United Kingdom) and North America, where they accumulate savings in foreign currencies before their visas expire and they are forced to return. As part of the 'internet generation', this young elite group of savvy Vhavenda use the worldwide web to maintain communication with each other and with those 'at home' who can access the internet – often through mobile phones. Whilst they and their families enjoy the economic and social benefits that come with upward mobility, their life experience marks them apart from the majority of young school leavers in Venda. For this latter group, rising unemployment has led to a dramatic decrease in successful attempts to find work of any kind, and an increase of suspicious envy towards those who do.

Introduction

Weekends in Venda are an ill-fitting mix of beer drinks, church services, football matches, and burials, whilst week nights are taken up with prayer meetings (*thabeloni*) for the deceased or with preparation for the funeral service and feast on Saturdays. This ritual activity centred on death is a grim reminder of the toll taken by the AIDS pandemic. Partly prompted by this health crisis and an associated moral panic, some groups of older men and women, at the forefront of a cultural revival undertaken with chiefly backing, have become ritual experts in initiation schools, closely mirroring those described by Blacking, through which they seek to reinforce social and moral order. Female initiation is particularly valuable in this quest because its ritual curriculum presents an ancestrally sanctioned system of regulations for the maintenance of health and fertility. The symbolic and material properties of menstrual blood are central to this system, and to the 'rules' (*milayo*) taught to initiates (*vhatei*) throughout the ritual process. The famous *domba* python dance and the other musical performances of girls' initiation have therefore been asserted as arenas for the propagation of traditional mores through which, some assert, the illness might be combated. Contesting this, peer educators assert their own versions of the musical tradition, as a means to inform the ignorant about the biomedical model of sexual disease transmission. Strategically utilised, contested, and refuted, different sets of values and ideas, each linked to its own set of practices yet also floating free of these, have come to the fore. These bodies of knowledge, and the people who promote them, compete with each other for legitimacy as they seek effective ways to overcome the disease.

Staying alive in such a setting, where financial insecurity is coupled with everyday reminders of death, is a matter of enduring a perceived crisis: it either leaves people adrift or leads them into complex webs of dependency and obligation. Funerals in South Africa are very costly affairs, often imposing substantial debt on the family of the deceased. In the absence of readily available employment, and with only partial uptake of insurance schemes, a death in the family increases the financial vulnerability of the poor. Financially unstable households are more susceptible to ill health, and in this context more likely to secure a basic cash income though quick-fix methods such as violent criminal activity or commercial sex work. This has the potential to create a grimly vicious circle, with death and financial insecurity mutually reinforcing one another.

Whilst Venda society is characterised by generational division, this dovetails with the separation of socio-political control along the lines of gender. In this patriarchal environment, young, unmarried women often strike up multiple concurrent 'transactional relationships' with 'sugar daddies': older, richer, and usually married men who may be teachers, civil servants, taxi drivers, policemen, or others with a disposable income. Such relationships should not be thought of as equivalent to prostitution or as characterised by promiscuity; indeed, in Venda, as in other parts of South Africa, they are often a socially acceptable means for women to make ends meet (Hunter 2002). This is in stark contrast, however, to women who practise beer hall prostitution or what Wojcicki (2002) has aptly named 'survival sex', who are generally not considered suitable for a transactional relationship. Those in both categories experience financial hardships, and both are liable to fall pregnant, becoming dependent on child welfare grants and on maintenance payments – often unreliable – from the father. A girl's giving birth drastically reduces a family's prospects of receiving bridewealth (*lobola*) but does not entirely remove the possibility of marriage, or of finding informal employment. If a woman does marry, she must learn the difficult skill of balancing her obligations to feed and clothe her children and spouse against her need to connect, mostly through the daily prayer sessions of her chosen church, with friends and female associates.

However, recent legislative change constituted a profound shift in the legal status of many South African women. Prior to the Recognition of Customary Marriages Act of 1998, 'customary' marriages, more frequently practised by black South Africans than the 'civil/religious' variety, were not legally recognised, but this has been reversed by the Constitutional Court. As a result of this fortification of so-called traditional cultural practices, women are in a stronger position to claim inheritance, negotiate divorce settlements, and gain access to child maintenance grants and pensions.

Groups of young men, denied the formal employment that was available to their fathers in mines or commercial farms, often find their way to the periurban areas of Sibasa and Thohoyandou (the former homeland's capital), often in search of an informal 'piece job'.[9] In such settings they are likely to be tempted by the rewards offered to those who engage in petty, or serious, crime. The fathers of these men, retired from their lives as migrant labourers, either spend time with church friends or in beer halls, but seldom do both. Older men and women, unable to rely on their sons' earnings as they had expected, depend on state pensions: a basic monthly income (R1,010 in 2009) that they increasingly collect along with a foster care grant (R680 in 2009) or a child support grant (R240 in 2009) for the care of their grandchildren.

In spite of the reality of adversity, often the difficulties of daily life are endured with a remarkably optimistic faith that gradually things will improve, as in the adage '*zwi do luga*' ('things will be all right').

---

[9] 'Piece jobs' generally consist of no more than a few days' work on a specific task for a set rate of pay – clearing a plot of land, helping to build a wall, picking at harvest time, and the like. Skilled labour is also recruited for piece jobs, such as car repair, plumbing, or electric work, for those who have experience of practical training but remain without formal employment.

For the second-smallest linguistic group in South Africa, Tshivenda speakers have produced an exceptional number of successful public figures in the post-apartheid era. These include the Reverend Simon Farisani (struggle hero and Speaker of the Limpopo Provincial House), Sydney Mufamadi (ex-Minister of Provincial and Local Government), Joel Netshitenzhe (former head of Government Communications, currently head of the Policy Unit, alleged during Mbeki's presidency to have had exceptional political influence [Calland 2006]), Cyril Ramaphosa (former NUM leader and now prominent businessman), and the late musician Lucky Dube.[10] Like other men who work 'in town', these individuals maintain strong familial connections in Venda. On visits home, they are known to address schools, community gatherings, and public holiday celebrations. Through this, they have become powerful role models for young and old Vhavenda who aspire to join the growing African middle classes. Possibly because of the visibility and inspirational character of these key figures, for every youngster in Venda who gets involved in crime there is another who has taken a loan and started a carwash, opened a small *spaza* shop from his house, fixes shoes or watches, sells phone calls and 'loose draw' cigarettes at taxi stops, braids hair, has started a non-governmental organisation (NGO), or offered his or her voluntary services to an existing one.

A sense of optimism is reflected in patterns of electoral support. The vast majority of Tshivenda speakers remain loyal to the African National Congress (ANC). In the area covered by the Vhembe District Municipality, under whose political administration the former homeland of Venda falls, over 75 per cent of votes were recorded in favour of the ANC in the 2000 municipal elections and in 2006 this increased to 86 per cent (IEC South Africa 2007).[11] The party's popularity, however, stemmed as much from historical allegiance and the lack of a credible political alternative as from the success of the strategies adopted by former President Mbeki. In the April 2009 elections, with Jacob Zuma at the helm, the ANC maintained its majority in Limpopo despite some success for the newly formed Congress of the People (COPE).

The mixture of optimism and hardship evident in Venda life is paralleled at the national level, where growth, stability, and prosperity are accompanied by unemployment and inequality. The ANC-led government has pursued policies of liberalisation designed to encourage international confidence in the South African rand: largely successfully if

---

[10] Whilst Lucky Dube himself claimed Zulu origins, his mother lives in a suburb outside Thohoyandou.
[11] Municipalities are subdivisions of local government that are divided into wards. They operate one level below provincial structures and two levels below national government. Since 1994, South Africa has adopted proportional representation as its electoral system; with three subdivisions of government to vote for this has proved to be an exceptionally complex and clumsy political arrangement.

one measures success in terms of economic growth and of the small but highly visible upper and middle classes that have benefited from the reforms. The turn towards neoliberalism was marked by a seminal shift in policy. This saw a move from emphasis on the 'people-centred', social-democratic Reconstruction and Development Programme (RDP) to the comparatively more conservative, 'top-down', macroeconomic Growth, Employment, and Redistribution Strategy (GEAR). This led to the privatisation of social services, reduction in social spending, and a liberalisation of trade relations.

Nonetheless, slow economic and social progress has been made since the dawn of democracy in 1994. In 1995 (using a poverty line of R462 per month) roughly 58 per cent of the population was living in poverty. In 2009, according to the South African Civil Society Information Service (SACSIS), this had been cut to 48 per cent.[12] Service provision, like poverty reduction, has been slow to get off the ground, and areas such as Venda have been sidelined in favour of more politically volatile regions such as KwaZulu-Natal, parts of the Eastern Cape, and various urban townships. Thus developments have been uneven, but progress has been made; and, although opportunities for some have not translated into opportunities for all, there has been a genuine attempt to redistribute wealth through the state apparatus. This is evidenced by South Africa's welfare system, exceptional among middle-income and developing countries. The combination of old age pensions, disability grants, and child and support grants has led some to suggest that policy may be veering back to the social-democratic principles of the RDP, or even that the ANC may be attempting to steer a 'third way' between the left and the right.[13] This has prompted commentators such as Seekings and Nattrass (2006: 314) to suggest that the post-apartheid state should be characterised not as neoliberal in orientation, but rather as a 'distributional regime'.

In a similar vein to the limited success of GEAR, policies promoting so-called black economic empowerment (BEE) have failed to induce a reduction in inequality, and South Africa remains one of the most unequal countries in the world (May et al. 2000: 26–8). BEE has achieved the promotion of some members of the African elite into positions of power, but by no means provided substantial gains for the majority.[14] Unemployment has remained at around 40 per cent since 1998 (Labour

---

[12] <http://sacsis.org.za/site/article/230.1> (accessed 12 February 2009).
[13] Daniel et al. (2005); Southall (2005: 458); Mbali (2004); Southall (2007: 1); Seekings (2005 in Nattrass 2007: 179).
[14] BEE has been defined as 'the increase of black ownership, control and management of state, parastatal and private activity in the formal sector' (Southall 2005: 457). 'African elite' refers largely to the class of African capitalists, many of whom were supported by the apartheid regime as a means to promote business in the Bantustans as a functional buffer between white capitalism and mass black poverty.

Force Survey 2004) and has been accompanied by the seemingly horizonless rising tide of crime and the highest per capita incarceration rate on the entire continent (Sloth-Nielsen 2007).

Daily life in Venda thus echoes national trends in post-apartheid South Africa. Both are experienced as a set of contradictions: the promotion of economic development is set against distinctly underdeveloped circumstances; the promise to provide basic amenities against the resounding failure to deliver; the reassurance of a 'better life for all' against the reality of a growing wealth gap; the experience of political freedom against the common occurrence of violent crime; extensive welfare provision against exposure to neoliberal policies and high levels of unemployment; the casting of votes in a democratic election against the reality of living under the influence of unelected traditional authority; the use of modern technology in the form of mobile phones, computer cafes, and solar panels against the pervasiveness of discourses on tradition; and the constant reminder to 'love life' against the increasingly frequent deaths of family and friends from AIDS.

AIDS and the Perception of a Crisis

It is difficult to imagine living in post-apartheid South Africa without experiencing the constant threat of HIV/AIDS in some shape or form. Despite ex-President Mbeki's now infamous claim never to have known anyone who has died of it, AIDS has sunk deep into the nation's collective conscience. Of course, this does not imply any uniformity in its comprehension. In another equally infamous statement, the current president Jacob Zuma recently championed the prophylactic properties of a postcoital shower, courting the fury of AIDS activists whilst playing to the sensibilities of an important constituency in the electorate. Many, then, do not accept the conventional scientific explanations, or act on them in recommended ways. But there is a profound sense that AIDS is here to stay, and that it is killing people.

Sex, the source of life and a ubiquitous source of pleasure, has become synonymous with death and distress. Previously healthy men, women, and children are becoming sick in increasing numbers, often hidden from sight by confused and frightened families. Political controversy surrounds the antiretroviral (ARV) medication that could help to hide the symptoms and quell the stigma of a slow, painful, untimely, and undignified death. Grandparents are bringing up their children's children, and there seems to be no stopping it: in the time it will have taken you to read this far, hundreds of South Africans have been infected with HIV.[15] In a very

---

[15] It is estimated that 1,500 South Africans are infected with HIV every day (UNAIDS 2007).

tangible sense, then, the epidemic is perceived as having brought about a crisis of sexual and social reproduction in South Africa.

As Bujra (2004) has demonstrated, using social reproduction as a conceptual framework to analyse AIDS highlights the impact that such individual suffering has on household and national economies. Agricultural modes of livelihood, and thus the reproduction of cheap labour in rural areas, depend on fit, productive bodies. Across Southern Africa, labour supply has been depleted as HIV infections manifest themselves as AIDS-related illnesses. Migrant labour, fundamental to the reproduction of capital in South Africa, and already in decline due to high unemployment in the wake of neoliberal economic reform, has been adversely affected. For Bujra, the rural households to which old migrants return and from which new generations emerge have long been the keystone in reproducing migrant labour in the region, but with the growing impact of HIV/AIDS, 'this transmission belt of new labour for old is fraying' (Bujra 2004: 631). However, a high rate of unemployment makes it difficult to establish the extent to which the AIDS epidemic has actually contributed to the current economic situation. Whilst some people cannot work because they are sick, for most people it is the lack of jobs that is the problem.

Still, illness is big business. Whilst AIDS is perceived as a crisis, this crisis has been converted into opportunities for the accumulation of capital. AIDS-related NGOs provide significant employment opportunities through national tenders and international donations. Palliative treatments are available, for a price, from international pharmaceuticals (increasingly now through the state – see Chapter 4) and traditional healers (see Chapter 6). Funerals are lavish affairs requiring the purchase of coffins, tombstones, undertakers' services, the hire of tents, seats, cooking equipment, food, and the like. These are generally provided locally, and someone will profit from them. Framing AIDS as a component in a wider crisis of social reproduction, then, should not be read as veiled Afro-pessimism. It does not preclude the analysis of innovative and resourceful ways in which many rural South Africans directly or indirectly make a living in the AIDS industry. Indeed, this rapidly growing business thrives off, and contributes to, the sense of emergency from which it sprang.

Each domain of investigation offered in this book represents an engagement in its own terms with localised perceptions of the crisis of social reproduction, and with manifestations of the liberalisation of the South African state and economy. The ethnographic accounts presented in the following chapters thus also represent a distinct, but connected, set of possible vehicles for regaining control over authoritative forms of knowledge and modes of producing value (cf. Comaroff and Comaroff 2004). In the everyday lived experience of rural South Africans, this relative stability is sought after, if rarely achieved, by establishing connections with what are taken to be essential, partially conflicting, sources of power: the state and chieftaincy; biomedicine and ancestral ('traditional') knowledge. Power's ambivalent qualities ensure that any values achieved in the process are at once reinforced and contested, marking out fractal points between generational and gendered experiences of daily life.

By situating AIDS education in the context of traditional authority in Chapter 2 and female initiation in Chapter 3, I demonstrate that the seemingly straightforward social processes involved in the acquisition of biomedical 'health-enhancing' knowledge belie various complexities involved in its dissemination. Progressive levels of analysis, in subsequent chapters, take you from the national level of policy formation to the micro-analysis of rumour and gossip, whilst the intervening chapters are designed to demonstrate how the two are connected. The focus is, however, not directed towards the South African government's previously controversial AIDS related policies: these have received extensive, possibly excessive, coverage in the literature (see Chapter 4). Instead, I am concerned with demonstrating the ways in which a seemingly less pertinent policy agenda, that relating to the political economy of traditional leadership in a democratic setting, has impinged upon AIDS-related discourse and the efficacy of prevention programmes. Clearly, the official response to AIDS in South Africa has been 'the most resounding failure of [ex-President] Thabo Mbeki's government' (Fassin 2007: xvii), and it is important to recognise this. It is, however, a turbulent time in South African politics. The recent decision by the ANC prematurely to terminate Mbeki's presidency has accompanied the government's apparent retreat from a so-called denialist stance on AIDS. The new Minister of Health, Dr Aaron Motsoaledi, has pledged to implement major shifts in AIDS policy, moving it towards the universal provision of ARV treatment. This potentially signals the end of a dark era in which the ex-President and the former Health Minister Manto Tshabalala-Msimang presided over a profoundly misguided national approach to HIV/AIDS. Given this wider context of political change, there is a need for new approaches to AIDS in South Africa. I demonstrate in this book that there are other, potentially more fruitful, ways of analysing responses to the epidemic: ones that need not resort to a continual reiteration of Mbeki's now infamous flaws.

Central to my approach, and fundamental to grasping the ways in which rural South Africans act to secure control over social and sexual reproduction, is the complex and fluid relationship between biomedical/scientific and ancestral/'traditional' conceptions of sickness and well-being. Here, it is impossible to make a clear-cut distinction between scientific and non-scientific modes of knowing: the science of AIDS has been incorporated into folk understandings, and attributes of the 'folk model' (Good 1994) are remarkably similar to scientific explanations.

Both explain HIV/AIDS in general terms of blood, semen, and the sexual transmission of disease, and practitioners of both will generally accept the reality that AIDS is responsible for the unprecedented frequency of funerals.

Despite these important similarities, however, the two bodies of knowledge employ contrary logics to explain the epidemiology and incidence of HIV/AIDS.[16] Scientific accounts, for example, now agree that HIV is most infectious in the months directly after the virus enters the human body, and they stress the high risk factors involved in multiple concurrent sexual partnerships (Epstein 2007). Some scientists promote male circumcision as a preventative measure, arguing that the thick skin that develops in place of the foreskin acts to some extent as a natural condom (Halperin and Bailey 1999). It has even been suggested that male circumcision become mandatory in regions with exceptionally high HIV prevalence, although such a policy perhaps underestimates the political and cultural significance of the practice (see Chapter 3).

Returning to non-scientific conceptualisations of HIV/AIDS epidemiology, a marked contrast is apparent. Folk models in Southern Africa place almost exclusive responsibility for prevention and contagion on women, through the regulation of menstrual blood, avoidance of contraception and abortion, and subsequent maintenance of fertility (see Thornton 2008, and Chapter 6 in this book). Ancestrally and chiefly sanctioned sex education, for example, is prominent in the songs and dances of the *vhusha* girls' initiation ceremony, analysed in Chapter 3. Thus, whilst peer educators mobilise 'tradition' in an attempt to secure legitimacy for the biomedical model, older women invoke authoritative notions of the past to support their stake in resolving the perceived crisis of reproduction.

AIDS has fitted easily into a wider complex of illnesses which are known, in the words of the old man in the introductory sketch, as *malwadze dza vhafumakadzi*, 'the illnesses of women'. Throughout South Africa's rural peripheries, this way of thinking about the pandemic takes on slightly different forms, but is propagated in largely similar ways: through ritual processes of initiation under the authority of elders and ancestors. Through the promotion of initiation ceremonies by chiefs and

---

[16] 'HIV incidence' is the new number of HIV infections in a population over a given period of time. 'HIV prevalence' is the actual percentage of the population that is infected. So, for example, whilst HIV incidence in South Africa seems to have reached a plateau, the number of infections continues to rise at a steady rate. HIV/AIDS statistics, however, are notoriously unreliable (see Pisani 2008): their variability within different demographic groups and across geographic regions can make it problematic to summarise them on a country-specific basis. Nonetheless, it is estimated that in 2006 20.7 per cent of women attending antenatal clinics in Limpopo province were HIV-positive, compared with 14.5 per cent in 2001. See the UNAIDS website, <www.UNAIDS.org>, for updated statistical estimations.

headmen throughout the country, non-scientific explanations of AIDS have experienced a surge of support in the post-apartheid era. The current revival of 'tradition' has thus placed gendered and generational divisions at the core of sociality, pitting men against women, young against old, as all strive to recover their capacities to act on the world, and blame each other for having lost them in the first place. Masculine expressions of concern for loose, polluted women and a perceived disregard for patriarchal authority are voiced in public, jockeying for position against AIDS educators' science of safe sex. Indeed, one of the conclusions of this book is that the political economy of traditional authority in post-apartheid Venda has created a highly charged force field within which biomedical AIDS education competes for legitimacy in the daily battle to secure social and sexual reproduction.

A second source of complexity, closely related to the first and discussed in Chapter 7, compounds the perception of crisis and confounds the difficulties faced by peer educators in the dissemination of scientific knowledge. It originates in the uneven and disjointed connections between HIV/AIDS education, on the one hand, and wider discourses that inhibit open, public conversation regarding causes of death on the other. In Venda, and across the wider region, there is a close connection between publicly expressed knowledge and assumed experience. Those displaying public knowledge related to witchcraft, for example, are likely to be branded witches. Similarly, those who know too much about a death are likely to be implicated in the fatality. Within this rationale, it follows that HIV/AIDS is bound into complex webs of secrecy and suspicion that prohibit its inclusion in open, public conversation.

Towards the end of the book, then, emphasis is placed on the importance of applying ethnographic approaches to patterns of speaking (and not speaking) about such taboo subjects. This is expressed in a model for understanding the current failure of AIDS education through a new way of conceptualising stigma and secrecy not as 'denial', but rather in terms of 'degrees of separation' which create and maintain distance between the speaker and immanent or actual death.

Before embarking on this story, however, I feel obliged to provide an explanation of my own relationship to Venda, central as it is to the analysis within these pages.

Researching AIDS, Politics, and Music

Not that long ago, it was claimed that 'nowhere is the failure of anthropologists to engage with the real world of suffering... more evident than in their absence from debate and action around the HIV/AIDS epidemic' (Barnett 2004: 1). Whilst a handful of anthropologists working in African contexts have since acted to fill this void (among others, Rodlach 2006;

Fassin 2007; Thornton 2008), Barnett's point remains relevant. Given the profound effects HIV/AIDS has on the societies we study, anthropology remains under-represented, and the use of its methods to analyse the epidemic is rare.

There are important reasons for this. It would take a particularly controversial interpretation of participant observation to ascertain the precise way in which people conduct sexual relations. As a methodology, anthropology may be ideally suited to harnessing at least some of the nuance required for an analysis of HIV/AIDS, but the transmission of HIV is not easy to research: sex happens between the sheets (or in the bushes) and people generally do not want to talk about it – or, for that matter, about AIDS.

It is rather the case, then, that some aspects of AIDS are more conducive to ethnographic study than others. Factors that can be seen as relevant in an epidemiological study, such as poverty and gender, have been analysed, and then used in the construction of general models that attempt to demonstrate how far these are causative in patterns of transmission. Such an approach allows the researcher, using tools such as interviews, focus groups, and surveys, to explore patterns of social behaviour which seem pertinent, but they are ultimately inadequate for assessing the complexities of social life.

The character of my involvement in Venda ritual, music, politics, and peer education dictated not only the subject of my research, but also its methods. Understanding the ways in which I gathered my data, my relationships with the main characters in the chapters that follow, and my status as a particular kind of insider/outsider, requires some knowledge of this situation. I have an association with the Venda region of 15 years' standing. My first visit, in 1995, was as a gap-year volunteer English teacher for an organisation known as the Project Trust. Realising that as a 17-year-old unmarried and childless youth it would be difficult to gain the respect of the adults I had been charged with teaching, I embarked on a joint English-teaching and Tshivenda-learning strategy: this proved a successful means of starting me on the slow process of getting to know the language. During my visit, I met and was befriended by an American Buddhist monk who had become a self-styled AIDS educator after nursing a friend who died of an AIDS-related illness. I became involved in several of his projects, distributing condoms and addressing village councils at weekends. He later established the Forum for AIDS Prevention (referred to above), an organisation with which I continued to be involved, but in a manner which combined activism with academic enquiry. Alongside my role in establishing projects and recruiting volunteers, I also conducted short spells of research with FAP volunteers for my undergraduate dissertation at the University of Glasgow. In sum, my analysis of the FAP and its peer education projects in Chapter 4 derives from a long trajectory of acquaintance, involvement, and observation.

Introduction

I also became the lead guitarist in a popular local reggae band. As a reggae musician, my involvement in the performance culture of this society so famous for its music, and my participation in the song writing and recording of this particular group, was a matter of intuition rather than strategy. After several years the band's success and popularity increased.[17] Like many musicians in South Africa, they are guaranteed at least twelve fully funded sell-out concerts every year, as they are enlisted to perform at government-sponsored celebrations on public holidays. I have been party to the band's rise to success and relative wealth in this short space of time, co-writing and producing two albums and performing live on a regular basis not only in Limpopo but in the Venda quarters of Soweto (*Tshiawelo* – place of rest). Through this I have become something of a minor celebrity in the Venda region.

As an AIDS educator, musician, and researcher, I have returned to Venda every year since 1995. Given my status as a foreigner with particular kinds of insider connections, it was no easy matter to convince people upon my return in 2004 that I was now a bona fide anthropological researcher. The memory of John Blacking, looming large in Venda and giving people a clear model of what an anthropologist should be, made matters worse. Given that the band's success had increased exponentially, it was increasingly difficult to maintain a background presence and I was identified primarily as a Rasta/reggae musician rather than as an academic.

This perception occasionally impinged directly upon my research agenda. Although I gained access to several female initiation schools through the mediation of King Kennedy Tshivhase, I failed to secure entry to their Christian equivalents. Never explicitly stated, a main reason for this was that, with my dreadlocks and adherence to Rastafarian ideology, I breached the fundamental requirements of ritual purity. Although many Christian friends who attended these churches and ceremonies understood my predicament, and although I gleaned much secondary information from them, ultimately they were unwilling to introduce me to their church communities through which I could have attempted to negotiate access.

My identity as a popular reggae musician did, however, have an advantageous dimension. It made my presence in male-dominated spaces such as beer halls and late-night music venues in Venda and Johannesburg safe, even pleasurable, and acted as a catalyst for amenable relationships with many groups of men from various backgrounds. Indeed, the

---

[17] I am not suggesting here that it was my inclusion in the band that instigated its success. The band in question, which performs under the name of the lead singer Colbert Mukwevho, has been a household name in Venda for well over two decades. Its recent success has been related to Colbert's ability to maintain government contracts for large shows, and his brother Mulalo's ability to produce radio-quality recordings from their modest recording studio, known as the 'Burnin Shak'.

tshilombe (plural: *zwilombe*) musician Solomon Mathase, whose song I analyse in Chapter 6, initially permitted my recording of his performances on the condition that I share the material with other producers in the music industry and promote his talents with a view to securing a record contract.

As an avid guitarist, I not only recorded the songs of Solomon and his peers, but learned to play and sing them. Musical repetition and innovation became a research tool through which I familiarised myself with the stylistic tendencies and the lyrical composition of *zwilombe* guitar songs. Venda *zwilombe* musicians' distinctive style of restringing and retuning the six-string guitar facilitates lengthy performances of songs which correspond to 'three chord tricks'. The marriage of my folk guitar finger-picking style with Solomon's distinct sound proved to be popular at our impromptu performances. In addition to being great fun, this brought me closer to Solomon and his group of friends. It facilitated my investigation, through the lyrical content of the songs we were singing together, of their attitudes towards sexual illness, traditional medicine, and sexual encounters, in a way that standard interview techniques, even if supplemented by participant observation, might not have done.

It was partly through my reputation as a popular musician that I became acquainted with King Kennedy Tshivhase, but my association with the king was immeasurably strengthened through my friendship with a trusted royal adviser, Mr Traugatt Fobbe. Mr Fobbe's father, a Lutheran missionary in Venda in the 1940s, had a close working relationship with the current king's father.[18] However, he was expelled from South Africa by the apartheid authorities under suspicion of involvement in so-called 'terrorist activity'. When the son, Traugatt, returned to Venda in 1993 to establish a tourist business, King Tshivhase honoured his father's memory by developing a close relationship with him. Mr Fobbe hosted the king and I at his house on several occasions in order that I might explain the objectives of my research, lobby for his support, and present a copy of my thesis.

My relationship with King Tshivhase presented a common ethical conundrum, typical of situations in which researcher and informant attempt to manipulate each other while partially concealing their true motives. Nonetheless, having studied anthropology as an undergraduate, he understood my intentions and supported my research in many ways: primarily by helping to organise accommodation in the village of Fondwe (see maps). From this vantage point, I was well placed to access the HIV/AIDS peer education projects that I had helped to establish in

---

[18] See Kirkaldy (2005) for a detailed analysis of the Berlin Mission Society in Venda between 1870 and 1900, and Chapter 2 in this book for details on the Tshivhase royal lineage.

Tshikombani and Ha-Rabali, and that I had now secured funding to investigate.

To help me assess the social dynamics of the projects, I employed as my research assistant Mr Mushaisano Tshivhase, whom I had first met in 1999 at the University of Venda. With Mushai, as in the broader Venda setting, I found myself in an insider/outsider relationship. As a person with some – albeit an incomplete – academic training, he had interests in common with my own, but there were limits to this commonality in two important respects. First, Mushai is in line to the Tshivhase throne, and often attempted to influence my interpretation of events and data in accordance with royal dogma which, to his disgruntlement, I initially rejected. As time progressed, however, I began to see the benefits of such an insight, so long as I recorded and used it in a highly contextualised manner. In this way, my fieldwork notes of events such as the installation of headmen (*vhuhosi* – see Chapter 2) cover my general observations alongside Mushai's interpretation of them as a royal insider. The same applies to my notes on the public sessions of female initiation, although, as I describe in Chapter 3, I attended the 'secret' sessions in the ritual hut (*tshivhambo*) alone.

The second reason for our occasional disagreement was his disapproval of my friends in the music industry. I spent a lot of time recording, producing, performing, and relaxing with the band and its entourage, but Mushai was never welcomed by them. In attempting to resolve the resulting tension, I learnt much about the convoluted politics in Venda. The members of the band are all of Mukwevho lineage, a proud group of Vhangona ('original' inhabitants of the area, also known as *Ngwaniwapo*) that trace their history to pre-Singo conquest (see Chapter 2). They regarded the (Singo) Tshivhase house as arrogant and authoritarian. The lead singer of the band made a statement to this effect at an award ceremony when, upon receiving an award for the promotion of the Tshivenda language from King Tshivhase, he refused to remove his hat. When asked explicitly to do so, he refused, replying: '*Misanda ha pfuki milambo*' ('chiefs don't cross rivers'), insinuating that this was not Tshivhase country. Mushai found this type of behaviour offensive and consistently encouraged me to spend less time with them. It became clear to me early on that the status of insider/outsider was not exclusively mine. Mushai was, by virtue of his royal blood, excluded from commoner cohorts. The band members, by virtue of their commoner identity and their celebrity Rasta status, excluded themselves from royal, and other, groups. This distinction between royal and common, of which I provide a detailed account in the following chapters, is fundamental to Venda sociality.

Whilst my split loyalties in these spheres of interaction allowed me some balance in my data collection and analysis, achieving balance in respect of my interactions with peer educators posed different challenges. While some of the older educators, who have known me for more than a decade, treat me more like a schoolboy than like a musician or an anthropologist, some of the younger ones, given my ongoing role in assessing the fluctuating demographic and economic composition of the projects through questionnaires, focus groups, in-depth and open-ended interviews, identified me as working 'for the (FAP) office'. Occasionally this acted to my disadvantage, in that it made people reluctant to talk honestly, but it also aided my research by enabling confessions of grievances in the hope that I would act in educators' interests, which I often did.

I spent a lot of time with peer educators both in and out of their working environment. This involved attending funerals and other ceremonies at weekends and at their training sessions and public performances. I became very close to many of them, and through this I gained the confidence to employ a more experimental methodology. I distributed diaries and asked them to make regular entries documenting their daily activities and work-related information (cf. Blacking 1964 in Venda; Jones 1993 in Cape Town) as well as village gossip, rumour, and scandal, not only specifically related to AIDS, but concerning general issues such as sexual networks, government mass media campaigns, witchcraft allegations, intra- and inter-village political rivalries, and the recent influx of illegal immigrants to the Venda region from Zimbabwe. They were asked not to reveal anything through which I could identify them personally, and I taught them how to use pseudonyms to conceal the identity of those they were writing about. This was, in general, a very successful approach which yielded considerable amounts of qualitative data.

I was granted yet further access to relatively invisible realms of experience by the educators' music. My focus on peer education songs in Chapter 5 was based initially on the observation that they spent most of their work time composing, practising, or performing musical renditions at public performances. My interest in this was compounded by the frequent claim that they 'sing about what they cannot talk about', and as early as 1999 I had embarked on a project to document peer education songs. In a similar way to my approach with Solomon Mathase, I employed my own musical ability as a research tool with peer educators. Many of the songs that I recorded, some of which are analysed in Chapter 5 and which you can hear at http://www.cambridge.org/us/9781107009912, were thus taught to me by the educators. The act of recording and listening back to the melodic patterns, harmonic structures, and lyrical content of the songs proved invaluable to my own learning. Again, through familiarisation with the lyrics, embodiment of the dance routines, and performance at practice sessions as part of their ensemble, I developed an awareness of, even an affinity with, the content that facilitated a comprehensive process of analysis. Learning and performing music undoubtedly reduced the social distance between researcher and researched in that I became the socially recognised *learner*. In this way I attempted to negate my identity as a popular musician in the process of learning about the songs, and the lives, of the peer educators.

My focus on music and the use of music as a research tool to some extent provided me with a means to uncover hidden realms of knowledge and experience, and the distribution of diaries augmented this. My observation of NGO volunteers followed on from my role in helping to recruit them and in monitoring them over a decade. Connections with royalty provided opportunities for investigation as well as demonstrating to me the intrinsically hierarchical and patrimonial character of Venda society. The peculiar character of my involvements in Venda, having shaped the subjects of my enquiry, also yielded the means of investigation in a manner that took me beyond observation and into participation.

2   The Battle for Venda Kingship

This chapter examines the context of a decision taken by the post-apartheid South African government to recognise one paramount king in each of the areas with a history of traditional leadership.[1] In Venda, this has given rise to a bitter succession struggle between the royal houses of Mphephu and Tshivhase that has reignited historically salient rivalries between the two. Notions of an African renaissance have become central to Kennedy Tshivhase's strategy for the consolidation of power, and it is this that has prompted the official promotion of tradition within his borders. I am thus concerned with the question of how far the recognition or imposition of culture by the state leads to a strengthening of traditionalist forces and visions within the local political arena (Oomen 2005: 25). In what ways has the state lent legitimacy to traditional leaders, and what have been the consequences of this 'on the ground'? I describe in detail the role of traditional leaders in the transition from apartheid to democracy in Venda. In doing so, I analyse the political origins of an official promotion of tradition, so that in subsequent chapters I can trace the 'folk model' of AIDS not only to the traditional/ancestral knowledge in which it is rooted, but also to the political processes through which it is mediated.

The Politics of Tradition and the African Renaissance

The concept of tradition, and the role it plays in rural post-apartheid South Africa, is central to the way in which I analyse the dynamics of AIDS discourse in Venda. Tradition has been invoked to reclaim a perceived loss of the capacity to control healthy social reproduction in the post-apartheid era. But this has played out in an uneven and

---

[1] There is some confusion in the literature, and on the ground, as to the correct terminology regarding the various rungs of traditional leadership in the post-apartheid era. I use the Tshivenda term *Thovhela* for 'king' (no plural). For chief, one level below *Thovhela*, I use the Tshivenda term *Khosi* (plural *Mahosi*). For headman, I use the term *Vhamusanda*. This is only used in the plural: the singular form of the word, *musanda*, refers to a royal courtyard. The term *Gota* (plural *Magota*) is interchangeable with *Vhamusanda*. For petty headman, the lowest rung of traditional leadership, I use the term *Mukoma*. See Figure 2.3 and Glossary.

contradictory manner, pitting generations and genders against each other in the abortive attempt to resolve the supposed crisis. Contemporary concern with a pre-colonial past, epitomised in the marketing of Limpopo Province as 'Africa's Eden' on the road to Venda, is by no means exclusive to South Africa: it is a truly global phenomenon. The revision of ethnic essentialism to include identity politics (to paraphrase Comaroff and Comaroff [1991: 1]) has taken on a multitude of guises in recent years, from New Zealand to Newfoundland, Amazonia to Australia.[2] A 'growing traditionalism' (Fuller 2003: 153) can be both helped and hindered by the potent forces of the state, and can involve the selective reclamation of older legitimating symbols as hedges against new symbolic orders (ibid.: 160). Vast numbers of people in post-apartheid South Africa are actively engaged, apparently independently of state policy, in processes that they consider to be part of a traditional, 'tribal' repertoire that is legitimate precisely because it is 'of the past'.

Whilst social scientists have felt compelled to deconstruct tradition by showing the complex forces that underpin it (cf. Ranger 1983; 1993), the fixity in time and inflexibility of tradition is what facilitates its manipulation as a political tool within global, rights-based discourse (Oomen 2005; Scorgie 2003). Tradition can appear as 'time present', encompassing the meanings of 'continuing', *and* a 'time past', carrying the meanings of previous and 'earlier times' (Cohen 1991). These different aspects are not mutually exclusive, and contemporary processes of traditionalism serve to blur any boundaries that may have separated them.

Examples of this can be seen in attempts to manage sexuality and curb the exceptionally high rates of HIV transmission among young people. Thus, a 'revival' in the practice of pre-marital virginity testing of girls in KwaZulu-Natal is justified by ritual experts explicitly in terms of the epidemic (Leclerc-Madlala 2001; 2005; Scorgie 2002). Likewise, the reintroduction of *Umkhosi Womhlanga* (the reed ceremony) by King Goodwill Zwelethini in 1991 was deemed necessary as a means to prevent HIV transmission by encouraging young Zulu girls to delay sexual debut until marriage. The Zulu king has made a controversial attempt recently to reintroduce male circumcision rites. He stated that circumcision amongst Zulus had been common until Shaka banned it in the 1800s, and that it was now necessary to reintroduce the practice in the fight against AIDS.

The notion that male circumcision can help prevent HIV infection has become popular in recent years. As mentioned in Chapter 1, some scientists have suggested that the thick skin that develops in place of the foreskin acts, to some extent, as a natural condom (Halperin and Bailey

---

[2] For examples, see Comaroff and Comaroff (2009), Bruner and Kirshenblatt-Gimblett (1994), Clifford (1988; 1997), Bern and Dodds (2002), Tonkinson (1997), Lindstrom and White (1993), and Robins (2001).

1999), and male circumcision is now a priority for American prevention strategies through PEPFAR (the President's Emergency Plan for AIDS Relief). Most research in support of this thesis has been conducted in Africa or India, however, and does not explain why Europe, where men are mostly uncircumcised, has one of the lowest HIV prevalence rates in the world. It is possible that the combination of many uncircumcised men and multiple concurrent sexual relationships has driven HIV infection rates upwards in sub-Saharan Africa (cf. Epstein 2007).

Growing evidence in support of the thesis that circumcision can help prevent HIV transmission could help to explain the extraordinarily high HIV prevalence in KwaZulu-Natal, estimated by UNAIDS to be over 40 per cent in 2006. Zulu men are generally not circumcised. Their Xhosa neighbours in the Eastern Cape, on the other hand, practise male circumcision widely during initiation rites. In 2006, they had a significantly lower estimated prevalence of under 30 per cent.[3]

The often violent historical rivalry between the two ethnic groups, and the aggressive nationalisms that have developed alongside this, endow physical markers of identity such as circumcision with powerful symbolic connotations. Zulu men's reactions to King Zwelethini's drive to reintroduce circumcision have expressed the desire for continuity over change: 'This is wrong,' said a young man interviewed by a national newspaper. 'We know this is a culture for the Xhosas... now they expect us [Zulu men] to accept a culture from other people. I cannot.'[4] It would thus appear that King Zwelethini, and others who promote circumcision as prevention, will face significant resistance to their attempts at promoting behaviour change through the reinvention of tradition. We saw in Chapter 1 that in Venda male circumcision is a mark of exclusion from ascendancy to the throne. Any attempts at promoting this apparently simple surgical procedure as a preventative measure against HIV transmission will have to take such factors into account, lest they be doomed to controversy, low uptake, and resultant failure from the outset.

Leaving aside the questionable ethics of such revivals, they are evidence that protagonists of 'tradition' have appropriated an idea of the past with which they seek to shape the present. Traditional leaders in Venda have made concerted efforts to promote 'tradition' in the region, stating that female initiation ceremonies, in their capacity to instil healthy reproduction, incorporate ancestral and biomedical AIDS education. Connections between the state and local politics are central to these ceremonial processes, although the people engaged in them may perceive their actions to be relatively independent of state influence.

Thus, tradition is never a mere expression of invariant knowledge. Rather, it is made up of fundamentally creative and interpretive acts on

---

[3] See UNAIDS Country Report, <http://www.unaids.org/en/regionscountries/countries/southafrica/> (accessed 12 February 2009).

[4] *City Press*, 24 January 2010, p. 8.

the part of the carriers of tradition which are intended to make it appear invariant, ancient, and primordial (Simpson 2002; cf. Fuller 1997). 'Cultural revivals' hinge on the collective, selective, and creative memory of distinct social groups whose recourse to specific knowledge ascribes to them a new-found social status, often as ritual leaders. Where such leaders make use of musical performance, the appearance of invariance and unchangeability may be particularly pronounced: Blacking remarked that musical symbols are especially resistant to change and that music 'can only confirm sentiments that exist but cannot create new ones' (1964: 108, 334). However, the ways in which peer educators incorporate traditional elements into AIDS education, described in Chapter 5, pose a challenge to this assertion.

In the South African context, the notion of tradition has a particularly unsavoury past. In the apartheid period as well as beyond it, a legally sanctioned politics of tradition has coexisted with a bureaucratic state and planning apparatus. The political and legal construction of tradition, in the guise of rural traditional leadership, resulted from its moulding by colonial forces into a form of 'decentralised despotism' in a 'bifurcated state' in which African people could be citizens outside of the homelands but remained subjects within them (Mamdani 1996). This represented an attempt to reinforce the legitimacy of the chieftaincy as one of the most reliable gateways to the state. And yet this coexisted with seemingly contradictory policies of 'racial modernism' (Bozzoli 2000; 2004) through which development interventions were planned and implemented, often through the structures of traditional leadership. In rural South Africa, invoked intentionally or otherwise by polysemic 'aspirations and intentions', notions of tradition and modernity roam large (Comaroff and Comaroff 2004: 330), but they have been shaped by contradictory combinations of primordial symbols, aspirations to economic growth, state planning, and chiefly aspirations.

Apartheid policy, then, was designed to cement ethnic identity and justify a programme of segregation (see, for example, Beinart 2001). Yet more recently, the politics of ethnicity has taken a different turn. Culture, tradition, and ethnicity are no longer propagated as barriers to engaging with the outside world (Oomen 2005; Comaroff and Comaroff 2009). Rather, they have become platforms upon which traditional leaders seek legitimacy in a democratic setting. Through the language and politics of tradition, local headmen, chiefs, and kings embrace national and global political processes, whilst mediating the frustrations, and occasionally the fortunate turns, of everyday life.

Key to understanding the continuities and transformations of the politics of tradition in post-apartheid South Africa is the phenomenon known as the African renaissance. Starting as an intellectual project, it rapidly attracted widespread recognition in South African public life, assuming an 'almost liturgical status' (Lodge 2002: 227). It has influenced

ANC policy significantly whilst informing research through newly established and well-funded institutes and academic networks dedicated to constructing a science that will provide 'African solutions to African problems'. The extent to which the African renaissance is based on essentialist assumptions and aims is epitomised by the key concept of *Ubuntu*, an allegedly 'African' variant of humanity towards others, the authenticity of which has exercised various authors (Msimang 2000; Vail and Maseko 2002: 125). I use the term 'African renaissance' as a descriptive, vernacular expression with a view to highlighting Venda traditional leaders' strategic alignment with wider ANC policy and the implications for the ways in which people understand AIDS.

Two predominant visions of the African renaissance have surfaced in public debate. The first is framed in modernist rhetoric and is symbolic of rebirth, in which regeneration will be achieved through liberal democracy, market economics, and a revolution in communications technology. In 2001, this assumed a strategic dimension through the New Partnership for Africa's Development (NEPAD) and drew significant attention (but limited funding) from the international community. NEPAD is based on market efficiency, good governance, and regional cooperation to support international investment, and is closely connected to the wider philosophy of the African Union (AU), of which Thabo Mbeki became the first president in 2002. The AU strives to create Africa-wide cooperation in trade, currency, security, aid, and diplomacy (Mills 2000: 139–84) and epitomises former President Mbeki's 'modernist' conceptualisation of the African renaissance, which embraces 'the economic recovery of the African continent, and . . . the restructuring of the political agenda in Africa' (Mbeki 2002: 159–60).

The second vision of the African renaissance is about African heritage. From this perspective, 'communities' succeed in 'reconstructing themselves around tradition, legacy, and heritage, around the values and relationships that characterised pre-colonial institutions' (Lodge 2002: 230). In this interpretation, there is an explicit call for the re-evaluation of African history and culture away from its colonial construction and towards a consolidation of the 'wealth of knowledge that Africans are carrying around in their heads' (Dladla 1997 in Vail and Maseko 2002: 128). This rhetoric can be traced back to the African nationalism of Marcus Garvey, through to Steve Biko and others who have promoted black consciousness. Intellectuals who have taken up this strand of the renaissance tend to be sceptical of the extent to which an increase in global trade will temper the historical disadvantage of the African continent, and call instead for development from within, beginning with a critical examination of consciousness on the basis of which a new African identity may burgeon and flower (cf. Appiah 1992).

This brings us back to the questions raised about the political uses of tradition. Commentators on the topic have questioned the practicalities and desirability of converting the 'African heritage' reading of the renaissance into policy (Ndebele 1997 in Vail and Maseko 2002: 129). They argue that uncovering 'mythical roots' is less significant than providing public amenities or employment. They suggest that, ultimately, the renaissance concept may represent a barrier to development and an unwelcome return to social classifications based on 'race' that have little place in a constitutional democracy for which many people paid with their lives. And yet, as academic debates ponder the commensurability of tradition and policy, often criticising the essentialist underpinnings of the renaissance, in post-apartheid South Africa there is a pronounced engagement on an everyday level with processes that are considered to be part of traditional repertoires, legitimised by their symbolic alignment with the past.

Traditional Leaders in the Democratic Dispensation

This contemporary concern with the past was evident at a recent event held at the Tshivhase royal palace in Mukumbani. The road leading up the mountains to the royal kraal was crammed as I forced my pick-up truck, laden with the local reggae band and our gear, through the dense sea of people. We were en route to perform at a ceremony organised in honour of the late King (*Thovhela*) Ratsimphi Frans Tshivhase, who had been posthumously awarded the ANC Luthuli Award for his contribution to the fight against white occupation of tribal land in the 1930s. Many in the excited crowd were hoping that the widely publicised event would feature an address by Nelson Mandela, and a rumour was spreading that he had arrived hours before with an army escort. As we inched into the packed forecourt, our entrance was announced over the loudspeaker and there was a brief bellowing of approval. The ground was at capacity, with men dressed in their finery and women in the bright kaleidoscope of colours woven into their traditional *minwenda* garments. Additional people had found perches in trees or on top of the huge grey rocks that surround and fortify the lush green forest that has hidden the Mukumbani mountain fortress from view for over two centuries. A large stage, draped in white shade-cloth and the ANC colours of black, green, and gold, had been specially erected and was protected by a troupe of men yielding submachine guns. The numerous dignitaries – who did not include Mandela – were arranged in three tiers on the stage with the most senior cabinet ministers and ANC elders towards the front. In the middle, an empty seat had been reserved in anticipation of *Thovhela* Kennedy Tshivhase, the current king, who was to receive the award on behalf of his grandfather.

On the back of the programme of events, an obituary explained how Ratsimphi Frans Tshivhase had ruled fearlessly from Mukumbani during the 1930s and 1940s. He had been prominent and influential in

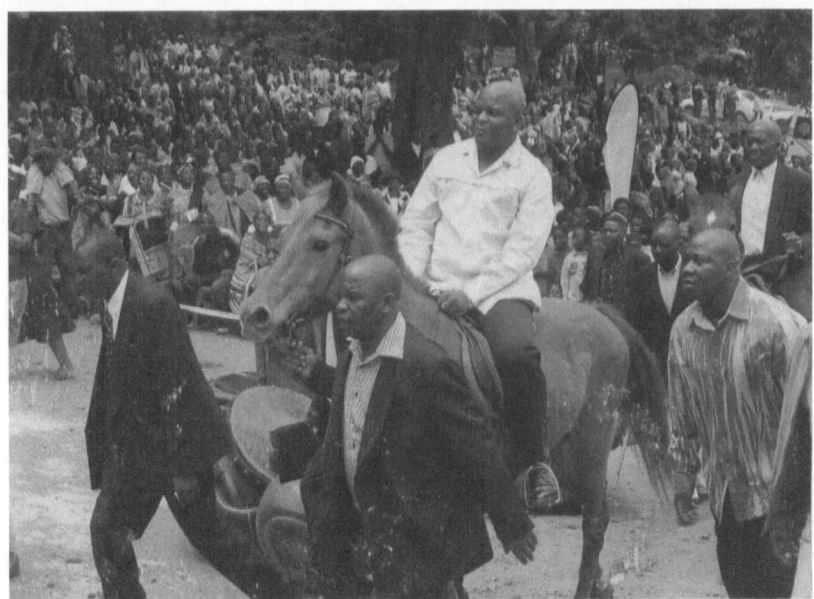

Figure 2.1. King Kennedy Tshivhase on his horse, 'Fly', riding into the arena at Mukumbani to collect the Luthuli Award on behalf of his grandfather, Frans Ratsimphi Tshivhase.

early struggle movements, and nurtured an allegiance to the Communist Party. His refusal to allow the fertile Tshivhase land to be demarcated for white farming projects initiated by the 1927 Black Administration Act had eventually led, in 1946, to his arrest. He was incarcerated north of Johannesburg at Hammanskraal, where he died in 1952: 'a pioneering hero of the struggle'.

In a dramatically executed and highly symbolic move, Kennedy Tshivhase arrived at the ceremony in a manner to which his grandfather would have been accustomed. Instead of his conventional entrance in a large entourage of blacked-out luxury vehicles, he surprised the crowd by riding up the winding road through the courtyard to the stage on horseback, clad in a bright white jacket, accompanied only by a handler (see Figures 2.1 and 2.2). It was a masterful stroke that guaranteed wide media coverage and placed him firmly at the centre of Venda's turbulent post-apartheid political arena, in which the royal house of Tshivhase has played a particularly interesting role.

What follows is an historical account of events leading up to the contemporary internecine dispute that has pitted the house of Tshivhase against its historical rival, the neighbouring house of Mphephu. Mphephu and Tshivhase both trace their descent to the same ancestor, Dimbanyika, as a result of which they consider themselves to be brothers.

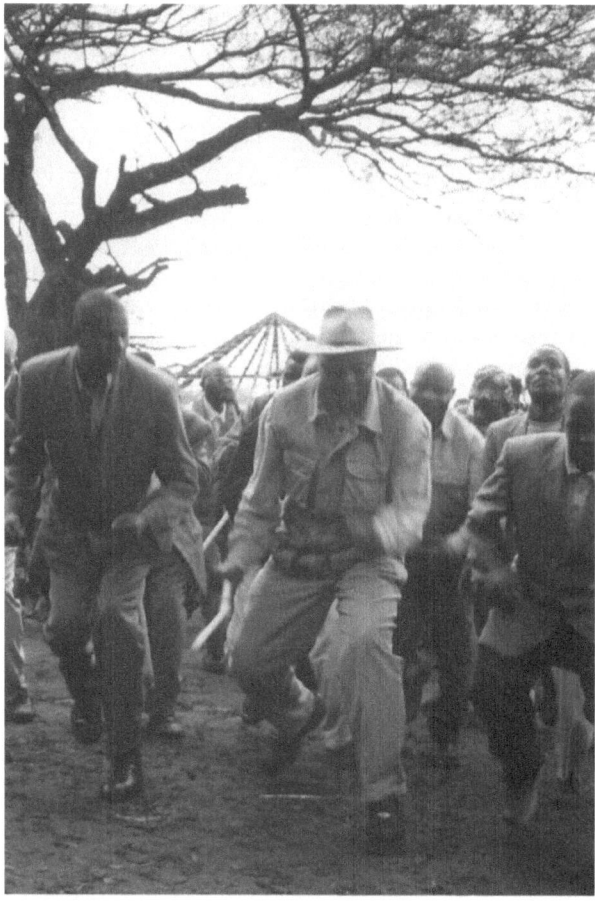

Figure 2.2. King Kennedy Tshivhase leading a *tshikona* at Mukumbani.

In the recent battle for paramount kingship, Toni Mphephu has emphasised his genealogical superiority as the widely recognised elder brother of the two. This dominance was reinforced by the apartheid government, which instated Toni's uncle, Patrick Mphephu, as paramount king and head of government in the former Venda homeland. Kennedy Tshivhase, as the younger brother, has been forced to seek legitimacy beyond the established genealogical record. His central tactic in this manoeuvre, illustrated in the narrative above, has been to accentuate the historical connections between Tshivhase leadership and the ANC. In so doing, he has strategically embraced the ANC-inspired African renaissance within his borders, prompting a cultural revival through which processes of female initiation, performances of traditional music, and the installation of *Vhamusanda/Magota* (headmen) in a ceremony known as *vhuhosi* have become regular features of daily life. In this way, Tshivhase's involvement in, and association with, the promotion of culture and tradition have been deeply rooted in politically strategic incentives.

Still, the incorporation of traditional leaders into the democratic dispensation has been controversial. The ANC-inspired uprisings against institutions of traditional leadership at the end of apartheid were indicative of a strong resentment against the extent to which kings and their henchmen had benefited from their association with the apartheid authorities. The social unrest seemed to indicate that any role given to structures of traditional leadership after the political rearrangements of 1994 would be extremely limited, giving way to a modernist vision of democracy.

And yet traditional leaders have made a remarkable return to the post-apartheid political arena. Whilst structures of traditional authority were certainly bolstered by the white minority government, they were not simply collaborators in running the homelands (Harries 2005: 3). On the contrary, CONTRALESA (Council of Traditional Leaders in South Africa), the umbrella body under which chiefs in South Africa collectively affiliate, called for the Bantustan system to be abolished (ibid.). Originally formed in 1987, CONTRALESA positioned itself largely in opposition to Zulu Chief Buthelezi's Inkatha movement which was, by then, well incorporated into the structures of homeland politics (cf. Mare and Hamilton 1987). However, the complexities of collaboration and resistance in spaces constituted by colonial and post-colonial orders do not lend themselves to a dichotomous explanation, in which some chiefs cooperated and others resisted. For example, Oomen (2000: 42; 2005: 226, 245) shows that in the cases of Kgoloko and Rhyne in Sekhukhuneland it has been possible for one chieftaincy, under the strategic guidance of a single leader, to change affiliation over time; it has managed to support, whilst being supported by, successive governments with opposed agendas (cf. Mbembe 1992 in Cameroon; Lan 1985 in Zimbabwe). Specific regional situations are complicated by particular histories of association and confrontation with colonial powers. In South Africa, this has hinged on pre-colonial arrangements that have taken on new significance in recent years as the boundaries between traditional authority and the state have been redefined by the ANC-led government in an attempt to reposition traditional leaders within the post-apartheid political sphere.

Several arguments have been put forward to explain this unexpected revival of royalty. Some have stressed the role of abstract, global forces in its contemporary comeback. Koelble and Lipuma (2005), for example, emphasise market forces (cf. Mayekiso 1996 in Ferguson 2006: 105). They argue that to maintain economic stability, transformative movements such as the ANC make 'two promises' at the dawn of democracy

(Koelble and Lipuma 2005: 77). The first promise is to adopt transparent, democratic policies, and to implement the liberalisation of the state and economy, through policies such as GEAR (see Chapter 1). The second undertaking is to implement institutions that 'remedy the injustices inherited from the past' (ibid.). They suggest that state attempts to deliver on this promise may be interpreted by 'the market' as a risky shift to the left, potentially decreasing the profit margin of investment and destabilising the national economy. In their analysis, traditional leaders are connected to, but not directly subsumed by, the state – and can thus apply projects that facilitate the redistribution of wealth without raising the suspicions of the abstract forces behind the market. For Koelble and Lipuma, then, structures of traditional authority in South Africa have enjoyed a comeback as a means to 'penetrate and integrate the hinterlands' with social justice (ibid: 92).

Whilst this argument flags up, and may partially explain, the role of traditional leadership in supporting development projects (see below), it ignores the significant expansion of the South African state, as a 'distributional regime' (Seekings and Nattrass 2005), into rural areas through service provision and welfare payments. Moreover, a focus on abstract global forces underplays royal agency. It cannot take into account the oscillating fortunes of rival houses, or the ways in which debts that were incurred during the struggle are now being settled through performances of solidarity at public ceremonies and through parliamentary appointments. There is more to this kingly comeback than a pandering to market forces.

Taking a similarly global but less economically deterministic approach, Oomen (2005) understands the post-apartheid resurgence of traditional authority in the context of a 'new world order' (2005: 4). Acknowledging the specific abuses of the South African past, in which successive governments reinvented tradition in the interests of racial segregation, she argues that in the last thirty years an erosion of the nation-state has led to the emergence of 'heterogeneous, network-like polities, operating locally, transnationally and internationally' (Oomen 2005: 7; cf. Meyer and Geschiere 1999; Young 1999). Culture and tradition, she claims, are no longer obstacles to modernisation: they are central means of engaging with it.[5] Claims to legitimacy and authenticity have been made on a truly global scale, for example through First Nations in North America, and indigenous rights groups in South America, Australia, and Botswana. In South Africa, where the right to culture is now guaranteed in Chapter 12 of the Constitution, the discourse of tradition has become integral to the practice of politics at every level. As guardians of culture, Oomen

---

[5] The extent to which tradition ever actually prevented Africans from engaging with 'the modern' has been questioned by several authors. See, for example, Vail (1989); Mamdani (1996).

argues, traditional leaders have taken to the stage in a powerful new guise. More than an extra arm of the state in the pursuit of rural social justice, kings have re-emerged as cultural icons in the new world order in which, she states, 'tribes [are] trendy and culture [is] cool' (2005: 4). Oomen consequently argues that traditional leadership in post-apartheid South Africa constitutes a new body politic that has grown to fill the void of the shrinking nation-state, and in this way chiefs and kings have gained popularity when most thought they would be sidelined (cf. Chabal and Daloz 1999; Mamdani 1996).[6]

Kennedy Tshivhase's strategic alignment with the African renaissance therefore echoes the politics of tradition on the global stage. And yet there can be little doubt that, despite the 'pulling back' of nation-states, national government sovereignty still trumps traditional authority. The bottom line here is that traditional leaders are employed by the state, and paid monthly salaries to exercise their duties – whatever they may be. Moreover, as we see below, the post-apartheid state has taken an active role in deciding who can – and who cannot – be a king.

Reflecting this state of affairs, the issue of how to incorporate structures of traditional leadership into a constitutional democracy has been a pressing one for the ANC-led government since the democratic elections in 1994. Although the process of drafting and implementing legislation was slow, Parliament finally passed the Traditional Leadership and Governance Framework Act in 2003. This edict covered a wide range of issues centred on the perceived need to restore the integrity of traditional authority institutions after apartheid. It was intended to mark a move away from the perception of traditional leaders as apartheid stooges or cultural guardians of the rural poor, and provide wider scope for them to operate, albeit in an auxiliary and advisory capacity, within the democratic process. Problems such as marginalisation of women, party political affiliation, remuneration, and relationships with other spheres of government were partially addressed, but much of this had already been settled in policy and legislation before 2003 (Oomen 2005: 55–6, 68–9). On the other hand, the Act was unclear on issues that urgently needed clarification, such as the precise relationship between traditional authorities and elected municipal councils, the extent of jurisdiction with regard to customary law, and the role of traditional leaders in the allocation of land. It did, however, offer some clarity by officially recognising three levels of traditional authority in the descending hierarchy of kings,

---

[6] Arguing that the position of chiefs in KwaZulu-Natal must also be seen as part of a longer history between the government and traditional leaders, Beall et al. take a similar stance. They argue, however, that the post-apartheid situation should be read through a 'politics of compromise' (2005: 757) in which the electoral influence of traditional leaders was central to maintaining security in that region.

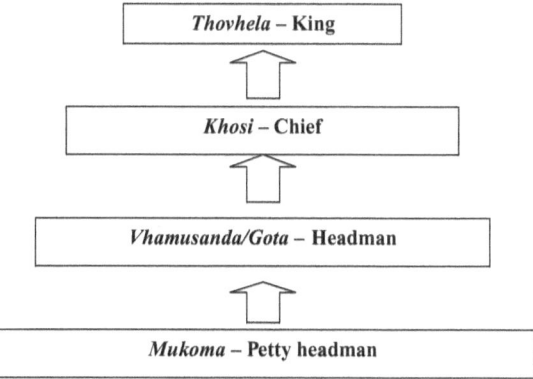

Figure 2.3. The hierarchical structure of a Venda kingship[7]

senior traditional leaders (chiefs), and 'headmen/women'.[8] In Tshivenda these correspond to the titles of *Thovhela*, *Khosi*, and *Vhamusanda* (see Figure 2.3).

Although the 2003 Act legitimised the existence of multiple chiefs and headmen/women under any king, it was clear that the government had the intention of establishing one king for each group with a history of traditional leadership. The motivation for this imposition is stated in the Act, and in subsequent reports, as a desire for 'uniformity'. The groups affected by this legislation are to be found throughout the country, in the provinces where South Africa's kings reside: North-West, Mpumalanga, Limpopo, Free State, KwaZulu-Natal, and the Eastern Cape (Oomen 2005: 56). The Act provided for the establishment of six Provincial Houses of Traditional Leaders, one in each of the aforementioned regions, from which the National House of Traditional Leaders in Pretoria, already established in 1997, would draw its representatives.

In recognising that several kingdoms were established, and others significantly elevated in status, by the apartheid state specifically to uphold the Bantustan system, the Act ostensibly sought to re-establish the

---

[7] There are 25 such tribal authorities structured in this manner in the Venda region. The arrows represent a strict flow of power, and direction of communication, which must be followed if an issue is to be raised with the king. A fine is imposed for taking an issue directly to the *Khosi*, and expecting him to raise it with *Thovhela*. As the diagram suggests, the positions are less numerous and more powerful as one moves up the hierarchy, culminating in a single monarch at its apex.

[8] The category of 'principal traditional leader' was reserved for kings who were in place prior to the 2003 legislation, but not recognised by the Nhlapo Commission (see below) as legitimate. However in government documentation, press releases, and final reports, the use of senior/principal traditional leader has been inconsistent, leading to some confusion over the actual meaning of the term.

accepted pre-colonial political order. In this way, it resolved to 'ensure that the legitimacy of those occupying positions within the institution of traditional leadership [was] beyond reproach' (Mbeki: 2003). Section 22 of the Act stated that the resolution of any disputes should be negotiated through the implementation of a commission that would hear evidence from as far back as 1927: the year that the Black Administration Act began official regulation of traditional leadership structures and defined in law the reclassification of African kings as chiefs. On 16 October 2004, the then government minister Sydney Mufamadi announced the members of the Commission on Disputes and Claims – which would become known as the Nhlapo Commission – and encouraged all traditional leaders with disagreements to refer them to it for adjudication (Mufamadi: 2004a).[9]

The formal announcement that the state intended to reclassify South African structures of traditional leadership, and recognise a series of single kings as paramount over all others in their respective 'traditional communities' (previously called 'tribes'), was not wholly unexpected. Nonetheless it caused considerable anxiety and intrigue in the corridors and courts of traditional power, not least because a paramount king (*Khosikhulu*) can expect an annual salary in the region of a million rand.[10] Moreover, as the title would be recognised throughout South Africa, and potentially beyond, there was substantial social and political kudos at stake.

The initial reports of the Nhlapo Commission were released in April 2008, and were intended to provide a comprehensive overview of the paramountcies that existed at the time of the 2003 Framework Act. These preliminary reports cite early anthropological and ethnological sources as evidence in their assessment of history, and demonstrate each claimant's desire to validate a specific set of historical events leading to the legitimation of royal status (South African Government 2008a; 2008b). The 2008 report identified 12 paramount kingships across South Africa, six of which it asserted had been artificially promoted during apartheid. These findings prompted a flurry of claims and counter-claims to the

---

[9] The Commission for Disputes and Claims was comprised of 12 advocates, academics, and politicians. It was chaired by the prominent lawyer and academic Professor Tandabantu Nhlapo, based at the University of Cape Town. In August 2007, Professor Nhlapo resigned from the Commission, to which Thabo Mbeki had appointed him in 2004.

[10] In 2005, a paramount king received a basic salary of R453,399, and a chief received a basic salary of R108,828. Both received a 'sitting allowance' of around R600 per day, along with subsistence expenses for attending the Provincial and/or National House of Traditional Leaders (South African Government 2005). A recent media report indicated that, in 2011, a paramount king receives R883,000 and a chief gets R162,000 per annum (*City Press*, 13 February 2011, p. 9). According to Koelble and Lipuma (2005: 76), the state spends more than R50 million a month supporting structures of traditional authority.

same positions, and the Nhlapo Commission embarked on a second whirlwind tour of South Africa's former homelands and self-governing territories, during which more claims to kingship were presented to the panel and submitted in legal documents detailing the claims of specific royal houses.

However, neat genealogies have not always settled quarrels over kingship. As anthropologists of South Africa have long recognised, royal succession can be a messy business. They have partly helped to make it so. On the one hand, it is partially fixed through established genealogy. Anthropologists and government ethnologists played a significant role in standardising the genealogies that would be used by successive governments – up to and including the current administration – to assist them in making decisions on traditional authority. Internecine disputes during the pre- and early colonial period were essentially open-ended, with flexible outcomes that depended largely on the extent of popular support and legitimacy (Schapera 1938; Fortes and Evans-Pritchard 1940; Comaroff 1974; Hammond-Tooke 1997). The extent to which any pre-colonial political order can be re-established in the present day, or any single line of paramount kings identified, is therefore limited. In the current political climate with well-established genealogies, as one of Oomen's informants has shown in the Bapedi case, "'you can't just claim paramountcy by pointing at history; you also need a following'" (2005: 221). In this fashion, contemporary battles for *Khosikhulu* throughout South Africa have often been complex affairs, hinging on diverse attempts to secure legitimacy through legal claims to genealogical superiority and assertions that historical wrongs are being righted. Significantly for the Venda case, contenders for paramountcy who are less senior genealogically were encouraged to stake their claims through other, more diverse means. The 2003 legislation has thus seen the legitimacy of traditional leaders tested on a national level through the concurrent scrutiny of the state, competing royal lineages, and the citizenry.

For some, the contemporary requirement of standardisation and uniformity has been relatively straightforward. The Zulu case, for example, states quite clearly that 'there was always only one king' (South African Government 2010: 191), and King Goodwill Zwelethini was declared king without contestation.[11] On the other hand, the claim made by Mpisane Eric Nxumalo as leader of the Shangaan 'traditional community' was rejected outright. The Nhlapo Commission judged their kingship to have been defeated long before 1927 – in neighbouring

---

[11] According to recent media reports, however, squabbles for the position of chief (one rung under paramountcy) in some smaller Zulu groups remain unsettled (see the *Sunday Times* [South Africa], 7 February 2010). In 2010, the government resolved to implement a new commission to settle disputes over positions of senior traditional leadership.

Mozambique – and as thus lying outside the Commission's remit. As a consequence, Amashangana have no kingship in contemporary South Africa.

Other cases have been more complex, involving protracted and very public spats between royal houses. The pronouncement on the Bapedi ba Maroteng paramountcy, for example, saw Kgagudi Kenneth Sekhukhune demoted from king to the position of principal traditional leader, making way for King Thulare Victor Thulare, who was judged the rightful heir to the Bapedi throne. Claims to the amaXhosa kingship were complicated by the apartheid state's creation of two separate homelands in the Eastern Cape; Transkei and Ciskei.[12] Paramountcy of Transkei was given to the amaGcaleka royal house, under King Zwelidumile Sigcawu, who was widely recognised at the time as the most senior of amaXhosa traditional leaders. In neighbouring Ciskei, the apartheid authorities promoted Archie Velile Sandile, head of the amaRharhabe lineage, to paramountcy. The Nhlapo Commission pronounced that this was an irregular creation of a dual kingship among the amaXhosa, and reinstated the lineage of amaGcaleka – under King Zwelonke Sigcawu – to paramountcy (South African Government 2010: 118–53).

In Limpopo Province, the situation was even more complex. Genealogical seniority and political legitimacy have been in contention over the course of two separate commissions. Matters were further complicated by the need to accommodate the members of several traditional polities: the former occupants of the previous homelands of Venda, Gazankulu (Tsonga/Shangaan), and Lebowa (predominantly Northern Sotho). The Ralushai Commission had been gathering data from 1996 to investigate 'claims by certain traditional leaders that they were irregularly deposed or not duly recognised by the previous government' (Mufamadi 2004b). The erratic methodology employed by the commissioners and the absence of terms of reference within which the data could be contextualised, however, led to general confusion as to what constituted evidence and who could submit it. The lengthy report of the Ralushai Commission was eventually submitted to the (former) Provincial Premier Ramathlodi in October 1998. However the findings were never published in full, reportedly because it was feared that the recommendations on the 244 cases (many of which had little to do with homeland disputes) would lead to widespread confusion (Mufamadi 2004b).

---

[12] Transkei was actually home to five paramountcies under apartheid, in the areas of east Pondoland, west Pondoland, Thembuland, western Thembuland, and Gcalekaland, all of which were subject to scrutiny under the Nhlapo Commission. Only three – those of amaThembu, amaXhosa, and amaMpondo – were recognised as legitimate by the Commission, securing their continued existence as paramountcies into the democratic era.

Although the recommendations remain secret, it is generally believed (thanks to gossip and press speculation) that Ralushai endorsed Mphephu's claim to the paramountcy on the grounds of the widely recognised genealogical seniority of his house to that of Tshivhase. Speculation aside, traditional leaders in Venda were forced to wait until the end of 2004 for the report's partial release. Each applicant was given a copy of the section that outlined his claim or complaint, but they were disappointed when it became clear that any recommendations made by the Commission were excluded from their heavily censored dossiers (*Limpopo Mirror*, 17 December 2004).

Picking up where the Ralushai Commission left off, the Nhlapo Commission held two rounds of hearings in Venda during December 2005, and a subsequent round in November 2008, during which submissions were made by legal representatives of the five claimants to the Venda throne: Mphephu, Tshivhase, Ravhura, Vhangona, and Mphaphuli. For reasons that will become apparent below, there were only ever two real contenders: Mphephu and Tshivhase. But they were not seeking similar recognition from the Commission. Mphephu's claim was to *the* Venda kingship. Tshivhase's legal team proposed that they be granted 'Tshivhase Kingship', as a subsection of the Venda 'traditional community' (South African Government 2010: 603). If genealogical superiority was to be given precedence, the title would go to Mphephu. If current political affiliations received priority, it would go to Tshivhase, in what would essentially be the official recognition of a dual kingship within Venda.

Pre-Colonial Expansion and Subjugation

My emphasis here is on how contemporary internecine disputes reproduce and reframe pre-colonial structures of political expansion and subjugation in post-apartheid terms (cf. Comaroff 1985: 18–19). Cleavages of power that were prominent before colonial contact set the scene for political rearrangements to follow, although they by no means dictated them. Since colonialism, some traditional leaders in Venda have sought power through association with white minority rule, whilst others have recently achieved influence through their previous support for resistance movements. For the royal house of Tshivhase, current popularity has lain in its emergence under a new leader untainted by the Bantustan system, with an accumulation of moral capital through ANC connections and a well-calculated association with the African renaissance. The rival house of Mphephu, on the other hand, has struggled to shake off a long association with apartheid-era politics, but maintains legitimacy in chiefly circles due to its pre-colonial genealogical seniority. The battle for *Khosikhulu* in Venda has thus been a bitter one, and has prompted a cultural revival that permeates practically every aspect of daily life within Tshivhase's borders. To grasp the dynamics of present-day politics, I now turn – as the Nhlapo Commission did – to accounts of the past.

The very notion of 'the Venda' is rooted in pre-colonial patterns of expansion and conquest. The current challenge for *Khosikhulu*, which was established as a result of that conquest, is based on a key form of social stratification: that between royalty (*vhakololo*) and commoners (*vhasiwana*).[13] The distinction between these two groups is fundamental to the political economy of traditional leadership in contemporary Venda, but the origins of the division are debated in contesting historical accounts.

A common Venda origin myth recorded in early ethnological accounts chimes with the oft-cited oral histories of royal elders.[14] Although their dates were often at odds with each other, they agreed in their accounts of great lakes, possibly in Tanzania (a notion supported by Wilson 1969: 169), a long journey through dense forest (said to be the Congo region), then drier lands (Zambia, Zimbabwe), until eventually they rested for a period of long, solitary, and unconquered confinement in the Soutpansberg Mountains (cf. Wessmann 1908: 10; Stayt 1931: 14). Government ethnologist van Warmelo (1932) recorded this oral tradition as part of a state-sponsored project to document genealogies specifically for use in solving succession disputes (Hammond-Tooke 1997: 112). He suggested that historically Vhavenda were shielded from foreign influence by isolation. In support of this now commonsensical belief, he pointed out the extreme northerly geographical location of Venda in South Africa, arguing that the Soutpansberg mountain range was a formidable barrier to the flow of contact with other groups in the region.

A more recent account, based on a detailed analysis of clans (*mitupo*; singular, *mutupo*) in Venda social structure, has refuted this. Its author, Victor Ralushai (1977: 17), formerly John Blacking's research assistant and responsible for the previously mentioned commission, argues that the significance of the Soutpansberg mountain range should rather be seen in military terms: through the lens, for example, of the successful defence it enabled against violent intruders during the *Mfecane*.[15] We saw in Chapter 1 how this story of Venda's cunning defence against Shaka's 'hordes' has been woven into the myth of Venda isolation, epitomised in the advertising campaign for 'Africa's Eden' on roadside

---

[13] For an in-depth historical account of this distinction, see Kirkaldy (2005: 203–11).

[14] The early ethnological accounts of Venda, and pre-colonial migration, can be found in Wessman (1908), Stayt (1931), van Warmelo (1932; 1948a–1948c; 1949; 1967), and Lestrade (1930a; 1930b; 1932; 1949).

[15] It was this strategic use of the mountain landscape that led to the building of royal households in steep, easily defendable gullies and on top of mountains, where their presence remains a distinguishing feature of the Venda landscape today. More recently, their symbolic significance has been hijacked by local Christian leaders who now elect to live in grand houses, on hillsides preferably above their churches.

billboards. Ralushai, while offering a more nuanced account of these military events, forcefully discredits the myth of tribal uniqueness, stating that 'Venda's geographical position between the Rhodesian, Mozambican, Northern Sotho, and Tswana (Botswana) areas, has made her a melting pot' (ibid.: 19). As evidence of this, he cites the frequent occurrence of both Sotho and Shona words in Tshivenda vocabulary, Venda architectural contributions to the wider area, and the presence of 'non-Venda' possession cults (*malombo*) and male initiation schools throughout the region. Blacking (1995c) takes this a stage further by identifying the various musical scales (penta-, hexa-, and heptatonic) characteristic of specific groups in the region, and analysing their infiltration into Venda musical practice over time.[16]

Although there is evidence to support a migration from 'the north', Ralushai argues that this 'north' reaches only as far as Zimbabwe, not to the great lakes region or the Congo basin. In this, Ralushai is joined by Blacking (1962; 1995b; 1995c), Marks (1975), and Nettleton (1992), who support the notion that in the early seventeenth century there were a number of aboriginal clans scattered over the Soutpansberg mountains, commonly referred to as Vhangona groups (singular, Ngona) with a degree of political centralisation in the ruling houses of Netshisevhe, Neluonde, and Netshiendeulu.[17] Archaeological evidence suggests that groups of Ngona were living in the Soutpansberg as early as the fifteenth century (Lahiff 2000: 60). These scattered clans had established exchange and kinship relations across the Limpopo River by the mid-seventeenth century, and shared significant social, cultural, and linguistic affinity with the Shona, Shangaan/Tsonga, and Northern Sotho. Moreover, they developed an extensive cosmology in which links to the Lobedu 'Rain Queen' (Modjadji) in the south-east were particularly strong (Krige and Krige 1943) and consolidated elaborate ritual cycles through which a specific musical tradition was born (Blacking 1995c). It is likely that this cosmological connection with Modjadji was influential in the tempering of Zulu aggression towards Vhavenda, given that Shaka passed through Lobedu territory with great deference to, and elaborate gifts for, the powerful queen who was widely believed to control the rain (cf. Krige and Krige 1943).[18]

---

[16] Kruger (1999) has conducted similar research tracing modern Venda political history through the regional variation in lyrical construction of a Venda genre, *Tshigombela*.

[17] The 'Vhangona Cultural Movement' announced its own contender for the position of *Khosikhulu* in the guise of *Thovhela* Tshidziwelele Nephawe. However, given that claims of irregular deposition were only recognised as far back as 1927 – and that Vhangona were defeated by Singo invaders – Tshidziwelele's case was easily dismissed by the Nhlapo Commission.

[18] This version of events was suggested by Zulu men in Johannesburg. Their account stated that Shaka was not defeated by cunning Venda warriors, but was being deferential to

Accounts show how the scattered settlement and cultural diversity of this loose collection of groups was to alter definitively with their conquest by invaders from the north. Around 1600, a progression of Singo clans from Zimbabwe, who were fleeing violence between the Shona royal families relating to upheavals in Rowzi society and the rise of Changamire dynasty, moved south across the Limpopo River and into Vhangona territory (Marks 1975). In the latter part of the 1600s, under the leadership of Dimbanyika, they reached a settlement, more commonly described as a conquest, building their headquarters at Dzata in the middle of the Nzhelele Valley (see Map 4).[19] The invading Singo clans had little to offer the Ngona culturally, but brought with them extensive skills in regional administration and the mobilisation of military power from the comparatively advanced Karanga civilisations. According to the historical record, they did not attempt to destroy what they found, but rather 'patronised the arts, made a pact with the priests, magicians and ritual experts, married local women and adopted some local customs' (Blacking 1995c: 140).[20] Singo clans quickly became the dominant political and military force in the area and established a level of political centralisation that reflected their power over the Ngona groups.

Their success in doing so is evident in the fact that most influential traditional leaders in Venda today, from the royal households of Mphephu and Tshivhase, trace their descent to the great Singo warrior Dimbanyika and his son, Vele-la-Mbeu (van Warmelo 1932: 6; Lestrade 1932; Ralushai 1977). However, there are 25 recognised kingships in Venda, not all of which are of Singo origin. The less powerful kings in areas such as Lwamondo, Makuya, and Manenzhe, for example, trace their lineage to Ngona occupancy (see Map 2). There are also less powerful Singo kingdoms, such as Khakhu and Rambuda. The Singo invaders, rather than waging war on the occupants of the Soutpansberg, allegedly incorporated elements of their political system, and thus the most important political factions, into their centralised system of government (cf. Kopytoff 1987). The socio-political division between 'royal' (*vhakololo*) and 'common' (*vhasiwana*) must thus be seen as the product of historical developments through which Singo invaders *became* royal and, in

---

Venda kings in recognition of their close relationship with Modjadji. Either way, both versions suggest that Venda remained 'untouched' by Zulu influence at the time.

[19] There is a dearth of historical research on the precise ways in which Singo invaders settled amongst Vhangona occupants of the land. Given that history is generally told by the victors, it is perhaps not surprising that there are no records of resistance by the Vhangona. However this should not lead us to conclude that the 'settlement' reached between the two groups was as peaceful as we have been led to believe.

[20] Blacking's poetic use of the term 'priests' belies the complexity of structures of traditional healing in Venda. See Blacking 1995c.

the process, subjugated the Vhangona occupants of the Soutpansberg Mountains, reducing their status to that of commoners.

Although it is not my intention here to provide a detailed historical analysis of Venda royal conflicts (see Ralushai 1977; South African Government 2010), a brief explanation is necessary. When the legendary leader and first paramount king, Dimbanyika, eventually died at Dzata in the early 1700s, he was succeeded by his son Vele-la-Mbeu. Ruling until the late 1700s, Dimbanyika's heir was in turn succeeded by Thohoyandou (early 1800s). Around 1870, Thohoyandou mysteriously disappeared, and a succession battle ensued. The *dzekiso* house (that of the senior wife chosen to produce the heir to the throne) had failed to give birth to any male children. However, Thohoyandou had fathered three sons: Tshisevhe, Mpofu, and Tshivhase (also known as Raluswielo) from less senior wives. As the eldest son, Tshisevhe was installed as king, but died soon afterwards. Tshisevhe's son – who was the rightful heir – believed his father had been murdered and fled in fear of his own life, abandoning his claim to succession. As the second eldest son, Mpofu (later to become Mphephu) inherited the throne. Tshivhase fled east to Dopeni (see Map 4), pillaging and torching villages on the way, and then to Phiphidi, where he became known as Midiyavhathu Tshivhase ('the one who burnt everybody's houses'). In search of secure headquarters during the *Mfecane*, he then migrated north-east to the mountains of Mukumbani (Ralushai 1977: 162) where the seat of the Tshivhase throne remains today and where the current king rode in on horseback to receive the Luthuli Award on his grandfather's behalf.[21]

Different royal factions are at variance as to what happened next. According to Mphephu history, after Tshivhase's migration east, the youngest brother attacked Mpofu twice in an attempt to usurp the paramountcy, but failed on both occasions. According to Tshivhase history, an independent kingdom was established at Mukumbani, which to this day has never been under the control of another traditional leader. It is this point of distinction which lies at the heart of Mphephu's current claim to paramountcy and Tshivhase's contention that the contemporary situation is essentially one of dual kingship. What is beyond doubt is that

---

[21] Van Warmelo (1932: 4–16) offers an alternative account of this historical transition, but similarly concludes that Mphephu is the senior royal lineage. Ralushai, however, offers a comprehensive and compelling critique of van Warmelo's account, pointing to important inconsistencies and their relationship to the inherent bias of his main informants. Of importance here may be a disagreement over the identity of the first paramount king: van Warmelo argues that Thohoyandou's grandfather was not Dimbanyika, but Ndymbeu (1932: 2). As Ralushai himself admits somewhat sheepishly: 'Besides, there has been so much movement and intermingling in Venda that it is impossible to know the truth' (1977: 30).

since this split between the two brothers the history of Venda kingship has been marked by dynastic struggles both within and between the houses of Mphephu and Tshivhase.[22] Subsequent episodes of royal division, as with other South and Southern African kingships, were largely mapped onto the schism between colonial collaborators and resisters (cf., for example, Delius 1996; Lan 1985), although the reality was much more complex.

The association between the Mphephu house and colonial structures of power began officially in 1925 during the leadership of George Mbulaheni Mphephu, but dates back to the arrival of the Voortrekkers in the region in the mid-1860s. In 1867, the legendary leader Makhado Ramabulana earned the title 'Lion of the North' by driving the Voortrekkers out of the Soutpansberg Mountains. In 1898, they returned to defeat Makhado's successor (Mphephu Ramabulana), who retreated into exile north of the Limpopo, only returning in 1902 to settle at Dzanani – where the current royal homestead of Mphephu remains. According to oral histories, Mphephu Ramabulana established several homesteads across the Limpopo in present-day Zimbabwe and instructed them to remain there as a safe periphery to which he could again withdraw in times of crisis. This is offered as an explanation for the small pockets of Tshivenda speakers to be found in Zimbabwe to this day, although it is not clear exactly how many of these groups trace their origins to the events of this historical drama.

Since its return south of the Limpopo, the Mphephu royal house has periodically fought, negotiated, and lived peacefully with white travellers, missionaries, traders, and settlers on the borders of Mphephu land (Giesekke 2004).[23] In 1948, George Mbulaheni Mphephu was succeeded by his son, Patrick Mphephu, who became the first president of the Venda Republic and whose nephew, Toni Mphephu, is the current king. The decision taken by the apartheid authorities to install Patrick Mphephu as 'paramount chief', initiating the political dominance of one royal family during the homeland era, had far-reaching consequences. The alliance between Mphephu and the apartheid state, and the tendency for neighbouring leaders with allegiance to Tshivhase to support liberation

---

[22] See also Lestrade (1932), Nemudzivhadi (1985), Ralushai (1977), Lahiff (2000), and Fokwang (2009) for extensive accounts of the Mphephu/Tshivhase division.

[23] Van Warmelo provides an account of settler leader Louis Trichardt's involvement in local political struggles in the area at this time (1932: 19–20). Kirkaldy notes that whilst German Lutheran missionaries were permitted to settle in the Tshivhase region from the 1870s, Mphephu (known at the time as Makhado) withheld permission for the establishment of any Christian mission within his borders as he believed that they 'prepared the ground for the Boers' (2005: 265). A close reading of the historical sources suggests that Tshivhase sought an alliance with the missionaries to compensate for his genealogical inferiority within the Singo clan (cf. Comaroff 1985: 29; White 1989).

structures, thus facilitated the continuation of pre-colonial political cleavages into the apartheid era.

Venda as a TVBC State: The Mphephu Chieftaincy and 'Development'

Intervening between mythical moments of origin and the *realpolitik* of the present, the most significant events affecting contestations over *Khosikhulu* occurred in the twentieth century. Since the 1927 Black Administration Act, the policies of successive colonial, apartheid, and Bantustan administrations have moulded political configurations in the areas reserved for black habitation. Having been seriously undermined during the course of the nineteenth century by military defeat and a subsequent loss of land, kingships were revived primarily as a new and convenient form of administration in the 'native reserves'. The many acts of legislation passed at this time provided for the appointment of kings (or chiefs, as they became known) and village headmen by the South African government. They were paid and held responsible for the collection of taxes, distribution of pensions, allocation of communal land, and the administration of customary law through tribal courts.[24]

The reserves of Transkei, Venda, Bophuthatswana, and Ciskei (known as the TVBC states) gained the status of 'independent homeland', but were far from autonomous and never recognised outside South Africa. They were, to a significant extent, funded and controlled by specially designated structures within the apartheid state. From Pretoria, the Department of Native Affairs (later Department of Bantu Affairs and endlessly renamed thereafter) maintained relationships of control and dependency by its administration and monitoring of funding through substantial loans or grants (Africa 1992; Egero 1991). Moreover, the department trained TVBC intelligence and security agencies to operate as remote extensions of apartheid surveillance networks, whilst the South African Police was able to operate without hindrance within homeland borders (Ashforth 1997; Herholdt and Dombo 1992: 85).

In this context, traditional authorities became one of the only gateways through which people, the 'subjects', could access the state, as 'citizens' (Mamdani 1996). For example, birth certificates were essential in order to procure a pass that permitted employment in white areas. To some extent, this remains the case today: 'Tribal Authorities' are inundated with requests for birth and death certificates, without which carers of children orphaned by the AIDS epidemic cannot receive their state welfare grants. The extent to which this is experienced as a bifurcation of

---

[24] For a detailed analysis of this, see Gluckman et al. (1949); Comaroff (1974); Comaroff and Roberts (1981); Delius (1983); Lahiff (2000); and Ngwane (2004).

citizen and subject under democracy, however, is less than clear. Such a distinction has been blurred by traditional leaders, like Tshivhase, who embrace democracy and seek legitimacy not only through royal ancestry but via the ballot box.

By 1948, with the coming to power of the National Party and the official establishment of apartheid, this system intensified. A central tenet of the Bantustan system was to provide rural bases for migrant workers, and to limit the extent of state welfare through reliance on extended family networks 'for the purposes of reproducing and exercising control over a cheap African industrial labour force' (Wolpe 1972: 450). Thompson (1985: 197) develops this point but recognises that the Bantustan system was underpinned by an ideological as well as an economic motive. He argues that the homeland policy also relied on 'racial theory in an extreme organicist form, likening races to organisms that have distinctive cultural as well as physical properties and characteristic courses of development'. The apartheid government, supported by *Volkekunde* ethnologists, maintained that Europeans were culturally superior to any 'Bantu race' and that in order for these courses of development to proceed the different 'races' had to be separated in as exclusive a manner as possible.

The bolstering of traditional structures of power and the construction of puppet governments in so-called homelands were thus intended to achieve much more than a convenient layer of bureaucratic administration in rural bases for migrant labourers. Within the wider ideological parameters of apartheid, the rejuvenation of kingship in rural areas was central to the process of 'retribalisation', intended to function as a hegemonic tool in the legitimation of racially motivated segregation (Vail 1989). In this way, racial identities and essentialised notions of 'culture' were mobilised to rationalise the policy through which Africans were supposedly shielded from outside forces of modernity by the codification of traditions in their own exclusive homelands. The term 'traditional leaders' is thus used here with extreme caution, in the knowledge that whilst such structures do have a pre-colonial past, they are to a significant extent a construct of more recent political forces (cf. Comaroff and Comaroff 1997).

Returning to the situation in Venda, the Bantu Authorities Act of 1951 involved the identification and subsequent creation of 25 separate Tribal Authorities, three Regional Authorities, and one Territorial Authority. Each of the 25 Tribal Authorities constituted a separate kingship, of which the houses of Mphephu and Tshivhase were widely acknowledged to be the most senior. Through these structures, the South African government implemented malleable forms of government in the homelands, and the seats of power in homeland government were generally taken by powerful traditional leaders. This was influenced by the assumption that they acquired allegiance and respect through patronage, ritual, and symbolic power (cultural capital, in Bourdieu's terms) as opposed to coercive force (Beall et al. 2005: 760). Of course, traditional leadership has never been accepted passively, and the apartheid authorities underestimated the extent to which chiefly power was in a continuous dialectical relationship with public opinion.[25]

Nonetheless, following this pattern, *Thovhela* Patrick Mphephu was appointed Chief Executive Councillor in the Thohoyandou Bantu Authority in 1962, which was granted partial 'self-rule' as the Venda Territorial Authority in October 1969. Self-rule was limited at this stage in that the apartheid authorities in South Africa remained in charge of security, economic policy, and foreign relations, and could veto any decision taken by the Venda government. Like the political leaders of other homelands at the time, Patrick Mphephu was 'not a comrade in the struggle against apartheid... [he] was an important black collaborator in the establishment and functioning of apartheid, and certainly one of its few black beneficiaries' (Koelble and Lipuma 2005: 74). Reflecting this in his inaugural address, Patrick Mphephu stressed the need for stronger cooperation between authorities in Venda and the Republic of South Africa:

[M]y councillors and I promise to work for the advancement of Vendaland. We have been cooperating with the [South African] government since the time of President Paul Kruger [1880s]... who gave us the reserves on which we are now residing. (Venda Traditional Authority – Minutes of the First Session, 6–9 October 1969, in Herholdt and Dombo 1992: 74)

The Territorial Authority was replaced by a National Legislative Assembly in 1971, and, by February 1973, Venda became a self-governing nation-state with two distinct political formations: the Venda Independence People's Party (VIPP), led by Johannesburg sociologist Baldwin Mudau, and the Venda National Party (VNP), consisting mainly of chiefs and headmen under the leadership of *Thovhela* Patrick Mphephu. Although the VIPP won the majority of 18 contested seats in elections to the Legislative Assembly in 1973 and 1978, the VNP held on to power through the support of 42 unelected chiefs and headmen, most of whom were selected from or were sympathetic towards Mphephu (Herholdt and Dombo 1992). In September 1979 Venda was declared an 'independent' republic and Patrick Mphephu was subsequently installed as paramount chief, head of government, and Life President of the Legislative Assembly: a title which sounded ludicrous but proved oddly prophetic when he died in April 1988 from suspected poisoning, shortly before the advent of South Africa's democracy spelled the demise of the Assembly itself.

---

[25] See Comaroff (1974) for a detailed discussion of this, and the ways in which chiefs were incorporated into homeland government in Bophuthatswana. See Beall et al. (2005) for a similar discussion regarding chiefs in the former homeland of Kwazulu.

Given the oppositional support for the VIPP during the Bantustan period, the Mphephu government was in a constant dialogue with the population in an attempt to maintain some form of legitimacy. Whilst their position of power hinged, ultimately, on unquestioned genealogical superiority, the role of unelected chiefs in the Legislative Assembly, and a monopoly of violence, the concern to maintain a veneer of legitimate government provoked particular strands of policy in the homeland. Most of this policy was 'handed down' to TVBC states from the apartheid authorities, and deployed by Mphephu in a manner that was seemingly in the best interests of 'his' people. To this extent, the Mphephu regime was characterised by the intercalary nature of traditional authority described by Gluckman et al. (1949). But in this process, as Kuper (1970) reminds us, there was also significant room for manoeuvre (cf. James 1990, for an example of chiefs in the Lebowa homeland who dispensed patronage through agricultural schemes). In this way, Mphephu's options were curtailed by the triad of influences, referred to above, from the apartheid state, the citizenry, and the kingship. Within this, he attempted to balance support and demands within his own royal house and as representative of 'the Venda' more generally – but, ultimately, although support from the citizenry was deemed preferable, it was never necessary: the pretence of legitimacy was closely shadowed by recourse to institutionalised violence.

This pretence, however, shaped the policy agenda of the time in terms of a pervasive approach to 'development'. This can be traced back to the Nationalist government of the 1950s, which enlisted the assistance of F. R. Tomlinson in constructing a strategy by which the human carrying capacity of the homelands, at that time known as native reserves, could be increased and sustained (cf. Beinart 2001: 161). The result was a comprehensive scheme for the rehabilitation of the reserves 'with a view to developing within them a social structure in keeping with the culture of the native and based on effective socio-economic planning' (Davenport and Saunders 2000: 392). Although the recommendations in the Tomlinson Commission were never implemented, the Verwoerd government embarked on a process of development that, it hoped, would facilitate the long-term sustainability of the racial segregation upon which apartheid was based (cf. Ashforth 1990). In this way, 'development' during the apartheid era was posited first and foremost as a potential solution to 'the native problem' and its implementation served to provide a façade of legitimacy: two birds with the one proverbial stone.

As a result, some decades after the non-implementation of the Tomlinson Commission, the Verwoerd government tried various strategies, with limited success. For example, some industrial enterprises were lured by large tax concessions to relocate to the borders between black and white areas. It was hoped that this would draw as many 'surplus' blacks as possible away from the white industrialised areas. Support schemes were established for the promotion and subsidy of large-scale commercial agriculture within the reserves. In addition to this, the government remained committed to the implementation of Tomlinson's 'betterment': a policy that pre-dated apartheid and was initially concerned with land conservation and the prevention of soil erosion in the reserves. Throughout the apartheid era, betterment was intensified. It became concerned largely with the macro-scale rationalisation and restructuring of land holdings and settlement patterns through which people living in the homelands were forced to live in grid-like villages with fixed allocations of land (between 0.5 and 1.5 hectares; see Lahiff 2000: 21) for subsistence farming (cf. de Wet 1995). The size of these plots, however, was widely held to be inadequate, and they provided at best a subsidiary source of food for the rural poor. Nonetheless, the apartheid regime continued to sideline subsistence projects in favour of support for large-scale commercial enterprises. There were some exceptions to this, such as the provision of smallholder irrigation schemes and support for private orchards run by community-based (that is, through the king) organisations (cf. Lahiff 2000).

In Venda, the policy of support for large enterprises was manifest in several forms. A forestry plantation was established in the mountains of Thathe Vondo. Two tea estates and a coffee estate were constructed in partnership with Sapekoe, a private firm with expertise in industrial cultivation of tea and coffee throughout Southern Africa. Firms such as Sapekoe were attracted to invest in the homelands primarily by the subsidies provided by the South African government and the vast pools of cheap labour. Throughout the Bantustan era, the tea estates employed a core staff of up to 1,000, while seasonal pickers numbered roughly 2,000. As Chapter 7 demonstrates, recently the Venda tea estates have been the focus of moral panic over a spate of alleged poisonings. Ultimately, however, they provided substantial benefit only for two relatively small elites: black managers and the small circle of white 'experts' imposed by Sapekoe who were paid vastly higher salaries for the assumed inconvenience of working in a remote black area.

When the South African government passed the Bantu Homelands Development Corporations Act (1965), it began the task of setting up development corporations, funded by the Southern African Development Bank, in each of the homelands (Davenport and Saunders 2000: 426). Some years later, the Venda Development Corporation (VDC) was established. Venda government propaganda at the time trumpeted the VDC as the 'most important public body in the homeland' (Bureau for Economic Research 1979: 8). Although the VDC was involved in maintaining large-scale projects such as the tea estates and canning factories, it was designed to assist the economic development of the homeland in more diverse ways. It was charged with generating 'sustainable employment' and began to foreground the promotion of tourism, arts, crafts, and leisure. In 1981, the VDC established Agriven: the Venda Agricultural Corporation Ltd. The main objective of Agriven was to provide support for medium-sized agricultural projects that were ultimately to be taken over by private entrepreneurs (Lahiff 2000: 88). Agriven increasingly became involved in joint ventures with private investors. Projects such as the packaging of fruits and nuts in on-farm factories throughout Venda were relatively successful in providing employment opportunities, but again provided substantial benefits only for the small elite of commercial farmers in the region.

In an attempt to achieve the desired diversity in economic development, the VDC became involved in several other projects. It coordinated the creation of an industrial estate at Shayandima in which clothing factories, bakeries, garages, and a brewery were established. It developed caravan parks, walking trails, and themed cultural routes, on which tourists (mostly white South Africans on their way to or from the Kruger National Park) could experience 'Africa' from the safety of their vehicles and, by arrangement with various tour guides, observe activities such as traditional dancing, wood carving, and certain stages of female initiation ceremonies.

Possibly the two most successful enterprises initiated by the VDC were the *Ditike* arts and crafts centre and the Venda Sun hotel. Both remain attractions in the area today, under a constantly changing private ownership. *Ditike* ('stand up on your own'/ 'support yourself') was strategically placed on the main road into the capital town of Thohoyandou, and was for many years a source of income and inspiration for Venda's many talented artists. A few of its artists, such as Noria Mabasa, Avhashoni Manganye (whose work appears on the cover of this book), and Mishak Raphelerani, have achieved international recognition from their early exposure at *Ditike*. During the homeland era, the Venda Sun Hotel was the jewel in the crown of the VDC. Boasting a large swimming pool, casino, cinema, air-conditioned en suite rooms, and conference facilities, the hotel was Venda's first concrete, consumable symbol of what development projects could achieve. It not only accommodated tourists or visiting officials to the area, but was regularly frequented by white South Africans who could indulge in gambling and, on Saturday evenings, view pornographic films: activities that were illegal in South Africa but, conveniently, permitted in the homelands.

Although this flurry of developmental activity may seem almost impressive, as indeed it was intended to, it does not appear to have made any significant impact on the homeland economy. Seekings and Nattrass (2005) provide a passing insight into the relatively homogeneous socio-economic profile of Venda at the time. They remind us that most income came from migrant labour remittances sent home by family members, state-sponsored businesses (such as agricultural wholesalers), and the regular incomes of civil servants (ibid.: 95–8). By the mid-1970s in Venda, this led to a situation whereby 46 per cent of the population had an annual income of R500–999, 4 per cent had R1,500–1,999, and only 3 per cent had R3,000–15,000 (ibid.: 119). This would suggest that in Venda, although there was extreme inequality at the time, the vast majority of people survived on broadly similar, albeit low, incomes.

Thus, whilst the Bantustan era was characterised by, even based on, 'retribalisation' and the fortification of essentialist, racist ideals of the 'tribal subject', there was a simultaneous, explicit attempt at legitimation that superimposed development or modernisation projects on a distinctly underdeveloped social reality (cf. Bozzoli's analysis of racial modernism in Alexandria [2000; 2004]). This seemingly contradictory set of processes brought about a peculiar socio-political arrangement whereby some revelled in resistance, some succumbed to the seduction of the ideological construct of separate development, and many others actively avoided politics; in the words of one elderly man: 'I simply tried to live my life and feed my family as best I could.' To be sure, this was a safety-first option given that the Mphephu regime was noted for political intimidation, allegations of torture, widespread corruption, and nepotism (Amnesty International 1983). However, despite the frequent abuse of violence, it is impossible to ignore the consistency of comments made by some who claimed they were 'better off during apartheid'. In the words of a popular reggae song by Khakhati Tshisikule, 'At least the traffic lights worked under Mphephu/When we worked on the farms/A job back then was at least safe/Oh! The sweet memories of employment!'

Nostalgic echoes in popular culture reflect and contribute to the perceived crisis of reproduction referred to in the previous chapter. Although this example primarily emphasises disillusionment with the current dispensation, it also illustrates how the puppet regimes of Bantustan states with their development projects secured a veneer of legitimacy that swayed at least some people. In this way, the paradoxical coexistence of contradictory discourses based on traditionalism and modernisation was the outcome of Mphephu's attempts to secure broad-based support.

For all its efforts, however, the Mphephu regime never achieved the popular following it desired. After his death in 1988, Patrick Mphephu was succeeded as Venda State President by his cousin Frank Ravele, previously Minister for Economic Affairs and Tourism, who was a close affine and ally in the VNP. Ravele's brief flirtation with the presidency was marred by allegations that members of the cabinet were involved in ritual murder, by student protests against corruption, and by widespread violence relating to a perceived increase in the practice of witchcraft. With the unbanning of the ANC and the release of Nelson Mandela in 1990, 'independent' Venda was rendered practically ungovernable by

> **Mushasha Commission** (Specific to Venda) **1991**: Abolished the position of *Khosikhulu* in Venda. Instigated by Brigadier Ramushwana's military regime towards the end of the homeland era.

> **Ralushai Commission** (Specific to Northern, later Limpopo, Province) **1996–8**: Established by Provincial Premier Ramathlodi to investigate irregularities in the course of apartheid-era influence on the institutions of traditional leadership in Limpopo Province.

> **Nhlapo Commission** (National) **2004–9**: Established after the 2003 white paper on traditional leadership to gather evidence and give a final, legally binding verdict in disputes over who should be 'Paramount Chief' – apparently oblivious to the Thohoyandou Court ruling that made this an illegal category.

Figure 2.4. Successive commissions that have shaped traditional leadership in Venda.

ANC supporters who, through widely successful strikes and demonstrations, demanded the end of apartheid and the Bantustan system (cf. Le Roux 1988 for Venda; Delius 1996 and Niehaus 2001a for other areas). State institutions such as the police, and representatives of traditional and generational authority, were targeted by groups of ANC Youth League 'comrades'. ANC supporters embarked on a spate of witch hunts in which several elderly people and police officers lost their lives, and which forced many chiefs and headmen to seek refuge in police stations. Under this unbearable pressure for change, Ravele relinquished power in a non-violent military coup led by Brigadier Gabriel Ramushwana of the Venda Defence Forces, supported by the South African Defence Force, in 1990.

Subsequent events, shaped by this groundswell of popular feeling, saw the institution of paramount chieftaincy delegitimised. In 1991, the military administration announced the Mushasha Commission to investigate the role of traditional leadership in the homeland (see Figure 2.4). Echoing an Institute for Race Relations annual report a decade earlier (SAIRR 1980: 334–5), the Mushasha Commission concluded that the position of *Khosikhulu* was 'unknown in Venda custom' – although to be more accurate the title had been vacant since Thohoyandou's mysterious disappearance from Dzata in 1870. Ramushwana promptly drafted legislation and abolished the position: symbolically removing the royal house of Mphephu from its position of unparalleled power and influence in the homeland. He also disbanded the Legislative Assembly and became chairman of a Council of National Unity, paving the way for four years of benevolent military dictatorship during which 'state structures and public services in Venda virtually collapsed' (Lahiff 2000: 73). In 1993, with the inevitability that Nelson Mandela would soon be President of the new South Africa, Ramushwana publicly 'crossed over' to join the ANC, and in 1994 Venda became part of the Northern (later Limpopo) Province of the newly unified South Africa.

Collaboration and Resistance

A fundamental task of Bantustan administrations, as the apartheid authorities saw it, was to collaborate with them in providing and supporting intelligence networks for the implementation of the South African Terrorism Act (1967), which allowed for extensive periods of detention without charge or trial. These networks were primarily involved in identifying 'subversive' (i.e. anti-apartheid) movements which, in Venda, were loosely but by no means exclusively associated with Baldwin Mudau's VIPP.

A widespread policy and practice of detention, torture, bribery, corruption, and violence continued to characterise the operations of the intelligence agencies and security police (Lahiff 2000: 72; Herholdt and Dombo 1992: 78; Fokwang 2009). After the suspicious disappearance of several members of the opposition under interrogation, and upon hearing the testimony of an exiled Venda Lutheran Dean, Amnesty International reported in a rare document – refreshingly frank given the strict censorship of the time – that 'the authorities in Venda should act without delay to prevent further possible abuses of fundamental rights, [and] . . . establish a formal inquiry into allegations of torture of political detainees and conditions of detention' (Amnesty International 1983: 3). After many of its members were intimidated and detained without charge by the security police during the 1984 elections to the National Assembly, for example, the VIPP took no seats and Venda effectively became a one-party state (Herholdt and Dombo 1992: 80). This became official in 1986 when Patrick Mphephu amended the constitution to make the VNP the only legal political party in the homeland.

This environment of political intimidation and violence nurtured rebellion. Most oppositional organisations, however, such as the United Democratic Front (UDF) and the church-based Movement for Democracy (MDM), actually operated outside of the VIPP and were largely unaffected by homeland politics. The UDF and the MDM, at varying degrees during different periods, acted in Venda as they did throughout South Africa as secretive, internal wings of the (then illegal) ANC. They sought to change minority rule by organising demonstrations, labour strikes, small-scale terrorist activities, and education campaigns amongst university students and school children. Importantly, the geographical position of Venda on the border of Zimbabwe and Mozambique rendered the area central in providing safe houses for members of the ANC crossing secretly in and out of South Africa. As a current ANC councillor told me:

[W]e were just told where to collect them by the [Limpopo] River, and where to drop them off. We *never* asked their names or their mission because the less we knew the better for everybody. Anyway they would not talk about that. Sometimes we did not even talk at all... only giving them food in the dark and a bed to sleep in... even my wife and children did not know and did not ask... yes, sometimes it was [frightening] because we did not know if so-and-so was [working for government] intelligence, but we were angry and determined to beat the system... that's what it was like back then. (Interview with P. M., 25 June 2005)

A middle-aged woman, also an ANC member and member of the Tshivhase royal family, recalled that:

[W]e did not talk about these things back then, even now you can find people telling lies to you, that they were not involved when you can find that they were [involved]... yes, the less you knew the better. I remember we beat a young woman at the [water] pump, in 1980 I think, because she was spreading gossip about spies sleeping in her neighbour's yard. She was lucky; you could have been killed for such gossip back then. We [ANC members] used to joke that we were the perfect witches, moving about at night and not being seen! (Interview with B. T., 12 April 2005)

Given the secrecy that continues to inhibit open discussion about individual involvement in these activities, it is difficult to plot the precise patterns of connections and oppositions, or of families' political affiliations or party membership, at this time. But the narrative of a broad division between resistant and collaborator chiefs such as Tshivhase and Mphephu has been replicated throughout South Africa: many 'great chieftains resisted manfully white intrusion' (Luthuli 1961 in Beall et al. 2005: 762) whilst others danced to the beat of the intruders.

Such a script should be viewed with caution, however. First, it should be underlined that enmity between so-called collaborators and resisters, more often than not, had a structural and historical element that predated colonialism and missionisation. This was the case, for example, in Tswana Tshidi chiefdoms. Montshiwa, leader of the 'traditional' royals, came into conflict with his less-powerful half-brother Molema who, having converted to Christianity, assumed a leadership role among the literate elite. 'Not only did this introduce an ideological contrast which was to give new voice to existing internal cleavages, it also became the basis of the renegotiation of power relations surrounding the chiefship' (Comaroff 1985: 30). Molema showed signs of mounting a challenge to his half-brother before his death, and his followers (the 'intelligentsia') continued to contest Montshiwa's followers' rights to office (ibid.: 33). But in the face of a common adversary (the Afrikaner National Party), the two united in opposition and neither the chief nor the intelligentsia cooperated with this new authority 'except in the most perfunctory manner' (ibid.: 39).

The Tshidi example demonstrates the historical importance of chiefly rivalry. Even if the missionaries or the National Party had bypassed them, Montshiwa would have remained at odds with his half-brother, but the forces of colonial power interrupted and influenced their pre-existing disputes; later they transcended these when they united against a common enemy. Any notion of collaboration or resistance must thus be problematised and situated in historical terms, where more fluid and fragmented arrangements reinterrogate and throw into question the banality of a dichotomous interpretation of historical process (cf. Mbembe 1992; Bayart 1993). The heroic 'struggle narrative', as in Lan's account of the Chiwese chiefdom in northern Zimbabwe (Lan 1985: 138), may obscure the complex ways in which chiefly authority interacted with colonial structures of power. Consequently, it would be misleading to suggest that every Tshivhase leader has been associated with 'the struggle', or that every Mphephu chief was a government stooge. The situation was much more disjointed.

Mphephu was more than an intercalary figure, torn between the apartheid state and the demands of his subjects (Gluckman et al. 1949; Kuper 1970). He sought, explicitly, to use his position of power to undercut the support base of his historical rival. During his corrupt and violent presidency, several of Tshivhase's headmen and chiefs were irregularly promoted to kings, some of whom were coopted into government structures. Many remained complicit through silence, and others were tempted into civil service positions by impressive salaries or other persuasive factors. The luxurious houses that were built at the time for cabinet members and senior civil servants remain a feature of the Thohoyandou landscape today, although the heated indoor swimming pools, jacuzzis, saunas, and double drive-in garages have fallen into disrepair.[26] In the village of Mauluma, home of Mphephu's friend and successor Frank Ravele, drinking water was piped into every home, outside of which flushing toilets and shower rooms were built. Less than ten kilometres away, in the village of Fondwe within the Tshivhase boundary, residents used 'long-drop' toilets and communal water pumps. Such inequalities persist today,

---

[26] In an ironic twist, King Kennedy Tshivhase recently renovated, purchased, and moved into King Patrick Mphephu's old government house in Thohoyandou, renaming it the Tshivhase Palace.

produced by and reminding subjects of the opulent lifestyles enjoyed by Mphephu and his allies.[27]

Patrick Mphephu clearly thought it wise to keep potential enemies close to him. He recruited actively among the traditional leaders connected to his rival at a time when many, but by no means all, were privileging material advantages over kinship and patron-political obligations. While political collaboration with Mphephu promised the accumulation of significant personal wealth, such a move was always a gamble, balanced against the potential loss of legitimacy in the eyes of those involved in the struggle.

As part of Mphephu's wider aim to marginalise and reduce Tsivhase's influence, several chiefdoms that border with – or are close to – Tshivhase were promoted to kingdoms. Influential collaborators who were brought into the fold in this way included (*Thovhela*) Muofhe of Tsianda, who was Minister of Communications towards the end of Mphephu's rule. Thus Chief Muofhe, along with several other traditional leaders, became a king under the Mphephu government. In a continual display of loyalty, Patrick Mphephu's portrait hangs in the royal council hut of Tsianda to this day. Another well-known collaborator, and one of the most influential members of the Bantustan government, was the notorious A. A. Tshivhase: Member of Parliament and headman (*Vhakoma*) in the Phiphidi region. He was a charismatic, controversial figure whose colourful political career ended abruptly in a ritual murder scandal during the late 1980s (cf. Le Roux 1988). As with many epochs in Venda history, this saga was documented in song. ANC supporters chanted a powerful call and response in *toyi toyi*:[28]

Alidzuli, Alidzuli	[His first name – meaning not to be seated]
A. A. Tshivhase, *Haa!*	A. A. Tshivhase, Ha!
O *via*	He has committed ritual murder
O *via na nnyi?*	Who was his accomplice in this?
O *via na Bobo, Haa!*	He killed with Bobo! (nickname of his close friend)

Although becoming a collaborator risked the loss of popular support, a standard had been set for high-ranking Tshivhase figures to side with

---

[27] The case of Mauluma, and the royal house of Ravele, is particularly interesting. Ravele leaders have recently cashed in on a land claim made on their ancestral home (*thavha*) at Levubu, a site that was incorporated into the old Republic of South Africa and developed into an exceptionally successful farming community. Instead of demanding the farming land, Ravele negotiated a share of its profits, from which they have benefited considerably. See Fraser (2007).

[28] *Toyi toyi* is a form of protest dance that became popular among liberation groups during the struggle against apartheid. It involves flamboyant and energetically rhythmic jumping from left foot to right, usually with clenched fists thrown into the air. McGregor suggests this was symbolic of the preparation for warfare (2005). I return to the music of the struggle and its contemporary relevance in Chapter 5.

Mphephu and the white minority government. Perhaps the most significant catch – his collaboration sealed Mphephu's grip on the traditional leadership – was John Shavhani Tshivhase. Shavhani was the regent in charge of the Tshivhase throne from 1970 until 1993, and he held several cabinet-level positions during his time in government. Kennedy Midiyavhathu, the current king, was originally enthroned in 1970 at the age of seven, but after threats were made on his life by rival contenders to the throne, the royal council relocated him to Pretoria, where he lived with his grandmother. His uncle Shavhani was installed as regent until Kennedy was deemed old enough to preside. That time came in 1993, and it took a Supreme Court ruling in Kennedy's favour to force his uncle out of power, and to herald a new, post-collaborationist era in Venda politics. It is the rise to power of *Thovhela* Kennedy Tshivhase, the most influential political figure of this new era, that I now consider.

The Emergence of *Thovhela* Kennedy Tshivhase

Tshivhase kings, overall, have had a history of opposing colonial and minority rule. Kennedy Tshivhase's Supreme Court victory over Shavhani in 1993 was thus more than a powerful assertion of his return, as a mature and educated young man, to claim the throne of the Tshivhase dynasty from which he had been excluded as a child. It was a highly symbolic move, through which he was honouring and reinforcing the memory of his father and grandfather, both of whom were renowned for resisting colonial influence through preventing white business interests from developing in the area.

Kennedy's father, *Thovhela* Prince Thohoyandou Tshivhase, died abruptly under suspicious circumstances in 1966, whilst at the pinnacle of his reign. He had been inaugurated in 1960, before Mphephu's ascension to Chief Executive Councillor in 1962 (see Tables 2.1 and 2.2) and took a radical stance against his rival's collaboration with white minority rule. Prince was deeply involved in supporting pro-democracy movements and worked in cooperation with several underground organisations. Many of these were covertly staffed by sympathetic Lutheran German missionaries, some of whom were forcefully expelled from South Africa for their involvement with him.

Previous to this, Prince's father, Ratsimphi (who died in detention in 1947), had been a personal friend of Nelson Mandela's: his involvement with the early liberation struggle later resulted in the posthumous presentation of the prestigious Luthuli Award. Ratsimphi was known locally as 'Mphaya'.[29] He reportedly gave himself this name after the British

---

[29] Ratsimphi was also known as '*phiriphiri mudifha namani*' ('the hot chillies that make meat tasty').

Table 2.1. Chronology of main political events during the Venda Bantustan era

Year	Political Development
1962	Patrick Mphephu appointed as Chief Executive Councillor in Thohoyandou Bantu Authority.
1969	Partial 'self-rule' granted to the Venda Territorial Authority.
1973	Venda becomes a 'self-governing nation state' with a Legislative Assembly and two political parties – VNP and VIPP.
1979	Declaration of Independence: Mphephu declared 'Paramount Chief' (*Khosikhulu*) and 'Life President'.
1988	Death of Mphephu/Ravele becomes President.
1990	Non-violent military coup led by Brigadier Gabriel Ramushwana following widespread demonstrations.
1991	Mushasha Commission abolishes position of *Khosikhulu* and symbolically removes the Mphephu royal house from power.
1994	The former Venda is incorporated into the new democratic South Africa as part of Northern (later Limpopo) Province.

Empire, to which he compared his own strength and influence. He has become a mythical figure in the Tshivhase area, and it is not uncommon to overhear elaborate tales of his wealth, cruelty, gargantuan marijuana (*mbanzhi*) consumption, and remarkable charisma.

The ANC/Tshivhase connection was recultivated in the post-apartheid era. It was endorsed symbolically at Kennedy's lavish reinauguration ceremony in 1993, at which struggle stalwart Walter Sisulu gave the keynote address. This, according to those present, turned the ceremony into an 'old-fashioned political rally' with the effervescence of a religious conversion. In recognition of this long relationship, Mandela graced Mukumbani with a presidential visit in 1997, thus uniquely privileging Tshivhase and granting the new king unparalleled moral capital in the region (cf. Fokwang 2009: 76). In a typically conciliatory move, however, Mandela then attended the inauguration of Tshivhase's arch-rival, Toni Peter

Table 2.2. Time-line of recent Tshivhase kings

Year	Political Development
1931	Ratsimphi installed as *Thovhela*.
1952	Ratsimphi dies in police custody.
1963	Prince (Thohoyandou), Ratsimphi's son, enthroned as *Thovhela*.
1966	*Thovhela* Prince dies.
1970	Kennedy Midiyavhathu (Prince's son) installed as child *Thovhela*.
1970	John Shavhani becomes regent.
1993	Kennedy wins Supreme Court order, and is reinstalled.

Mphephu, at Dzanani in November the following year. Toni Mphephu's predecessor, his brother who was named after the legendary Dimbanyika, had been on friendly terms with Kennedy Tshivhase until his death in a road accident in 1998. They attended functions together, and Kennedy played a leading role at his funeral.

During the 13-year gap between the death of Ratsimphi in 1947 and the installation of his son Prince in 1960, the Tshivhase royal council was engaged in attempts to prevent governmental interference in selection of the Tshivhase king. Before his death, Ratsimphi had responded to demands that traditional leaders dispatch the heir to their throne for 'government training' by sending Muzila Tshivhase, who was not in line to the throne, as a decoy.[30] Upon his return from government training, Muzila was installed only as *Vhamusanda* (headman), and deployed by the royal council to Muhuyu: a village far from the centre of power at Mukumbani. Upon Ratsimphi's death in 1947, Muzila Tshivhase was placed on the throne by the National Party government, but was not recognised by the royal council as *Thovhela*. He received no installation ceremony: his term in office was imposed from outside the royal council. Muzila remained on the throne, at the behest of the government in Pretoria, until his death in 1959 under mysterious circumstances.[31] Prince Tshivhase, the genuine heir, who had been waiting in the wings, was rapidly installed as *Thovhela*. Thus, whilst Muzila was a 'collaborator' in terms of his government training and illegitimate seizure of power, the Tshivhase royal council resisted the extent of his command by refusing him the title of *Thovhela*, and keeping him, literally, at a safe distance from the seat of power in Mukumbani. During this time, the royal council was effectively controlled by a group of 'resister' elders, who continually stalled the transfer of land into white hands. In this context, the 'collaboration/resistance' dichotomy takes multiple forms simultaneously; seen in its starkest terms, it does not adequately reflect the power dynamics of the time.

During the four-year gap between the death of Prince in 1966 and the installation of Kennedy in 1970, Tshivhase royal affairs were again organised by the royal council, which worked to decide who the next king should be. Factional disputes that exist to this day originated at this point. A significant minority opposed the ascension of Kennedy on the grounds of a significant technicality: his mother had not been chosen,

---

[30] Muzila Tshivhase's father was indeed Ratsimphi, but Muzila was born to a wife taken by Ratsimphi before he was installed as *Thovhela*, and so not in line to the throne. Prince Tshivhase, also Ratsimphi's son, was born after his father's installation and so was a legitimate heir.
[31] There are unsubstantiated rumours that Muzila's life was actually ended prematurely by a radical faction within the Tshivhase polity.

as dictated by convention, by the *makhadzi* as the mother of the *dzekiso* house, and thus of the future king.[32]

Despite, or perhaps because of, internal factionalism, Kennedy Tshivhase's well-timed entry into the public sphere during the early 1990s was shrewd and strategic. Having been absent from homeland politics during the 1980s, and coming from a royal house with a history of alignment against the homeland authorities, he emerged innocent of connections to the unpopular political and traditional leaders of the era. In a perspicacious publicity stunt designed to emphasise this dissociation, he funded the circulation of thousands of T-shirts with his image in the ANC colours of green, black, and gold (see also Fokwang 2009). This political alignment has allowed Tshivhase to form alliances with potentially unsupportive politically active groups such as the civic associations. These had developed under the leadership of young males during the 1980s, largely as an alternative polity to apartheid-sanctioned government and traditional authority (cf. Ferguson 2006: 104–5). As a widely recognised 'comrade' with well-publicised liberation credentials, Kennedy has been able to resolve local-level disputes by bringing many of the civic structures in the region to the negotiating table with regional headmen and elected councillors.

One of his first actions as the newly installed *Thovhela* was to reconfigure the Tshivhase Tribal Council (TTC), which he renamed the Tshivhase Territorial Authority (TTA). This was based on an apartheid-era construct which involved a weekly meeting of headmen and chiefs at the royal headquarters in Mukumbani. In Tshivhase's opinion, the TTC had grown weak in the twenty years or so since 'collaborator' John Shavhani had been regent. He believed that it lacked influence or relevance, and had been reduced to a group of 'yes men' through his uncle's nepotistic tendencies. Tshivhase's diplomatic skills were put to the test. The group that opposed his succession on technical grounds joined forces with the faction that had been brought into the fold by Shavhani. A significant coalition was formed between these two groups that staunchly opposed Kennedy's return to power in fear of being removed from their comfortable positions of status within the council. However, in a move which mirrored Mphephu's earlier co-opting of the Tshivhase regent into the homeland government, Kennedy chose to keep any potential enemies close to him and did not remove any of his potentially rebellious opponents from their positions.

---

[32] The *makhadzi* of a royal family is the eldest paternal aunt to the king. She decides which royal wife (*mutanuni*; plural *vhatanuni*) will mother the next *Thovhela*. She is, theoretically, *Thovhela's* closest adviser and often the most trusted royal councillor. The *Makhadzi* plays a central role in any Venda royal council (see Stayt 1931: 167–71, 249–50). She not only chooses the mother of the next king (which is not simply a hereditary calculation), but has significant influence in ancestral worship rites and at all levels of the decision-making process.

The new king initiated a change of direction intended to transform the TTA into an effective and relevant institution through which democratic governance and municipal policy was to be mediated, and if necessary resisted, by the rural poor. Perhaps showing some bias, Fokwang (2009) argues that this has made the TTA a shield against market forces.[33] This supports Koelble and Lipuma's argument that traditional leaders have survived the transition to democracy by demonstrating their potential use in promoting social justice. The TTA, unlike neighbouring traditional authorities who have little influence over the civics, has used its political clout successfully to oppose several unpopular municipal policies such as a blanket charge for the collection of refuse and a drastic increase in the price of allocating plots of land. The new TTA abolished equally unpopular fees imposed under the regent for access to services and resources such as burial in a public cemetery, the collection of firewood, and development of small agricultural projects.

Significantly, in a move inspired by the new constitutional rights of women, Kennedy cancelled the regulation under which women were permitted to apply for land only through a male relative, thus freeing all women to make applications on an equal basis (Fokwang 2009). Although this caused major ripples of discontent among many prominent figures in the Tshivhase hierarchy, it has become an accepted procedural norm in the TTA, and Tshivhase gained some support from NGOs and local women's rights movements for it. Such a 'progressive' stance by traditional leaders with regard to gender in the post-apartheid era has yet to be recognised by authors on the topic, who continue to exclude the Venda region from their analysis (cf. Beall et al. 2005; Beall 2005).

Kennedy Tshivhase has continued in this vein, becoming one of the most influential and dominant new political figures in Limpopo Province. As head of the Tshivhase Territorial Authority he also serves at the local level (Vhembe District) as chairperson of CONTRALESA (Council of Traditional Leaders). In 1995, he was deployed by the ANC to the National Council of Provinces, South Africa's parliamentary upper house in Cape Town, and is head of the Roads and Transport Portfolio in the Limpopo Provincial Legislature. He is provincial chairperson of the South African Charter of the African Renaissance, and has sat on several other boards and advisory panels at the national, provincial, and local levels of government. Moreover, following many of his ANC colleagues, his interests spread into the private sector when he was appointed as Executive Chairperson on the board of Soutpansberg Petroleum (SBP).[34]

---

[33] Fokwang presents what could be termed a 'Tshivhase-centric' account of historical and contemporary processes. As I discussed in the introductory chapter, the micro-politics of conducting research in the Tshivhase region can be revealing, but the researcher must take care not to be seduced by the mythical heroic nationalism at the core of the polity.

[34] SPB went into administration in 2008.

During an interview in mid-2005, he told me that he hoped to become a South African ambassador to the United Nations, an ambition that he may yet fulfil, given that he was recently deployed by the ANC to serve as a South African representative to the Commonwealth Secretariat.

The Battle for Paramountcy

Having established the dominance of the Mphephu royal house during the Bantustan era and explained the post-apartheid emergence of Kennedy Tshivhase as the region's most powerful and influential traditional leader in the democratic dispensation, I now return to the contemporary battle for paramountcy (*Khosikhulu*). This will involve looking at the specific strategy adopted by the TTA in this potentially epoch-making struggle for the consolidation of power. As outlined above, the royal house of Mphephu can rest assured that it should secure the paramountcy by virtue of the fact that its lineage, directly descended from Thohoyandou's eldest son, is the most senior. This was recognised by a majority of Venda chiefs in February 2003 at a meeting organised by the provincial Department for Local Government when the assembly of traditional leaders (opposed only by Tshivhase) voted that, by this right, Mphephu should be installed as *Khosikhulu*. Later that year, the 24 chiefs filed a case at the Thohoyandou High Court on behalf of Toni Mphephu, in which they asked the court to overrule the findings of the Mushasha Commission (see Figure 2.4), and Brigadier Ramushwana's 1991 abolition of the title, to re-declare Toni Mphephu as paramount chief.

In a bizarre decision, the High Court ruled that Ramushwana had acted legally in 1991 when he passed legislation that abolished the position of paramount chief, and the chiefs lost their case. It would thus seem that the national government, in the 2003 legislation on traditional leadership, has instigated a competition for what is, according to the Thohoyandou High Court, effectively an illegal category. This pleased the Tshivhase camp, in that it seemed to pave the way for a dual kingship among Venda traditional leaders. Tshivhase later stated that, in his opinion, the meeting of traditional leaders had in any case been 'illegal', and was reminiscent of apartheid-era politics, when decision making was controlled by 'people who want to feed their own stomachs' (*Limpopo Mirror*, 28 February 2003).

Tshivhase's case, on the other hand, is bolstered by his recently achieved power and influence, with which he has attempted to promote popular support by engaging in an (unofficial) campaign for the consolidation of power. In the knowledge that well-established pre-colonial genealogy firmly supports the interests of his closest rival, Tshivhase has attempted to influence the decision of the Nhlapo commissioners with a different strategy. Principally this has involved attracting popular and political backing through his endorsement and promotion of the wider ANC agenda of development and the African renaissance. At the same time, statements made to the press, such as 'the Tshivhase are kings in our areas, and the Mphephu are kings in their areas' (*Limpopo Mirror*, 9 January 2006), have indicated that Kennedy, like the Thohoyandou High Court, is unsure as to the ultimate legitimacy of a paramount chief. Moreover, the Nhlapo Commission in Venda heard that the house of Tshivhase 'has never and never could' be ruled by Mphephu, as it would symbolise a return to the oppression of the Bantustan era (ibid.).

The wider significance of Kennedy Tshivhase's dramatic entrance to the ceremony in honour of his late grandfather can now be grasped: it represents his performance of legitimacy, simultaneously speaking to the kingship, the state, and the citizenry. To enact the spirit of Ratsimphi on horseback in front of leading ANC colleagues who would undoubtedly have influence in lobbying commissioners of the Nhlapo enquiry was clearly a calculated, if opportunistic, decision, executed to maximum effect in front of a capacity gathering in the spacious grounds of Mukumbani. Moreover, the address was intended to drive a wedge between the traditional leaders (including those under the old Tshivhase order) who tarnished their reputations by collaborating for many years with the apartheid regime, and those like himself who emerged from structures of the struggle with impeccable credentials, to protect and lead the rural poor into the democratic dispensation. Although his acceptance speech was drenched in populist rhetoric, it was also aimed at the ANC dignitaries, and the intention was obviously to leave them in no doubt that he should retain the title of king in the Tshivhase region.

As he outlined in the address, Tshivhase's priorities in the run-up to the Nhlapo decision have consisted of three closely connected elements; the inauguration (*vhuhosi*) of more headmen under the chiefs in his region, a dynamic engagement with the African renaissance, and the promotion of development.

Tshivhase's Strategy for the Consolidation of Power

With the genealogical record going against him, Kennedy Tshivhase has been forced to seek legitimacy in other quarters. An increase in the inauguration (*vhuhosi*) of headmen/women since the announcement that Venda would again have a *Khosikhulu* has been vital to this strategy. Although a minority of these, such at the *vhuhosi* of *Vhamusanda* Ratshitanga at Ngulumbi in August 2005, have been conducted to install a single headman after the death of a predecessor, the majority have had a more strategic goal. This has often involved multiple installations, such as at Dopeni in 2003, when six petty headmen/women were promoted to the position of *Vhamusanda* (headman/woman). Similarly, in July 2005 at

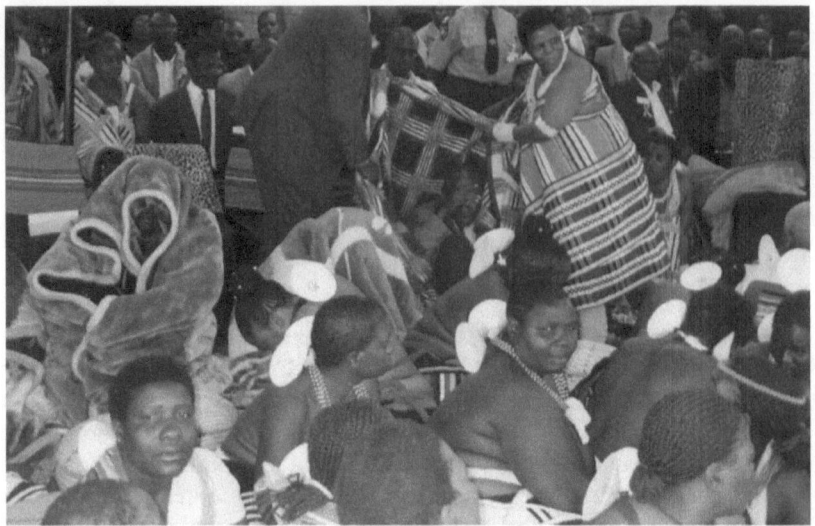

Figure 2.5. *Vhuhosi* ceremony at Ngwenani ya Themeli. The new headmen crouch under blankets waiting to be unveiled by a senior royal.

Ngwenani ya Themeli, five headmen were promoted from petty headman to headman in one lengthy session (see Figure 2.5). Most of the newly installed headmen previously held a less prestigious position of responsibility in the hierarchy of traditional authority, and all of them belong to a royal family in the areas where they live. Upon inauguration, they are allocated a location over which they will preside, a (male) 'assistant' (*ndumi*), and a *makhadzi*. Historically, the allocation of an assistant and a *makhadzi* has been reserved for a newly installed chief (*Khosi*), but these roles have now been redistributed to lower levels in the hierarchy.

The importance of this is to be found in the terms of the 2003 legislation, in which the government recognised only three tiers of traditional authority. Whereas *Vhamusanda/Gota* (headman) is officially recognised by the state as a legitimate office, *Mukoma* (petty headman) is not (see Figure 2.3). In the context of the overwhelming support given by the majority of chiefs to Mphephu, it has been in Tshivhase's direct interests to entrench as many headmen as possible under his authority. As a result, in the dossier presented by the Tshivhase house to the Nhlapo commission, the number of *Vhamusanda* under the TTA was stated as 80, whilst Mphephu registered only 50.

The official 'party line', however, is quite different. With a growing population in the former homeland, members of the Tshivhase Territorial Authority point out, there is an urgent need to 'restructure our systems of rural governance so that the people can be properly represented at all levels by committed, transparent traditional leaders'.[35] This restructuring, however, has by no means translated into more accessible traditional authority for the rural poor. Rather, it has often resulted in chaotic duplication of the simplest tasks. Moreover, jealousies and rivalry between the newly appointed leaders and the older, more established ones has in places developed into a scramble for jurisdiction and crumbs of power.

In such contestations over boundaries of authority, 'the people' have often been forgotten. A good example of this is a recent attempt to build a community pre-school for children infected or affected by HIV/AIDS at Tshikombani (see Map 4). After the project organisers had applied in the appropriate manner, via the lowest rung of traditional leadership, permission to occupy and build was eventually granted by the TTA. After several weeks, however, the builders were instructed to halt proceedings as the newly installed *Vhamusanda* had not been informed of the building, and had other plans for the plot of land. He took his complaint to the TTA, which initially upheld it and only later allowed building to recommence, after the dispute had been settled and borders had been confirmed.

In Tshivhase's wider strategy, the installation of headmen/women is as important for its symbolic value as it is for the numbers of officially recognised leaders it produces. The *vhuhosi* ceremony follows a conventional structure; it is a grand public spectacle accompanied by long speeches, traditional dances, and ceremony. The new headmen must crouch on a stage, hidden under a thick blanket, and endure intense heat whilst the crowd gathers (see Figure 2.5). An entourage of luxury vehicles with armed guards in trench coats and shades heralds the arrival of the king and the opening of the ceremony. As he steps out of the car, he is engulfed by a large and loud *tshikona* group that escorts him regally to the throne upon which he presides over the occasion.

After several hours and numerous addresses, the king performs the main duty of the day, unveiling the new headmen by removing the blankets and announcing their names. They are then asked to state the identity of the assistant and *makhadzi*, which is done with much ululation and praise calling. *Tshikona* is again sounded, and only after the removal of the blankets will Kennedy lead the assembly of men in the dance, followed closely (in a strict hierarchy) by his royal council, the newly installed leaders, and then male spectators of the general public. In this way, *vhuhosi* has been engineered so that the unveiling of the new headman is eclipsed by the dramatic arrival of the king and his participation

---

[35] Interview with King Kennedy Tshivhase, 2 July 2005.

in leading the *tshikona*. The extravagant opulence of the occasion is indicative of its contemporary political importance, and the performance of *tshikona* at *vhuhosi* can be read in both functional and symbolic terms.

Despite the celebratory tone of such occasions, the king's strategy for the consolidation of power has not escaped criticism. Whilst the main attraction at *vhuhosi* is centred on the *tshikona*, the king, and the actual unveiling, there were distinct voices of dissent to be heard around the periphery. Most conversations on the fringe of these events voice a general discontent at the 'donations' made by every homestead in the village to fund the event, and point to the bureaucratic confusion that was bound to ensue. This was reflected in an exchange I overheard between two elderly men at *vhushosi*: 'This isn't right; you can't just make a headman out of nothing. We have too many as it is' – to which his friend replied, 'Well, they say it's a democracy now, so maybe we shouldn't complain'. This was also true of the Luthuli award ceremony at Mukumbani. Every household on Tshivhase land was instructed to donate up to R20 for the provision of food, entertainment, accommodation, transport, and 'security' for the dignitaries: an obligation to which many objected. This dissent was symptomatic of a frequently voiced opinion that King Kennedy is in the process of accumulating a dubious and substantial personal wealth, but this seemed to reinforce deference towards him as often as it led to his being dismissed as a corrupt politician. Clearly, acquiring popular support from the citizenry is a key element of his strategy, but Tshivhase is engaged in a balancing act between this and the accumulation of *Vhamusanda* that are intended to support his claim for paramountcy in the eyes of the state.

As provincial chairperson of the South African Charter of the African Renaissance, the inauguration of so many new headmen in the region has certainly provided Tshivhase with an opportunity to promote the virtues of Venda culture (*mvelele*) and tradition (*sialala*). Although the 2003 legislation represented an attempt to create spaces for the wider participation of traditional leaders in the democratic dispensation, Tshivhase encourages his new traditional leaders to remain as 'guardians of culture'. The consistent rhetorical references made to the 'importance of preserving our traditions' and 'living the African renaissance, as the people can only make it happen when their leaders inspire them!' are generally reciprocated in the responses by the new headmen. Interestingly, and in support of Oomen's position, much of the discourse of these exchanges is framed in rights-based language. The new *Vhamusanda* at Ngwenani, for example, asserted in his inaugural speech that:

[A]s it is my right to be crowned headman here, in my area, it is your right to dance *tshikona*, to go to initiation schools, to enjoy Venda culture, to have a job, to water in your house and to electricity... we will work together, as Vhavenda, towards these goals. (Ngwenani, 12 July 2005)[36]

Tshivhase's relationship with the African renaissance has not been restricted, however, to a 'reculturation' of newly installed headmen. Fokwang (2009) reports that his preoccupation with socio-cultural activities has led to the notion amongst his subjects that Kennedy is a champion of tradition. Traditional dances such as *tshikona* have been structured into regional league tables, competing in annual contests. The promotion of female initiation has been central to this process, and it is in this context that Tshivhase has claimed that AIDS education has been incorporated into the ritual curriculum: an assertion to which I return in the following chapter.

In a broadly similar way, a concern for legitimacy in the eyes of the citizenry has framed post-apartheid concern with 'development' in Venda. This has been formalised recently in the Tshivhase Development Trust (TDT), through which Kennedy has propagated and assimilated the popular ANC discourse within his borders. The TDT originated as a modest and small-scale but reasonably successful attempt at lobbying; it raised and managed funds for community-based projects that were designed to provide employment, promote health and education, and develop agricultural initiatives. With Tshivhase's political clout behind it, however, the TDT has attracted attention and mushroomed into a more prosperous and ambitious organisation. It has assisted in the construction of several schools and a library, and has provided solar power in remote areas. It currently operates banana and timber plantations.[37] Another opportunity for expansion was taken when the TDT inherited the land which the two moribund tea estates had occupied since the 1970s. The closure of the estates between 2005 and 2008, to which I return in Chapter 7, sent shock waves through the community. The TDT, at this time, vowed to phase out the tea and maintain employment opportunities by introducing a commercially viable macadamia nut farm. In 2008, with the help of substantial government subsidy through a parastatal known as the Agric Rural Development Corporation (ARDC), the TDC reopened the tea estates, although the macadamia plan was never brought to fruition. By 2009, the tea estates were running at a profit, selling their produce under the newly branded 'Midi' tea (from Midiyavhathu – the king's royal name).

[36] The Tshivenda word for 'rights' is *pfanelo*, also meaning duty or obligation. This term has been widely translated into discourses of 'female empowerment' so that posters can be seen to read *'Pfanelo dza vhafumakadzi ndi pfanelo dza vhathu vhote!'* (Women's rights are human rights!).

[37] According to Fokwang (2009) the TDT acquired land for the banana farm from the Mphephu-era Venda Development Corporation (VDC), but it is unclear what the VDC used the land for.

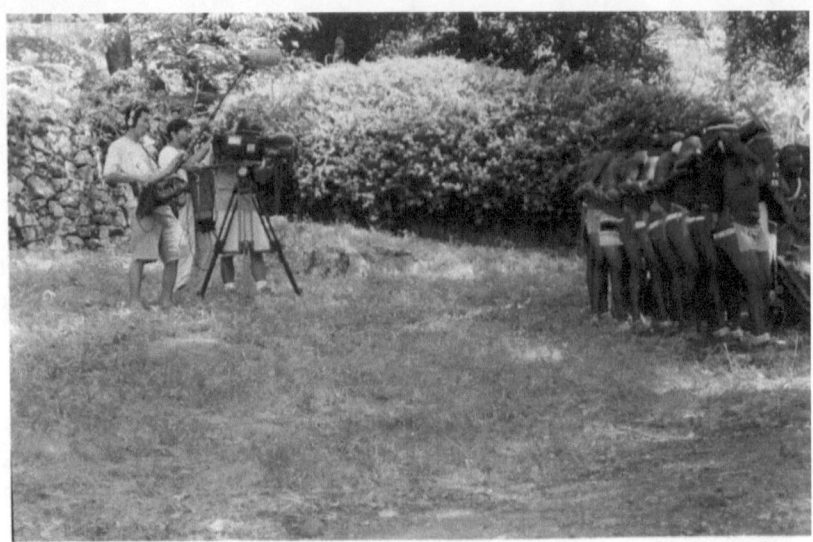

Figure 2.6. A Japanese film crew records initiates at Mukumbani during a staging of the *domba* python dance.

The TDT has also sought to encourage tourism to the region. Most importantly, an overnight camp has been established on the nationally famous and internationally marketed 'Ivory Trail' in close proximity to Mukumbani, which is utilised as a checkpoint for off-road challenge races that periodically blast through the mountains and villages of central Venda, and attracts tourists who prefer to be 'off the beaten track'. The camp has also been frequented by numerous film crews from Japan and Australia, and from exotic location specialists like the *Lonely Planet* and *National Geographic*. These crews come mostly in search of 'authentic' *domba* footage with which to contextualise documentaries or travel guides, and chiefs under Tshivhase are more than happy to negotiate a deal with them (see Figures 2.6 and 2.7; cf. Bruner and Kirshenblatt-Gimblett 1994).[38]

The combination of Tshivhase's active engagement with the ANC rhetoric of African renaissance and development against the background of impeccable liberation credentials made him confident that he would retain the title of king within Tshivhase borders. In this competition, however, Tshivhase lacked the backing of the majority of chiefs in Venda,

[38] During fieldwork I acted as a translator and guide for several of these film crews, mostly in the Tsianda region where a genuine *domba* was taking place, although most of them would have been happy with actors going through the motions. Fees charged by chiefs for filming a *domba* ranged from R3,000 to R15,000 (in 2005/6), which is a substantial sum of money for attending the public session of the initiation.

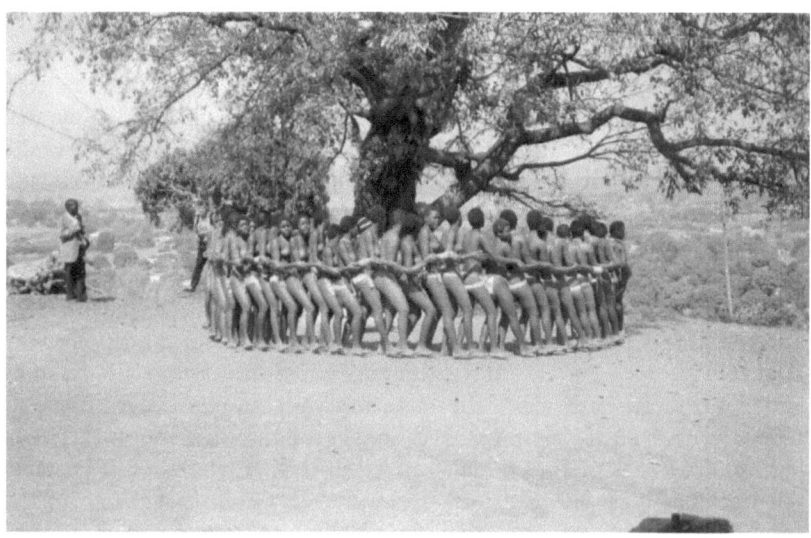

Figure 2.7. Early morning staging of the *domba* python dance at Tsianda for a National Geographic photographer. Note the photographer to the left of the circle. He requested they stage the dance in the morning so he could capture it in good light. As part of the ritual curriculum, this dance would usually be performed late in the evening.

who, despite recent history, have little option but to defer to Mphephu as head of the senior lineage of the Singo clan. The battle for *Khosikhulu* in Venda not only brought historical frictions to the fore, but also remoulded them in terms of the modern democratic dispensation. Despite Mphephu's clear-cut genealogical advantage, the delay in publishing findings of the Nhlapo Commission suggested that Tshivhase's strategy had been successful.

Conclusion

In late 2010, President Zuma announced that the Nhlapo Commission had made a decision regarding the Venda kingship: the line of paramountcy in Venda will – again – be traced through the house of Mphephu Ramabulana (South African Government 2010: 603–39). Kennedy Tshivhase had failed in his attempt to convince the Nhlapo Commission that he is head of an independent sector of the Venda 'traditional community', or that Venda should have a dual kingship. The government chose to recognise genealogical superiority over political connections. In doing so, they were seemingly oblivious to the Thohoyandou High Court ruling in 1991 – after the Mushasha Commission – that the position of paramountcy in Venda was an irregular appointment by the apartheid government. Still, whilst Tshivhase's strategic alignment with the African renaissance and his cultivation of ANC contacts may not have earned him a kingship, he did receive a prestigious deployment within the party as South African representative to the Commonwealth Secretariat.[39] As in the cases of Kgoloko and Rhyne in Sekhukhuneland (Oomen 2000; 2005), it has been possible for the Mphephu chieftaincy to change affiliation over time, and to support, whilst being supported by, successive governments with opposed agendas.

In recounting this chronological narrative, parallels between the apartheid and post-apartheid eras have been striking. The politics of culture have been played out in both eras under increasing state scrutiny and control. In both cases the state has insisted on recognising only one paramount leader among 'traditional communities', but rather than letting structures of traditional leadership decide who should be king, the state has imposed decisions 'from above'. Given that the historical record demonstrates clearly that pre-colonial internecine disputes were often open-ended affairs, in which established genealogy was considered along with popular following and political cleavages of the time, it is by no means clear how the Nhlapo Commission has served its primary goal of 'righting historical wrongs'. It would be more accurate to assert that, in a continued desire for 'uniformity', the post-apartheid government has relied upon, and thus reified, vigorously contested versions of specific historical events.

Moreover, whilst the political and ideological intentions have diverged over time, the policy priorities of traditional leaders have been very similar. This has facilitated the coexistence of two seemingly contradictory roles. Development and modernisation combined with culture and traditionalism in a quest to establish and maintain legitimacy with and for 'the people', the state, and the kingship.

Throughout the apartheid and post-apartheid eras, the multifaceted roles of culture and tradition have been integral to the implementation of traditional leadership. This raises some important questions. To what extent is 'tradition' experienced any differently to how it was in the past? Is 'culture', in the context of the African renaissance, now a means of engaging with and actively attempting to solve the perceived crisis of

---

[39] In late 2010, Tshivhase spent most of his time travelling the African continent fulfilling the duties of this deployment. Whilst the judgement of the Nhlapo Commission officially categorised him in the position of 'senior traditional leader' (chief) it is highly unlikely that this will change the perception of his subjects that he is indeed the king of Tshivhase. As my research was conducted in his area, with his blessing, I will continue to afford him the respect of the title *Thovhela* (king) throughout the book.

reproduction that characterises life in rural, post-apartheid South Africa; and if so, then for whom?

In the next chapter I take up these questions with an ethnographic account of female initiation within Tshivhase's borders and an investigation into the claim that AIDS education has become a part of the ritual curriculum.

3 A Rite to AIDS Education? Venda Girls' Initiation, HIV Prevention, and the Politics of Knowledge

> Ritual knowledge, unlike science, is antithetical to change. It is conceived of as the property of the ancestors, the founders of all social life. It must be handed on, not tested, altered, improved or even discarded. Since it supports experience and validates the seniority of elders, it is not surprising if they throw the weight of their secular powers behind it. (La Fontaine 1985: 189)[1]

In this chapter I develop the argument that state interference in the political economy of kingship has been integral to the promotion of 'tradition' in post-apartheid Venda. I address the ways in which this is connected to a recent increase in the frequency of female initiation, and analyse the dynamics of King Tshivhase's assertion that ritual elders, in his region, have incorporated HIV/AIDS education into the ritual process.

At the initiations I attended in the village of Dopeni (see Map 4), I expected to find ritual experts following Tshivhase's instruction to include HIV/AIDS education in the curriculum. On the contrary, however, there was a violent reaction against its inclusion in the ceremony, which ended with ritual experts punishing the initiates (*vhatei*) for singing about condoms and antiretroviral (ARV) medication. Through the expulsion of AIDS knowledge, biomedical AIDS knowledge, the elders were acting to entrench positions of privilege in a ritual hierarchy by protecting a monopoly on ancestral knowledge. Biomedical explanations of the epidemic, introduced to the ritual by the initiates, were interpreted as a threat to the established order in which the authority of ancestral knowledge is absolute. This reveals that although structures of chiefly power have recently been bolstered by national government, they remain relatively powerless to penetrate and influence the hierarchical structures upon which female initiation depends for its performance and regulation. Moreover, the evidence presented in this chapter demonstrates that

---

[1] Following La Fontaine, M. G. Smith, and others, I maintain a distinction between *power* – as coercive force whether as a result of physical, political, or economic pressure – and *authority*, as the right to recognised command, legitimised by appeal to principles which are part of the moral order (La Fontaine 1985: 17).

if biomedical AIDS education is to be incorporated into female initiation ceremonies, then elderly women (as ritual elders) must either be as fluent in the nuances of scientific explanation as are their younger counterparts, or at least be accepting of this source of knowledge.

Both sides in this account represent attempts to re-secure healthy social reproduction in a time of perceived crisis. In the context of rising unemployment, declining domestic income, rampant crime, and daily deaths, ritual elders and initiates have experienced an 'intergenerational disarticulation' (Comaroff and Comaroff 2004: 337). The clash of values between young and old obscures, however, a common desire: to restore knowledge and techniques which have the power to re-establish an equilibrium in social relations between young and old, men and women, rich and poor.

In the ritual that I describe below, the elders' intention was to reinstate respect (*thonifha*) in younger generations. Like other groups of elders throughout South Africa (see Scorgie 2003 for an example of this in KwaZulu-Natal, and Ngwane 2004 for another in the Eastern Cape), they believe the erosion of generational deference is responsible for an attrition of moral rectitude – and a correlated increase in sexually transmitted infections – among young people. In the case of Venda girls' initiation, the AIDS epidemic has been interpreted by elders not through scientific explanations, but though ancestral ('folk') knowledge. As such, AIDS is believed to be rooted in the build-up of pollution in female bodies that do not adhere to the *milayo* (rules/laws) of the initiation school. In contrast, the young initiates at the ceremonies I attended were familiar with bio-scientific explanations for the recent abrupt increase in AIDS-related deaths. By recounting the safe sex slogans they have learned from local NGOs – to which I turn in the following chapter – the initiates brought biomedical solutions to the crisis into the ancestral arena. In this highly prescriptive context, the two bodies of knowledge were mutually exclusive, and the biomedical approach clashed with the established ritual curriculum.

The increasing frequency of inauguration ceremonies (*vhuhosi*) has been accompanied by a drive to encourage new headmen/women (*Vhamusanda*) in order to promote 'Venda culture' in their areas, as discussed in Chapter 2. Since it is considered inappropriate for a king to interfere directly in internal affairs of *Vhamusanda*, this recruitment drive has largely been implemented indirectly through addresses made by Tshivhase at inauguration ceremonies or other public occasions. During these speeches, new leaders have been encouraged to endorse Venda traditions, and to 'preserve customs' (*u vhulunga sialala yashu*/'to save our culture'). In this way, the newly installed leaders and their subjects learned that 'the people respect and honour a chief by dancing *tshikona* for him and a chief returns that respect by leading [being the head of] the people's *tshikona*'.

It is important to recognise in this statement, and countless others like it, how the performance of *tshikona* is symbolically linked to – and represents – harmonious social relations between the ruler and the ruled. I have already shown that *tshikona* is central to the *vhuhosi* ceremony. Moreover, the extent to which it is understood to epitomise Blacking's famous connection between 'humanly organised sound and soundly organised humanity' (1973: 3), at least for males, should not be underestimated. In this way, the significance of *tshikona* in the post-apartheid era is inseparable from Tshivhase's attempted balancing act to secure legitimacy: between the state, structures of traditional power, and the citizenry. 'People enjoy dancing *tshikona*', he once told me. 'It makes them proud to be Vhavenda.' And yet *tshikona* did not simply disappear during the Bantustan era. It was, like other forms of communal performance in Venda, both appropriated by the authorities *and* used as a vehicle for the expression of discontent.[2]

At the 'cultural projects' initiated in the Tshivhase region the perception was repeatedly voiced that the authenticity of culture had been in decline through the Bantustan era. Clearly, in the absence of reliable historical records, it is difficult to assess the frequency and scale of events such as *tshikona*, *tshigombela*, or *domba* over long periods of time. Nonetheless there can be little doubt that they suffered to some extent from negative associations with the homeland political authorities, which attempted to manipulate the historic and symbolic significance of these events to create the illusion of popular support for the dominant political powers of the time (Blacking 1965: 37). Some categories of performance, such as *mabepha* (singular, *bepha*) musical expeditions between ruling homesteads, disappeared altogether after Blacking recorded their initial demise in the late 1950s (Blacking 1962). In general, the call to preserve cultural activities, and the recent increase in female initiation ceremonies, should be understood in terms of an ideological attempt by traditional leaders to rebrand them, exorcise their associations with or memorialisation of apartheid, and infuse time past with positive associations of a healthy, thriving future.

---

[2] At this juncture, I do not want to engage with the debate as to whether forms of musical expression reinforce hegemonic power or create spaces for resistance (Blacking 1973; 1985; Kruger 2002; 2006; Wulff 2006; Waterman 1990; Erlmann 1996; Coplan 1994). Clearly, there has been a move away from this dualistic opposition and the performance of music and dance has a dual capacity to function as both (cf. James 1999; 2006). For example, the female *tshigombela* and the male *tshikona* both conform to and resist structural arrangements, depending upon the context in which they are performed, by whom, and for whom. This line of thought will be taken up in Chapter 5, with a focus on the music of HIV/AIDS peer group educators.

Vhuhosi and the Promotion of Female Initiation

The association between Venda girls' initiation and AIDS prevention has not been based – like male circumcision – on scientific inference, but on the extent to which ancestral knowledge, conveyed in its unquestioned entirety, can be invoked by ritual elders to stem the epidemic. Ancestral knowledge is released gradually, over the course of several years, at the progressive stages of female initiation. Ideally, a girl's first initiation, *vhusha*, is held at a headman's kraal, following which *domba* is held in the courtyard and ritual hut of the chief's royal palace (*musanda*). A chief (*Khosi*) should host a *domba* soon after inauguration and thereafter conduct the initiation every three to five years. The first *domba* hosted by a king is known as *domba la tshifularo* (*domba* 'of the first count') after which he is entitled to a bride from the graduates (Blacking 1969c: 149) and during which he may join in the famous 'python dance' with young men who are encouraged to attend the later stages of *domba* and scout for potential wives.

Domba has a symbolic register for females similar to that which *tshikona* has for males.[3] Blacking has argued that some stages can be understood as figurative re-enactments of successful social reproduction and sexual intercourse in which boundaries between ancestral spirits and human beings are blurred in the interests of maximising conditions for the promotion of fertility and the reproduction of 'the Venda nation' (Blacking 1969d; 1985). This is not academic abstraction. Certain stages of *domba* are explained to initiates explicitly in these terms, and ritual objects worn by certain initiates transform the girls, at different stages of the ritual, into powerful female ancestors from their royal lineage (see Figures 3.1 and 3.2). In this sense, a chief's responsibility to host a *domba* soon after inauguration goes beyond the instrumental demonstration of political power. *Domba*, like *tshikona*, facilitates the control and maintenance of a healthy cosmological – and thus social – order, without which conditions for prosperity would be impossible, and through which solutions to the current crisis of reproduction are sought.

Venda girls' initiation is ideally experienced as a continuum, and a girl should attend *domba* only once she has graduated from *vhusha*.[4]

---

[3] You can listen to a rendition of the 'Great *domba* song', recorded at Tsianda in May 2005, at http://www.cambridge.org/us/9781107009912.

[4] Blacking (1969a: 13, 18, fn10; 1969b: 72, 82) provides examples of initiation being attended in alternative orders, largely for pragmatic considerations. In the discussion here I do not go into any detail about the brief intermediate stage, reported in previous accounts, known as *tshikanda*. This has been subsumed into late stages of the *vhusha* and early stages of the *domba*, and its primary role of teaching the royal initiates the songs of the commoners' *vhusha* would appear to have been sidelined in the interests of efficiency (cf. Blacking 1969e). Similarly, I have chosen not to discuss *musivheto*, a school run for girls between the ages of 7–11, mostly by Northern Sotho men, in which varying degrees

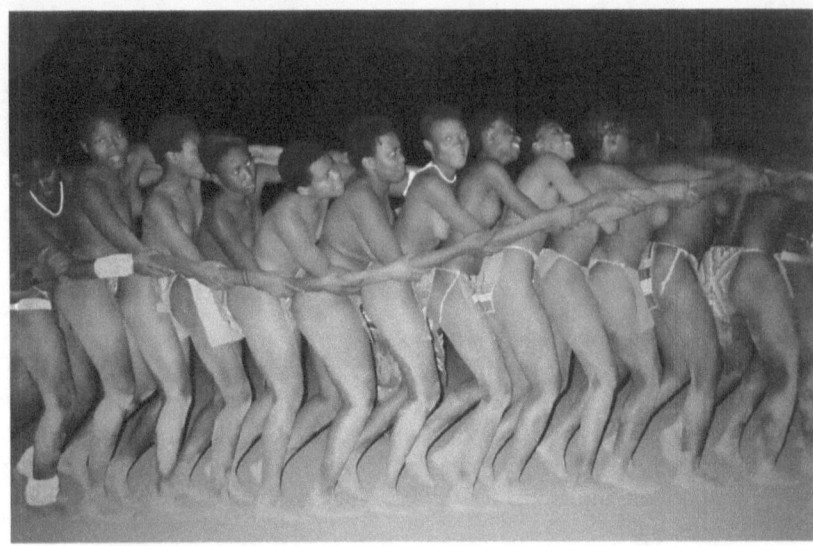

Figure 3.1. The *domba* python dance at Tsianda. Note the ritual aprons (*mashedo*) on the initiates and the white beads marking royal status.

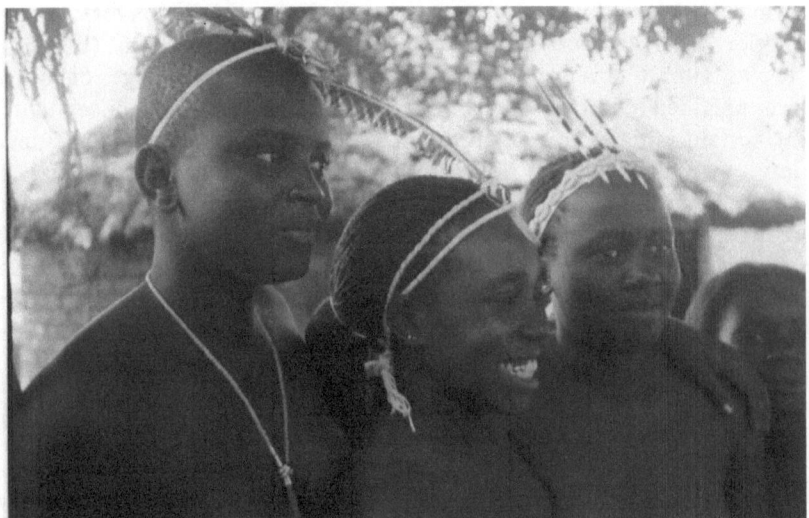

Figure 3.2. *Domba* initiates at Mukumbani with porcupine feather headbands. The porcupine is part of a complex system of totems in Venda genealogy, and is symbolic in this case of the royal, and thus ancestral, authority that these initiates held over the other participants in the initiation.

To produce enough girls who are ready to dance *domba* at a given time it is thus essential that *vhusha* initiation ceremonies are conducted in headmen's homesteads. Conversely, the more headmen who are inclined to conduct *vhusha*, the greater the expectation that a chief will complete the process by later hosting *domba*. In this way, the increasing numbers of newly installed headmen in the Tshivhase region – charged with the role of preserving traditions – have yielded, correspondingly, a sharp increase in the frequency of *vhusha* initiation ceremonies.

As if to lead by example, to 'set the ball rolling' in a confident assertion of his power, Kennedy Tshivhase hosted the first stage of his *domba la tshifularo*, in which over 2,000 girls participated, at Mukumbani in the summer holidays between 2001 and 2002. In order to get this number of initiates he effectively poached girls in various stages of *vhusha* from traditional leaders in his area. Many girls who danced had reportedly never even been to *vhusha*. A similarly flexible attitude to traditional expectations was evident when Tshivhase stated publicly that, as he already has three wives, he would relinquish his right to choose a virgin bride from the graduates, reiterating his assertion that AIDS education would be incorporated into the curriculum. In taking this stance he projected an image that combined respect for tradition with a modernising zeal, making him the ideal candidate for paramountcy. To some extent, however, this backfired on the young king. Tshivhase's refusal to select a fourth wife from the initiates led many traditionalists in the Territorial Authority to question the efficacy of the ritual before it had even started. According to the dissenters, *domba* will appease the ancestors – and thus reach a conclusion – only once the king marries a graduate. Tshivhase's refusal to do so, according to this faction, may actually have disrupted the cosmological order with potentially undesirable consequences.

Nonetheless, the ritual proceeded. The *mme a domba* ('mother of the *domba*')[5] of Tshivhase's *domba la tshifularo* at Mukumbani was Noriah Lowani Mbudziseni Ralinala, a highly respected traditional healer and ritual expert from the village of Dopeni. At that time, Noriah was also the *makhadzi* to the chief at Dopeni, *Khosi* Khakhathi Silas Ralinala. In 2003, Noriah's achievements as a ritual expert were recognised officially when she was installed as a headwoman (*Vhamusanda/Gota*) at an inauguration ceremony along with five other relatives, and given responsibility for a subdivision of the village. In further recognition of her new-found

---

of genital mutilation are reportedly practised. It is not at all common for parents to send their children to *musivheto*, nor is it associated with traditional authority.

[5] Paradoxically, the ritual name given to the leader of the *vhusha*, a position that is always occupied by a female, is *nematei* where the *ne-* signifies male ownership. In contrast, the elderly male who presides over the hearth of every *domba* is known ritually as Vho Nyamungozwa, where the *nya* signifies female ownership.

influence, Noriah was encouraged by the Tshivhase royal council to form a centre for tradition (*sialala*) on a plot of land in her district of Dopeni. Funding was arranged through the National Arts Council, and the *Dopeni Vhulungani Sialala* ('Dopeni preserve your traditions') was established in June 2004. The Dopeni project is an example of how Tshivhase has sought to combine development with a cultural revival, dovetailing the simultaneous existence of modern and traditional in one enterprise. The aims of the project were threefold: to provide employment and income generation; to promote cultural activities; and, most importantly, to disseminate ritual knowledge amongst the newly inaugurated traditional leaders in the Tshivhase area.

Noriah's first objective was to write a booklet. In this, she recorded selected details of female initiation, *thevhula* (rites of the ancestor cult performed annually on royal ancestors' graves), *malombo* (possession/*ngoma* rites of affliction), *luambo lwa musanda* (the language of the royal homestead), and *mafarelwe a lushie* (the handling of a new-born baby). This booklet was approved by a council of royal elders and, according to Noriah, was circulated to every headman and chief under King Kennedy.

For the official opening of the project, a small leaflet was produced to advertise the 'courses' which were available:

Dopeni Vhulungani Sialala

Vhulungu	R600	Bead making
Mitshino ya sialala	R150	Traditional dances
Vhusha / Domba	R300	Female initiation
U gudisa mahosi milayo na luambo lwa musanda	R500	To teach laws and the royal Venda language to chiefs
U gudisa vhatununi milayo na luambo lwa musanda	R500	To teach laws and the royal Venda language to chiefs' wives
U gudisa vhana milayo na luambo lwa musanda	R500	To teach laws and the royal Venda language to royal children
Zwidade	R100	Children's games, riddles, counting songs, fairy tales

The Dopeni Project

By the time of the official opening of the Dopeni project, I had been spending three or four days a week there for some months. I was introduced to Noriah by Mr Fobbe (see Chapter 1), who explained to her that I was interested in *mvelele* (culture). Most of this time had been spent recording and translating her exhaustive repertoire of ritual knowledge, focusing on the rites of female initiation. Having read Blacking's extensive works on the subject, I was keen to record my own inventory of *vhusha* and *domba* songs, from which I was planning to make a comparative ethnomusicological analysis.

In the period leading up to the official opening, however, I abandoned my recordings and offered the use of my pick-up truck (*bakkie*) to assist in the transportation of tents, chairs, food, water, and guests. Although exhausting at the time, this provided a means whereby the 'social distance' between researcher and researched was reduced by working together towards a common goal. The secluded front cab of my blue Nissan pick-up was the venue for many informal interviews: people seemed at ease talking, gossiping, and joking in the relative privacy of the *bakkie*, where they knew others could not overhear them.

I arrived at 5.30 a.m. on the morning of the opening. King Kennedy had confirmed that he would attend, and so every traditional leader in the region was expected to follow suit. Noriah was keen to impress them and promote her business, whilst I was anxious to impress her and increase my chances of attending the *vhusha* ceremony due to take place at the project in the following months. I had been charged with the task of supplying the king's refreshments for the day (he requests Chivas Regal whisky: the name has echoes of Tshivhase) and I had been on a tour of Venda nightspots to procure it, getting slightly distracted along the way. Several migrant workers had returned for the ceremony and had decimated the supplies of maize beer (*mahafhe*)[6] intended for the guests. Large, open tents had been erected dangerously close to the pit-latrine toilets and the speaker system I had acquired from a local musician had somehow been misplaced. I walked into the *tshivhambo* ritual hut[7] to greet Noriah, and found her hunched over a mound of smouldering herbal medicine (*mushonga*), coughing profusely and praying loudly to her long line of ancestors for a successful passage through the day. She had recognised the wail of my fan-belt in the cold of the morning, and so did not have to look up to know who had entered. 'Aaa, good morning Thitupulwi

---

[6] *Mahafhe* is known as 'traditional Venda beer', or *halwa*. Made from fermented maize corn, it is brewed by many elderly women who sell it from their homestead, sometimes providing music and seating for customers. It varies greatly in quality and strength but is readily available and very cheap. Homesteads which sell *mahafhe* advertise their wares by flying a white flag from the gate: the flag is said to be symbolic of the empty maize sack, and is only hoisted when the beer is ready for consumption. In 2009, a jar of *mahafhe* sold for between R4 and R6.

[7] The design of a *tshivhambo* hut (from *u vhamba* – to stretch cow skin over a drum or to crucify) has important symbolic value. The symbolism of the skin is incorporated into several female initiation rites, in which the initiates are 'hung' upside down from a pole behind their knees and attached to the *tshivhambo* door, to 'stretch' the body. The design of the poles (*matanda*) on the inside of the roof is also specific to *milayo* (rules) of initiation through which girls memorise ritual knowledge.

[my Venda name], don't worry, everything will be fine!' Unconvinced, I said a quick prayer of my own, and set about repitching the tents.

Miraculously, by the arrival of the first guests at 11 a.m. (only one hour late) everything was in order. Royal bodyguards had been loitering since around nine, and culinary representatives had been dispatched from Mukumbani to monitor the preparation of food for any suspicious activities that might suggest poison. As was expected, they regularly asked the cooks to taste from the huge, bubbling pots of meat and porridge (*vhuswa*), and several young children volunteered themselves for the job, securing a hearty breakfast in the process. My last task was to collect a red carpet across which the entourage would walk to enter the royal tent which, thankfully, given the changeable weather conditions, was now further away from the toilets. Roughly 300 guests, and throngs of uninvited spectators, were entertained by performances intended to advertise the prowess of those involved in teaching traditional dances at the project. In between dances, long addresses were given by prominent local politicians, chiefs, and traditional healers.

By the time Noriah's slot in the programme arrived, the crowd of onlookers and passers-by were growing restless, being curious to witness the praise calling (*zwirendo*) for which she is renowned and has won several prizes. She is a powerful woman, possessing both ample social status and a formidable physical frame (see Figure 3.3). Dressed only from the waist in the colourful Venda women's cloth (*nwenda*, plural *minwenda*) and wrapped in the long red rope (*thahu*, worn by girls and women attending initiation and also to signify ritual impurity during menstruation), Noriah took the microphone and walked into the middle of the dancing arena, standing directly on the worn-out spot upon which the main drum (*ngoma lungundu*) had just sounded the heartbeat of a *tshikona*. She performed the recital as if her life depended on it. Sweating profusely and eventually in tears on her knees, she called out elaborate praises for the long succession of chiefs and kings in the Tshivhase lineage from Dimbanyika up to the present day, pausing only to inhale deep wheezing breaths before continuing relentlessly for perhaps a quarter of an hour. The crowd seemed genuinely impressed by her oratory. As she came to a close, punching the earth until a cloud of dust rose around her, we fell silent. With this by way of an introduction, King Kennedy arose to deliver his speech. Women bowed down to ululate and men crouched into the respectful *losha* position, mumbling his praises:[8]

---

[8] Praises (*zwirendo*) for the king are not formulaic and can be improvised on the spot. There are several, however, which are in common circulation, some of which I have cited in the text. *Zwirendo* are a mixture of outlandish compliments and statements intended to scorn and ridicule the king; not to disrespect him but to elevate his status by comparing him to unworldly creatures and seemingly impossible events.

Thovhela muhale!	Great King, our hero!
Mbila u lume!	My Highness!
Khakha u mela!	Something so great that it should not be there!
Thindi ndia mila,	Dense fillet of meat
Ndi kundwa nga shambo	Swallowed without hindrance of bones!
Muthomboni wa Dzata!	Honourable one of Dzata!
Tshiulu tsha madini!	Mound of soil in the water
Gole mutumbuka vhathu!	Creator of people!
Ndau ya nduna!	The biggest male lion!
Vele la mbeu!	Great ancestor![9]
Lutiti luna dzhasi!	Small birds wear long robes!
Tshizwa tsha bête ndi tshuhulu!	A cockroach's thigh is big!
Zulu muthombee!	Even Zulus surrender!
Vhafa lini ra wana vhatanuni?!	When will you die so we can get the Queens?!
Iwe une we ifai wa fa!	By a just word from your mouth we will vanish!

The king opened the address with comments on various topics of the day, asserting that the current disputes over land claims were futile as all the soil belonged to him, and proceeding to champion the role of women and children in a democratic society. Many of the young girls from the project were placed in front of the royal tent, dressed only in ritual aprons (*mashedo*; singular, *shedo*)[10] with their arms crossed and heads respectfully bowed. He continued:

[Y]es, our traditions must be preserved, but this must be conducted in the correct/authentic way! These young girls should not be seen here, in public, wearing only *mashedo*. These things are secret, sacred of the ancestors, and this project has been charged with preserving these things! Girls, get inside! We support *Dopeni Vhulungani Sialala* in the spirit of the African renaissance, so that our Venda traditions are not forgotten and our traditional leaders are well trained in their responsibilities... but our traditions and culture must not ignore problems of today... problems like unemployment, HIV/AIDS, which is why we have these things as a part of our initiations... so that our children can grow correctly/authentically whilst protecting themselves.... They are the future! (Translated from Tshivenda)

After this rebuttal, the young girls in *mashedo* who had been scheduled to close the ceremony with a brief performance of the *domba* python dance

---

[9] Vele is a well-known mythical hero in the Tshivhase dynasty, and appears in folklore throughout the region. As related in Chapter 2, he was the son of Dimbanyika, who led the Singo clan across the Limpopo River around 1700.

[10] *Shedo* is the small apron worn around the waist of an initiate during the *vhusha* and *domba*. It is usually made from the colourful *nwenda* cloth (see Figure 3.1).

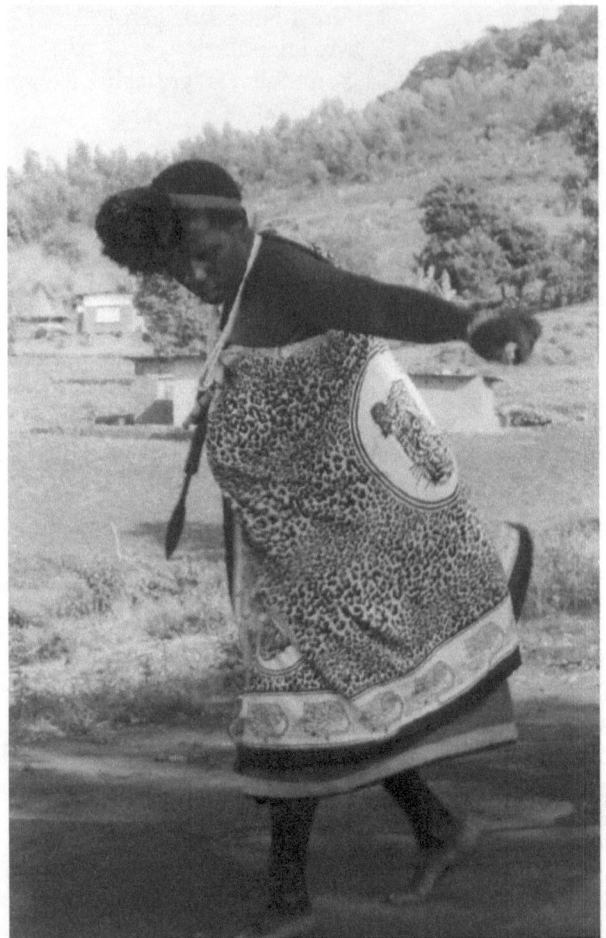

Figure 3.3. Noriah Ralinala performing the rites of *malombo* possession, at Phiphidi village. Note the ritual spear in her right hand. She is wearing a black and white blanket, in contrast to a red headband.

were hastily bundled into the *tshivhambo* hut and the award-winning *tshikona* group from Ha-Khakhu swarmed into action around Noriah, who retreated from the dancing arena. In a symbolic stamp of approval on the opening of the project, King Tshivhase rose to lead the *tshikona* dancers in his trademark, charismatic style, posing for photographs and video footage on the way. The opening – despite Kennedy's rebuke – had been a success, and the dignitaries retired to eat at Noriah's elder sister's homestead.

Negotiating Access to the *Vhusha* Initiation

My assistance in coordinating the official opening of the Dopeni project was largely motivated by the hope that my efforts would be repaid. I knew there was a *vhusha* ceremony scheduled at Noriah's homestead in the coming months, and I wanted to attend it. The decision granting my permission to enter the *vhusha* was eventually taken at two levels. Initially, King Tshivhase – although he had studied anthropology at the University of the North during the 1980s and was generally sympathetic to my project – was sceptical of my proposal to 'sit in' at the initiation. I took the opportunity to raise the issue with him at Mr Fobbe's daughter's christening in Sibasa, some weeks after the opening of the Dopeni project.

At the christening, Tshivhase sat at the head of the royal table, flanked by two bodyguards and his inner circle of councillors. After everyone had eaten, the usual long line of people who hoped for a word with the king took a seat and waited for the place next to them to become vacant. In this way, a brief conversation with him could be secured without going through the hierarchically arranged array of headmen and lesser officials described in Chapter 2. His bodyguards maintained the circulation of hopefuls by limiting each conversation to no more than ten minutes. I joined the table, and commented that the *malende* drumbeat of our entertainment reminded me of a *domba* recording that John Blacking had made in the 1960s. This sparked a lively discussion which had captivated the royal table by the time I rotated to a seat next to the king. Two of the men at the table had known Blacking personally as young boys, and were keen to elaborate on the impact they had had on his research.

Indicating my desire to speak, I took up the *losha* (submissive/respect) position and the men at the table followed suit. On being given an opportunity to speak, after lavishly praising Tshivhase for his *domba la tshifularo*, I explained my intention to interview a random selection of the *midabe* (graduates).[11] The royal table found this suggestion highly amusing and broke into a roar of laughter. Clearly this would be very difficult, the king explained, as it is taboo (*zwia ila*) for the graduates to discuss their experiences there. Was not I just looking for a wife, he joked, in which case he could make the necessary arrangements? Mr Fobbe then suggested that I should attend a ceremony to 'witness the thriving culture of Tshivhase' first-hand. I had planted this idea with him beforehand, and he knew that a *vhusha* was imminent at Dopeni. The table fell silent as the proposition was considered. 'Do you know that we do AIDS education there?' the king asked, to which I shook my head. 'You Western academics should

---

[11] In terms of the statistics course I had recently undertaken, if $n = 100$ or more, then a random sample from this could facilitate statistical generalisation from a group to a population (in this case $n = 2,000$). I later abandoned this project.

enjoy that! It is not impossible [for you to attend], Fobbe can take you to the project at Dopeni, but the final decision will be made by Noriah, not me!' He was, then, referring me back to the acknowledged ritual expert whose authority over the Dopeni project he had recently authorised and endorsed. He appeared to be deferring to her authority, in seemingly disingenuous ignorance of the extent to which it reflected on his own.

Kennedy's decision to 'send' me to *vhusha* invoked the ethical conundrum of reciprocal manipulation that I discussed in the Introduction. To be sure, it was a tactical move which he hoped would facilitate the projection of his engagement with the African renaissance, through my coverage of the affair, to a wider audience. I, in turn, wanted to grasp a very rare opportunity for a male – a foreign, white male – to witness first-hand Venda girls' initiation. I had little intention of assisting his case for the paramountcy, being more interested in the micro-politics of the rites. We both understood this potentially mutually beneficial situation, although it was never acknowledged as such. Noriah, for her part, granted permission for her own specific reasons. After my assistance with the official opening and continued presence at the project, she held a meeting with the senior project members at which it was agreed that I would be permitted to attend the *vhusha*. The conditions attached were that I would effectively sponsor it with some food and soft drinks for the initiates, bottled beer and *mahafhe* for the elders, and a large tub of snuff for one old lady who was particularly opposed to my attendance.

Noriah was enthusiastic, as though preparing for her moment of fame. She told me to come with cameras, videos, and microphones. For Noriah, to have *her vhusha* recorded and documented would make a significant contribution to Venda heritage, an accompaniment to her widely circulated booklet and, as she told me, help people 'to remember her legacy'. It was thus important that every detail was recorded accurately (making it necessary for me to return several times over the next year), and she delegated a literate assistant to sit next to me and provide a running commentary during the ceremonies. A contract was drawn up in which I agreed not to share 'the secrets of the *tshivhambo*' with anyone who was not initiated, with the exception of my 'research to be written in England', and Noriah received a copy of my videos and photocopies of my notes.[12]

In this way, my attendance at the *vhusha* had political significance in a number of ways, and I was acutely aware of the endeavours to manipulate my presence there. Several women who turned up to participate were

---

[12] The quality of the video turned out to be exceptionally poor. The fire inside the *tshivhambo* constantly drew the focus of the video from the initiates to the light of the flame. Nonetheless, the microphone captured the sound, allowing me to transcribe the songs as they were performed. I also recorded audio material on a cassette recorder.

shocked to find a white man in the corner, preparing to record the proceedings on a video camera, asking questions and writing down secret, ritual knowledge into a notebook. Noriah appeased them by explaining that I was working for her, and pointed them to the refreshments which I had provided. I was invited to the ceremony four times, under more or less the same conditions.

Having invested many hours hanging around the project and talking with Noriah, I was familiar with most of the initiates, their families, and most of the initiated women. Nonetheless, my presence might have influenced proceedings in subtle ways of which I am unaware and which I was thus powerless to change. For example, it is possible that Noriah omitted or modified certain elements of the *vhusha*, and that the initiates and older women reacted differently in my absence. Similarly, having attended the ceremony and documented proceedings, I know that Noriah intentionally excluded much esoteric content from her booklet which could have been read by uninitiated women or men. For example, passwords for entry into the *tshivhambo*, ritual names for body parts and clothing, and many proverbs and anecdotes told to the initiates during certain dances were omitted intentionally. However, she chose to include the well-known elements such as colour symbolism and the focus on 'preparation for marriage', with issues relating these to sexual health in terms of Venda aetiology – more of which below. These things considered, I now turn to the ceremony.

The *Vhusha* Initiation

Blacking (1969a) has described the *ideal* sequence of events which lead up to a girl entering the *vhusha*. Upon her first menstruation (*u vhonna nwedzi* – 'to see the moon') a girl should inform her maternal aunt, who informs the headman. Once a small group of girls has been reported, the headman should then call in female ritual experts, who are not necessarily related to the royal family, to hold a *vhusha*. The venue should be the homestead of the headman or woman, and whilst not engaged in the business of her initiation, a novice is a source of labour for the women who live there, although she must not leave the boundaries of the homestead. In addition, the stages, songs, and dances that should be performed at *vhusha* in ceremonies that could last up to a week have been documented extensively by Jeannerat (1997), Stayt (1931: 106–10), van Warmelo (1932: 37–52), Blacking (1969a; 1969b), and by Noriah herself in my field notes.

Given that historical variations can be influenced by regional differences and personal preferences, the specific order and detail of the ritual can take various forms (cf. Barth 2002). This was accepted by the ritual leaders at Dopeni, who told stories of certain ritual experts who privileged specific elements of *vhusha* over others without affecting its overall efficacy. Much literature on female initiation in Southern Africa (Richards 1956: 55; Comaroff 1985; La Fontaine 1985; Rasing 1995; Turner 1967) has noted the adaptation of rites of passage to the time constraints of modern life: as their duration decreases their content is condensed. In Venda, in much the same way as boys' circumcision takes place during the winter school holidays, female initiation has been tailored to fit with the school week. *Vhusha* at the Dopeni project thus took place over the course of a single weekend, from Friday afternoon until Sunday morning. It provided an abridged course in which the ritual leaders maximised efficiency by minimising the overlap between subjects taught and by stressing only what they asserted to be the core elements.

This condensed ritual format, combined with the bureaucratic framing of the event to fit the National Arts Council's requirements and the list of other cultural activities from which initiation can be purchased, give the post-apartheid *vhusha* a distinctly 'rationalised' feel. The commodification of culture is a global phenomenon, with particular characteristics and consequences in different historical settings (Comaroff and Comaroff 2009). In Venda, this was reinforced by the attempts at standardisation through Noriah's booklet, to which my video was to become an appendage. In this way, I was an active participant in the rationalisation of the ritual: one intended to be yet further augmented through the use of information technology. Noriah had asked me to teach her to use a database through which she could document the number of 'clients' that the project had 'generated', using the nearby computer café at Tshikombani. It was her intention, in storing data in this format, to give her future funding proposals the edge over those of any competitors. A more vivid image representing the modernity of tradition is hard to imagine.

Overall, it became clear that *vhusha* was a practice undergoing a particular kind of revival rather than one in which continuities were evident. It was, in 2004–5, by no means common practice for girls to attend *vhusha*, and it would be misleading to suggest that a majority of parents send their daughters 'to be sung for' (*u imbelwa*) at a leader's kraal. The recent drive to promote initiation is an attempt to reverse the falling off in attendance: a drive in which the political pressure on newly installed headmen to support their chief's *domba la tshifularo* has played no small part. Kennedy Tshivhase's bid for influence, and his insistence on his headmen's loyalty and their ritual complicity, has added a sense of urgency to the incorporation of young girls into *vhusha*. At the same time, these headmen have their own political, economic, and cultural reasons for enthusiastic participation in the project.

As Jeannerat (1997: 100) has pointed out, young girls' views on the merits of initiation often diverge from those of elder women. Many, she argues, refuse to attend because they believe *vhusha* to be 'cruel and senseless', are opposed to the way in which it 'invited them to engage in sexual relationships', and are convinced that it 'does not help for their future' (ibid.). Whilst these quotes from young, uninitiated women shed light on some opinions held toward *vhusha*, it would be mistaken to seek in these comments an explanation of why such girls do not attend the initiation. The decision is taken not by the potential initiates, but by their parents, who will pay the initiation fees on behalf of their child or make the promise to do so in the future. Whilst the resolution not to send children to initiation may be influenced by the historical association of culture with Bantustan authorities or notions of the modern set against 'time past', the crucial motivational factor in this decision is church affiliation which, in turn, is closely associated with social class.

From fieldwork conducted in the 1960s, we can ascertain that this has been the case for some time. Blacking (1964b: 158) demonstrates that girls who attended the Lutheran church at that time, and who by definition did not attend female initiation or any other such traditional activities, had distinct – and distinctly privileged – life stories and life courses. Non-Lutheran girls who participated in 'traditional' activities were subject to social stigma and dubbed 'salempore girls' by contemporaries who, as mission church affiliates, considered themselves modern Christians in comparison.[13] The stigma attached to salempore girls was exacerbated by the divisive spatial politics of Lutheran missionisation, which was characterised by the 'insistence on their converts' almost feudal subordination' (Delius 1983: 160–78; cf. James 1997).[14] Along with this spatial segregation of Lutheran converts – many of them moved to live in or around mission stations and symbolically distanced themselves from chiefs and other centres of traditional religion – there was a doctrinal concern that African Christians must abandon cultural practices. As such, Lutheran missionaries in Venda sought to convince converts that institutions such as initiation were 'schools of the Devil' (Kirkaldy 2005: 213). Church affiliation, as I show in the following chapter, remains an important marker of identity, and (non-) participation in various practices can be read off from this. The HIV/AIDS educators who are members of mission/mainline churches (such as Lutheran or Methodist) cited purely religious grounds for refusing to send their daughters to *vhusha*.

[13] Salempore is the material used to make the Venda female dress *nwenda* (plural *minwenda*). It is also used by Shangaan women for a similar purpose. It is of Indian origin and its presence in Venda dates back to early Indian traders from roughly 1890. The standardised length and width of *minwenda*, that gave rise to the style of wrapping it around the waist several times to secure a fit, is the product of early tax regulations under which certain measurements were exempt from import duty (cf. Hobsbawm and Ranger 1983).
[14] See Comaroff (1985: 30) for alternative spatial dynamics of missionisation among Tswana; Mayer and Mayer (1961) for an example of self-imposed geographical separation among 'red' (traditionalist) and 'school' (Christian) Xhosa in an urban environment.

Blacking's main character in the biography of Dora, a Lutheran schoolgirl, associated the salempore girls with a backward and uncivilised lifestyle. It is unfortunate that Blacking did not procure the parallel biography of a non-Lutheran Christian or a salempore child, as this would have provided us with a more comprehensive historical picture from which we could have built an understanding of how class formation relates to church affiliation in the region. As in other regions of South Africa, membership of a mission or mainline church in Venda has been associated with the middle classes or the petite bourgeoisie (Kiernan 1977). Conversely, membership of the African Independent Churches (AICs) tends towards the poor and illiterate peasant-proletariat, with the massively popular Zion Christian Church (ZCC) appealing in particular to migrant labourers and female domestic workers (Comaroff 1985: 188–9; cf. Garner 1998).[15] However, the post-apartheid era has seen a changing dynamics of class in South Africa. As I demonstrate in the following chapter, religious affiliation may not be as accurate an indicator as was previously thought.

Despite these recent forms of boundary blurring, attendance of girls' initiation in contemporary Venda is decided largely along the fault line of religious affiliation. Complicating this picture, and not mentioned in Blacking's rendition of Dora's story, is the apparently contradictory phenomenon of believers' Christian initiation schools. There are two categories of initiation that girls may attend in the post-apartheid dispensation: *vhusha ya vhatendi* (*vhusha* of believers/Christians) and *vhusha ya musanda* (*vhusha* of the royal kraal).

The *vhusha ya vhatendi* is conducted regularly but exclusively by women's groups within the ZCC. The ZCC is divided into two camps (*ya tshinoni* – of the bird; and *ya naledzi* – of the star), each of which is presided over by a grandson of the founder, Bishop Engenas Lekganyane. Both camps in Venda are known to practise female initiation that, to a large extent, is a direct re-enactment of *vhusha ya musanda*. There are three key differences: it is conducted on the premises where church meetings are held; the initiates are fully clothed in the process; and some songs have been replaced by church hymns. As Comaroff (1985) has demonstrated

---

[15] Of course, there are exceptions to these general trends. To clarify: by mission/mainline churches I am referring to those with mainline orthodox theology and a history of missionisation. In South Africa these are Anglican, Methodist, Presbyterian, Lutheran, or Roman Catholic. Membership of these churches constitutes just over 30 per cent of South Africa's population. By African Independent Churches (AICs) I am referring to those churches that provide an 'African articulation of Christian doctrine and symbol' such as the Zionist or Apostolic, which also make up just over 30 per cent of the (black) population (Garner 2000). The ZCC is the most popular church in South Africa, with over 11.1 per cent of the total population (US Government 2006). The 'I' in AIC can also represent 'initiated' or 'indigenous', but these refer to the same phenomenon. Whilst Pentecostalism has become increasingly common in some parts of Venda, its influence has remained relatively peripheral to that of the ZCC.

A Rite to AIDS Education? 91

among the Tshidi Rolong in the Mafeking region, Zionist churches characteristically blend pre-colonial ritual systems and symbols with the lived experience of modern life (see also Rasing [1995] for a discussion of contemporary *Chisungu* female initiation among urban Zambian Roman Catholics). The *vhusha ya vhatendi* is an example of this hybridisation: it includes pre-colonial elements in modern forms of religious practice.

Hearsay confirms these suggestions about both the continuities and the differences between the form and content of the two rituals. Although, for reasons outlined in the Introduction, I was unable to attend a Christian *vhusha*, I did glean information from secondary sources which suggested that it thrived in the Bantustan era when the royal initiations had become unpopular, and continues to thrive today. I conducted numerous semi-structured interviews with women who participate regularly in Christian *vhusha*. Initially, although I was very well acquainted with many of them, they refused even to discuss the matter with me. But when I demonstrated my own ritual knowledge, passed on to me by Noriah, they became more inclined to talk, possibly out of curiosity to discover how much I actually knew. Despite these differences, the corpus of ritual knowledge appears to be almost identical in the two kinds of initiation school, although several ritual objects are different and each stage in the Christian version opens and closes with a prayer.[16] It is significant for my argument in subsequent chapters that Zionist churches in Venda incorporated and have retained female initiation. This is not least because of the vast numbers of girls who are initiated there, and thus the many ritual experts who have a vested interest in the promotion and understanding of sexual illnesses through an aetiology of ancestral knowledge.

To add to the complexity, there is one further subdivision within the non-Christian *vhusha*. This is between the *vhusha ha vhasiwana* (for commoners) and *vhusha ha vhakololo* (for royalty). The following account is of the commoner's *vhusha*, which was also attended by royal children (this is a lopsided situation, since commoners may not participate in the royal ceremony). There is no singing at the royal initiation, and esoteric codes are given in the royal language, *luambo lwa musanda*.

In this wider context, then, King Kennedy's drive to promote female initiation necessarily had a selective uptake, with participation being decided partly along the lines of church affiliation. Through Kennedy's campaign to retain his kingship, a tension has begun to develop between the desire of newly installed headmen to recruit *vhusha* initiates and the lack of parents willing to send their children to *vhusha ha musanda*. It is

---

[16] There is a focus on black tea or *Trekker* coffee and condensed milk, which are used to represent the colours black and white in the construction of moral lessons. I did not hear of any Christian substitute for the colour red; in line with *vhusha ya musanda*, initiates are covered in red ochre and models of the human body are used with red, white, and black clothes painted on.

not at all clear what measures the king might take to resolve this pending problem, or how this tension will play out in the future. Seen in terms of his ongoing balancing act to achieve and maintain legitimacy, however, it is not necessarily the actual number of initiates which is of immediate importance. The public promotion of initiation, at least for Kennedy, is what brought him directly into line with African renaissance discourse and thus to the heart of ANC ideology. Nonetheless he continues to promote new traditional leaders, creating an excess of ritual experts and a deficiency of potential initiates. Given the nature of ZCC affiliation – its leaders and members have remained resolutely apolitical during both apartheid and post-apartheid eras – it seems highly unlikely that there will be a movement from the Christian *vhusha* to support any African renaissance. Rather, the Christian *vhusha* has maintained a steady and unfluctuating group of adherents.

Such a claim of continued popularity has been repudiated by Buijs (2003), who states that 'First missionary and later state education has meant the virtual end of female, if not yet male, initiation rites [in Venda by the late 1990s]': a statement which may be applicable to *vhusha ya musanda* but is an invalid representation of ZCC practices. Whilst the royal *vhusha* lost popularity during apartheid, the Christian *vhusha* seems to have flourished. My informants explained this explicitly in terms of the non-political stance taken by the ZCC during the Bantustan era. As I was told during an interview: 'I started with the ZCC because they didn't talk politics there... I could sing for my daughter [have her initiated] there without worrying about these young boys [ANC Youth League] that watched people going to the chief's kraal.' This suggests that there was a movement from royal to Christian *vhusha* under apartheid, and raises other issues – for a different discussion – about the role of the Zionist church in the practice of passive resistance.

As I now describe, a secondary tension has developed that Tshivhase did not preempt. This is between the buttressing of ritual experts' authority and ancestral knowledge through the official promotion of female initiation and the initiates' interpretation of illnesses through the biomedical model.

Milayo (Laws) and the Stages of Initiation

During the *vhusha* initiation, initiates memorise certain rules and laws (*milayo*; singular, *mulayo*). Blacking (1969e: 21) defines *milayo* as 'kinds of instruction... in particular [with] songs, dances, symbolic acts, and explanations of these'. Van Warmelo (1989: 222) translates *milayo* as 'a formulation of what is traditionally right... exhortation in support of traditional standards of behaviour... as taught in initiation rites'. A significant proportion of *milayo* are embodied through the performance of physically demanding and painful *ndayo* dances that are intended to stretch (*u vhamba*) the body. Although the pain is supposed to be excruciating, the girls are not permitted to express any indication that they are in discomfort (cf. La Fontaine 1985; Blacking 1969a; 1985; Wulff 2006). Some *ndayo* are designed to demonstrate and practise sexual positions in preparation for marriage (cf. Beidelman 1997: 182; La Fontaine 1985: 116). It was because of their association with fertility and reproduction that Tshivhase believed they presented a potential opportunity for ritual leaders to include HIV/AIDS education in the ceremony.

At the Dopeni project, the progressive stages of *ndayo* were performed throughout the course of Friday and Saturday nights, beginning at sundown and ending just before sunrise. All of the rites were performed inside the *tshivhambo* hut around a blazing fire, and youngsters were employed to keep inquisitive passers-by from excessive prying. Initiated women sat in an outer circle on the bench incorporated into the *tshivhambo* wall, and the initiates occupied the space between them and the fire, with ritual experts moving between the two at will. The different *ndayo* took between 30 minutes and an hour, after which the girls were covered with blankets and told to lie down silently, whilst the initiated women told stories, drank *mahafhe* beer, and recounted memories of their initiations. The contrast between the intense levels of noise produced by the drums and singing of the *ndayo* rites with the quiet and stillness of the breaks was of important symbolic value. The initiates were repeatedly told that they should 'find comfort in the silence' (*u wana khuthadzo kha phumudzo*) and that this should stay with them throughout their married lives. In other words, reinterpreted from a post-feminist position, 'accept your position and don't complain about it'.

During the performance of *ndayo* that I witnessed, Noriah specifically emphasised that I must understand a certain sequence that was performed at the end of the first night. This was usually between 2 and 3 a.m., by which time smoke from the smouldering fire had reduced me to tears. The sequence took roughly one hour, and whilst it was accompanied by drumming, lyrics seemed to be added only sporadically by the initiated spectators, who were preoccupied with humiliating and insulting the initiates.

The first of these rites – a variation of what Blacking calls *dzole* (1969a: 14) – started with an initiate putting a small bundle of hardened corn (*mavelle*) on the far side of the fire. One after the other, the initiates approached the corn on their knees with their joined hands pushed into the air behind their back. Bending down towards the corn, raising their arms higher behind them, they carefully caught one piece of corn in their lips. They then shuffled around the fire, with the corn as close to the ground as possible, and deposited it in an empty broken pot (*kali*) at the other side of the fire until the original bundle was gone. Noriah shouted across the fire, '*Sa mmbwa! Sa mmbwa!*' (Like dogs!), suggesting the association between this *ndayo* and the embodied experience through which a wife should satisfy her husband in various sexual positions.

As if to reinforce this, the second *ndayo* in the sequence involved a specific drum (*murumba*) being placed onto the initiate's shoulders while she crouched on hands and knees. An initiated woman then leaned over onto the *murumba* and transferred all her weight to the small of the initiate's back. Holding this position through support of other initiates, the initiate slowly crawled backwards, clearly in great pain. In the third lesson, initiates squatted in a row like frogs, keeping heads bowed, backs as straight as possible and their arms crossed in front of them. A thin, dry twig was then fed through their thighs by a ritual expert and the girls were 'taught' to bounce in this one position on the balls of their feet, without losing balance or breaking the twig. Again, Noriah shouted at me across the fire, 'You see, now they are learning to make it with the wife on top!'

Several initiates broke down in tears, being scorned after failing to perform the *ndayo* adequately. When this happened, the initiate's 'ritual mother' (see below) covered her with a blanket, comforting her in a dark corner whilst the initiated women howled with laughter and obscene taunts. Finally, Noriah taught the initiates a form of masturbation in what was known as *bububa kha i gwanda mabvu*, the literal meaning of which is obscure with no direct translation to English, but has reference to the marking of a cow's hoof (*gwanda*) in the earth (*mavu*). The *vhatei* lay face down, with their hands above their heads. An elderly initiated woman slowly walked over their buttocks, grinding their pelvises into the floor. Noriah informed them that this 'is for when the husband is away... like raiding a village for beer and cattle after it has been burnt down!' (in other words taking something, in this case pleasure, from nothing).[17]

Although the performance of these *ndayo* dances seemingly presented the ritual experts with several opportunities to include AIDS prevention in the ritual curriculum, not one was taken.

Ludodo: The Introduction of Biomedical Knowledge

There are wide discrepancies in the early ethnographic literature regarding the details and occurrence of the stage known as *ludodo*. Van Warmelo describes its performance every night at *domba* whereby 'there are no fixed formulae (*milayo*)... anything may be said, the object being to accustom the young folk to the use of obscene language' (1932: 56).

---

[17] This raises questions as to the extent of genital mutilation performed at the *musivheto* ceremony, in that it would seem pointless to perform such an act in the absence of a clitoris.

Writing in the same era, Stayt (1931: 113) suggests that it happened only on the second night as an inaugural stage of the *domba* and is concerned only with the pragmatics (but not *milayo*) of pregnancy, marriage, and childbirth. Adding to the uncertainty, Blacking (1969b: 89) asserts that *ludodo* was a *mulayo* performed at the end of *domba*, which took the form of a structured story in which a young girl is impregnated and must reveal the father; in this account, the rite is referred to not as *ludodo* but as *muvhudziso* (the interrogation). As discussed above, this suggests a regional and historical fluidity of initiation practices.

In Dopeni, as part of the rationalised initiation programme, *ludodo* was the very last performative stage of the *vhusha*. The initiates were ordered to sit down in a row, each between the legs of the girl behind her and grabbing the girl in front of her around the waist. To a medium tempo, they moved forwards collectively by rocking on either buttock. Like the *ndayo* outlined above, this caused the girls considerable physical discomfort and their struggle to achieve unison was mocked loudly by the elder women. Wulff (2006), following Blacking (1969e: 154), has suggested that this pain is intended to accompany 'the interrogation' and embody the discomfort of childbirth in the initiates.

As the girls formed a line and were taught the movements, my commentator (who was clearly animated by the prospect of *ludodo*) explained that 'it [*ludodo*] is for the initiates to use sex words and insult people'. I could already hear this from Noriah, who towered above the line of girls, brandishing a large blunt drum stick (*tshiombo*) with intent. She was instructing them to verbally abuse each other with obscene words in short snaps, and demonstrating what she meant with the help of some of the elders. For every two movements forward, they all sang 'Eeee! Eeee!' (counting one, two), and for the next two beats (and progressions) one of them would continue the narrative, which was again punctuated with 'Eeee! Eeee!' and so on. They progressed anti-clockwise around the *tshivhambo* fire, and I sat in the outer circle. By this stage of the evening most of the initiated women and ritual experts were drunk and all were clearly enjoying themselves with yarns of their own ritual expertise, sexually explicit stories (some of which were clearly intended to tease me), and general laments for the 'good old days'. They variously insulted and humiliated the initiates at their leisure, scorning them for transgressions such as loss of posture, talking, or daydreaming.

It took the initiates about half an hour to master the harmonious progression of the melody in unison with the movement. It was a remarkable scene, with the initiates laughing nervously at the prospect of being explicitly rude in front of elders (many of whom were relatives), and the elders scorning them for the laughter, encouraging the insults. After some encouragement, the improvised narrative of sung speech began rather clumsily – led by Noriah's younger daughter Fhatuwani, as a child of the royal kraal in Dopeni and one of the initiates.

Uyu hannengei	That one over there
U na tumbu	She is pregnant
Ndi mishumo ya Khotsi a Mashudu	It's the work of Mashudu's father
Ndi musidzana	It is a girl
Khotsi awe vho fa vhege yo fhelaho	The father died last week
Vhana vha hoyo muvhundu	And the children of this village
Vhokhotsi avho vha do fa!	Their fathers will also die!

They continued after a brief pause, this time taken up by the initiate directly behind Fhatuwani, her school friend and neighbour:

Fhatu o ya thavhani	Fhatuwani went to Mukumbani,
U vhulaha mmbwa nga mulimo.	To poison the dogs there.
O u wanaho ha vhabvannda. [Indians/Zimbabweans]	She got the poison from outsiders.
U di ita vhutali.	She thinks she is so clever.
Na vhabebi vhawe	Even her parents
Vha a zwi tikedza!	Supported it!

This round of *Ludodo* was met with loud ululation and laughter, and the initiates seemed encouraged by this response to their controversial improvisation. It would normally be unthinkable to accuse a neighbour of using poison at King Tshivhase's kraal in Mukumbani, and the suggestion that Fhatuwani's mother (Noriah) was complicit in this made it all the more shocking.[18] They continued:

Ho ula u dzula Phadzima	That girl lives at Phadzima
O nyovhiwa nga kholomo	She was fucked by a bull
Na zwino o gonya muri!	And she is pregnant by it!
U do beba hani?, lunwe!	How will she give birth to it? So big!
A si na thaidzo.	She won't have a problem.
A si tshifevhi?	Isn't it that she is just a slut?
Khou uyu, ndi tsheri	Look at this one
Ya Vho Fraize!	She is Fraser's girlfriend!
U do takala a tshi pfulutshela	She wants to migrate
Shangoni la zwikotshi	To Scotland.
U do shavha hayani, lunwe!	She will run away from home!
Hu pfi o ambara sa mukhuwa.	They say she dresses like a European.
Mpengo!	She is mad!
U funesa malegere!	She likes sweets (sex) too much!

[18] This is significant for the argument to be made in Chapter 7. In response to the instruction to be rude and say things that would normally be prohibited, they instantly began improvising around the topic of death and poisonings.

The narrative developed along these lines for around half an hour, sometimes including references to my presence, and weaving between the topics of death, immoral sex, illness, witchcraft, pregnancy, and poisonings. The initiates were clearly enjoying the moment, and the older women reciprocated the joviality. They had all taken a turn to lead the improvisation, and Fhatuwani, who had started it in a clumsy, off-beat blunder, signalled her intention to have another try:

No no vhuya na zwi pfa naa	Did you ever hear,
Zwo ambiwaho nga ha	About what was being said
Ula musidzana nga ha aidsie?	About that young girl having AIDS?
Ndi mudziazwitshele!	She is the worst gossip in Dopeni!
O da fhano vhege yo fhelaho.	She was here just last week.
U na aidsie!	She has AIDS!
Ri a divha uri o iwana hani,	We know how she got infected,
Hone, u do fa lini?	But when will she die?[19]

With this, Noriah slammed the thick drum stick into Fhatuwani's thigh and the back of her neck, scorning her loudly. I did not hear what was said, because Noriah's words were drowned by Fhatuwani's scream and an old lady to my left shouting 'Who the hell sent her here? Control these royal daughters of yours!' But the initiates were still going:

Ri songo la	We must not eat (have sex)
Nga uralo!	Like that!
A lifholi!	There is no cure!
Ndi ARV fhedzi!	Just antiretroviral treatment!
Ndi kwine u di tsireledza,	It is better to protect yourselves,
Kha vhanwe vhatukana,	From some young boys,
Vha no ri a huna Aidsie,	Who say there is no AIDS.
Ri fanela u khondomisa!	But we must condomise!
Shumisani khondomu Wee!	Use Condoms!

With this second round, any remaining joviality turned to open hostility and the *ludodo* chain broke up completely as the girls were subjected to stick lashings and exceptionally harsh rebuttal from the elder women. I was unceremoniously elbowed out of the way by the furious elders beside me who croaked and heckled in a chorus of disapproval, 'What is meant by this?... Where is her elder sister? Sort this out!' One old woman grabbed my cassette recorder and threw it onto the ground. Noriah, conscious of the fact that I was (trying to) record the incident, tried to rectify the situation by starting another round of narrative but

---

[19] Again, in the context of Chapter 7 about the politics of speaking and not speaking about AIDS, note that talking about AIDS leads to the girl being infected with it.

her voice was drowned by the older women's protestations. I looked for the youngest ritual expert, an AIDS peer educator who was also Noriah's eldest daughter, but she had left the ritual hut. The initiates, like me, seemed to be genuinely confused by the controversy they had caused. It was the end of the second night and they were exhausted. A few were in tears after being beaten, and they all huddled in a corner covering themselves with blankets as the assembly of women dispersed into the night, kicking and spitting on the initiates as they walked past them, shouting loudly about returning at dawn for the final stage at the river.

It was 3.30 a.m., and I remained seated on the ground in the now eerily silent and dusty *tshivhambo* hut, the only noise coming from the crackling of the fire and the whimpering, weeping initiates. I was writing notes frantically and checking my video recorder by the light of the flames, when Noriah joined me. 'Did you get everything?' We watched a few minutes of the *ludodo* through my camera, and she walked with me to my *bakkie*. 'Don't worry', she said, 'you will come back and see it done properly next time'.

Ritual Stratification and Authority

The drama outlined above occurred at my second visit to *vhusha*, and there was no subsequent mention of AIDS in either of the following two I attended. The embodiment of disciplined sexual technique in *ndayo* presented, at least for me, a potential strategic point at which AIDS education might have been introduced into the initiation. In hindsight, this opportunity arose on several different occasions during 'lessons' in which red, white, and black are used to convey an aetiology of sexual health based on the build-up and removal of pollution and blood-related taboos (see below). Although King Tshivhase had stated that 'his' female initiations incorporated AIDS education, the ritual elders at Dopeni continued to omit it from the curriculum. Why, then, when it did appear, couched in biomedical discourse by the initiates, was it extinguished forcefully through ritual beatings and severe verbal abuse? To answer this question, I look in closer detail at the role of ritual knowledge and experience in the construction of the hierarchy upon which *vhusha* is based, and the role of esoteric *milayo* (rules/laws) that are integral to this (cf. Blacking 1969b; Jeannerat 1997).

At the Dopeni project, the ritual experts are a tight-knit group of between eight and ten matrons and elderly women. All have royal connections and profess to be adherents of ancestral religion rather than Christianity. Some of them are related to Noriah, whose eldest daughter is the youngest expert at 35 and a longstanding acquaintance of mine from the HIV/AIDS peer education project which operates in and around the village. There was a clear-cut distinction between this group and those at the next level of the hierarchy: the ordinary initiated women of all ages and social categories who came and went during the course of the ceremonies depending on who was being initiated and on other commitments such as funerals or domestic chores. Despite this clear hierarchy of command, both ritual experts and the rank-and-file initiated women took part in debates over the form, content, and sequence of various rites. Moreover, authority within the ranks of the latter group was strictly prescribed by age (more precisely, by when they danced *domba*). In recognition of this status, older non-experts were deferentially offered *mahafhe* before the younger experts.

The initiates (*vhatei*) at the ceremonies I attended were a combination of royal and common children from Dopeni and the surrounding villages of Shanza, Tshikombani, Tshivhilidulu, or Tshirenzheni.[20] They had all been sent there by their families, but only a handful had managed to pay the fee of R150 (in 2004/5). Some parents could not afford the minimum deposit of R50, and so committed their daughters to settle the debt through labour in the headwoman's orchard. Others, who had the cash, refused to pay it all on the grounds that participation in the ritual was vastly overpriced; they seemed to be in continuous negotiation with Noriah over this issue. Indeed, the 'steering committee' of the Dopeni project agreed to cut the price of initiation to R100, but this was scrapped when those who had already paid began to demand their money back. It is expected that some payment should be made for *vhusha*, but the suspicion that Kennedy is amassing a dubious fortune has tainted the project; people gossiped that the exorbitant fees go into the king's pocket, and that government subsidy funds have been 'eaten' by those running the project.

Independent of payment politics – discussion of which was restricted to adult conversation – small groups of between three and five initiates were going through different stages of the initiation simultaneously. *Vhusha* incorporates girls at three stages of the initiation process, all of whom are stratified with different ranks performing specific duties (see Figure 3.4). In apparent contradiction to Victor Turner's classic works on initiation, the girls undergoing this phase of liminality do not experience a levelling sense of communitas. Instead, throughout *vhusha* and *domba*, the explicit stratification of initiates is integral to the ritual process. For this reason, *vhusha* is usually performed by each initiate three times. In the 1960s, initiates often waited months between the stages (Blacking 1969a: 8),

---

[20] At one ceremony, the single *mutei* was a grown woman who had come from Pretoria after a consultation with an *inyanga* revealed to her that the source of her bad luck was that she had not 'been sung for' as a child.

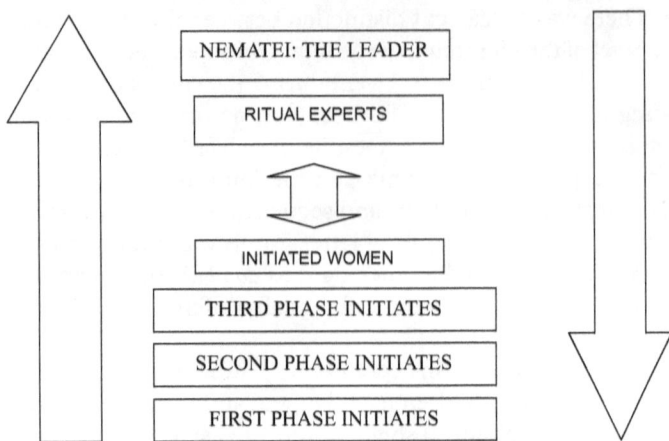

Figure 3.4. The hierarchy of authority in *vhusha*. The arrow on the left represents the direction of deference and the accumulation of experience, whilst the arrow on the right represents the flow of esoteric knowledge and authority in the *tshivhambo* ritual hut. The arrow in the middle represents the blurred boundary between experts and the rank-and-file initiated women who often debated the exact form, content, or sequence of the rites.

but in Dopeni in 2005, the sequence was completed on successive days over the course of the weekend.

The first stage, *muhulu* ('the growing person'), involves ritual beating, nakedness, shaving of hair, being covered in red ochre, poor food, taunting, and the strict observation of taboos such as avoidance of washing, salt (all things white), and men. A girl's second attendance, *u lata matavha* ('to wash away the dirt'), at which she is referred to as *pfunzi* (teacher), brings a gradual release from taboos and a responsibility to prepare food for first-timers. Girls at this stage help with the ritual instruction of first-timers, but remain under the authority of girls attending for their third and last time as initiates, those undergoing the final phase of *tshikhwakhwatho* ('the finishing'). These girls, on their last visit, are known as *midabe* (graduates) (sing: *mudabe*). It is intended that they become involved in fictitious kinship by taking a 'ritual child' from the incoming group to whom they provide comfort and assurance during stage one. According to Blacking (1959; 1969a: 5) this relationship should endure into adulthood, but *midabe* to whom I spoke cast some doubt on this.

As La Fontaine has argued:

The legitimacy conferred on ritual officiates is that of traditional knowledge: the information, understanding and experience needed to ensure the correct performance. The ritual... contrives to demonstrate the effectiveness of their knowledge and confirm their authority as legitimate. (1985: 17)

Bearing this in mind, attempts to understand initiation through the role of 'collective memory', formed when a group undergo painful experiences (Beidelman 1997; Reily 1998 based largely on Blacking 1985: 86–7), would appear to underestimate the extent to which female initiation is as much 'for' the initiated as it is 'for' the initiates. In this way, the 'laws' of initiation, gradually revealed, serve not only to facilitate the initiates' progression into adulthood through their acquisition of knowledge and secrets, but equally importantly to uphold and bolster the authority of the elders and the initiated (and by extension, of the ancestors) in the context of ritual performance (cf. Bloch 1974; 1992).

Theoretically, all women who have been through *vhusha* are members. Upon demonstrating knowledge of passwords and signs, grips and tokens, they can enter the *tshivhambo* hut at any stage, share the traditional beer, and join in the coaching and mocking of the initiates. Evidence that someone 'has been sung for' comes in the form of knowing the esoteric code learned at *vhusha*, in which objects from the *tshivhambo*, wild animals, and the natural world are associated with human body parts at various stages of sexual intercourse, pregnancy, birth, health, and sickness. For example, if an initiate is told 'the door is just open, you can see the light peeking through', she must answer 'A woman who cannot have intercourse soon after giving birth'. The poles in the roof, the small window frame, the ashes of the fire, the seeds from the grass, et cetera are all coded in this way into a complex secret language that permits or restricts access to the initiation. These laws are not only presented to the initiates through *ndayo*, but in a variety of song words, poems, riddles, and counting games. Moreover, a variety of ritual objects such as clay models of people, huts, and wild animals are used as didactic aids in the commitment of *milayo* to memory (see Figure 3.5; cf. Nettleton 1992).

Female Initiation and the Venda Cosmology of Sexual Health

Although *milayo* often have no obvious meaning for the initiates, a significant proportion constitute what might loosely be called a 'moral code' that outlines ideal female behaviour. These reflect conservative patriarchal values such as virginity at marriage, obedience, and endurance. A central theme running through *milayo*, and fundamental to *vhusha*, is the promotion of sexual health and fertility, mostly through symbolic associations made between the colours red (menstrual blood/pollution/danger/female), white (semen/purity/milk/safety/life/male), and black (menopause/ashes/death) (see Figure 3.5; cf. Turner

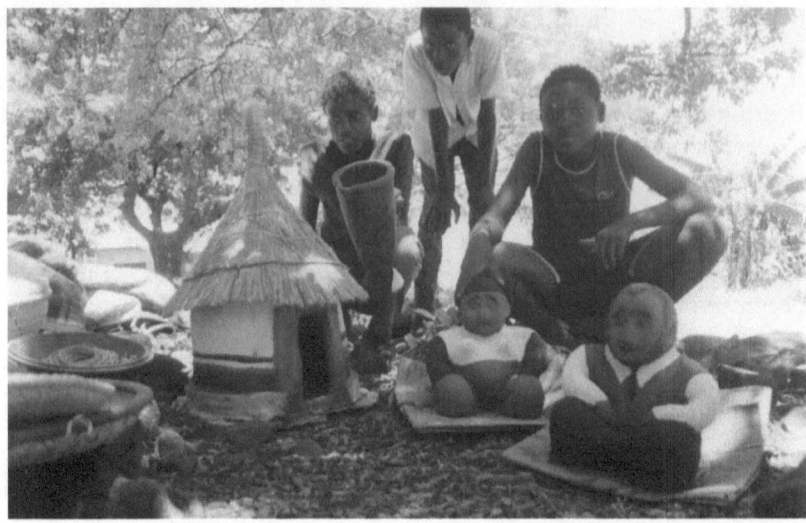

Figure 3.5. Ritual objects of the *vhusha* and *domba*, used as didactic aids during initiation. Note the male figure on the right, the female in the middle, and the miniature version of the ritual hut (*tshivhambo*) on the left. They are painted in the symbolic colours red (for danger, heat, pollution, blood, female), white (for safety, cool, semen, bones, male), and black (for post-menopausal women, ashes, death).

1967; 1969a for Ndembu; Blacking 1969c: 158 for Venda). The clay sculptures mentioned above are always painted in these colours, as are the beads used for other rites and the dried corn used in the *ndayo*. These are woven into many complex and often abstract narratives about people and animals (and creatures that are a combination of the two) that have breached blood-related taboos and subsequently experience problems with sexual health through a build-up of pollution (red), ending with a loss of fertility (black). This is encapsulated symbolically in the timing of the *vhusha* (immediately after the first menses) and the changing terminology of the noun used to refer to girls who are 'sung for'. They are transformed from being *musidzana* (little girl) to *khomba* (dangerous girl). The danger is inherent in a girl's potential to get pregnant, and thus the potential to become polluted if the menstrual blood is not regularly managed in a hygienic manner by thorough washing of the body and the use of disposable cloths or rags as tampons (*miserwa*; singular, *muserwa*).

This is enacted by the first-stage initiates in the morning during *vhusha*, when they are ceremonially immersed to the waist in the river (*u kamisa*) by elder girls, and by the ritual experts whilst singing the song of the second stage, *u lata matavha* ('to wash away the dirt'). The 'dirt' in this

A Rite to AIDS Education? 103

sense is not only the red ochre that has been smeared all over the initiates the night before, but also the menstrual blood (of which the ochre is a symbol) that the initiate has been producing for this first time in her life. At Dopeni, this happened on the Saturday and Sunday mornings. On the Saturday the initiates were immersed for up to four hours, whilst on the Sunday they were treated less harshly. The water, early in the morning, was very cold, and they were clearly being made to endure this pain as the symbolic embodiment of the importance of washing thoroughly whilst menstruating. The cold of the river, I was told, acts to neutralise the dangerous red heat of menstrual blood.

Early accounts of female initiation, perhaps restricted by prudish conventions of the time, reported this in less explicit terms. Stayt thus explains that:

A menstruating woman... was always strictly taboo... [during *vhusha*] a great deal of time is given up to sexual teaching.... [T]hey are taught that... marriage is not a game but the precursor of child birth, and, as such, must be properly understood, so that the resultant children will be strong and healthy, uncontaminated by dangers and diseases resulting from improper knowledge and broken taboos. (1931: 110–13)

Similarly, van Warmelo (1932: 45) writes about 'the soaking' of initiates during *vhusha*. Van Warmelo published his accounts of Venda ritual with the full text in Tshivenda, as provided by his informants. In this account, we read that the initiate '*u ya u tambiswa. ... A tshi vho ya lwa vhuvhili vha ri "O lata matavha, o ima"*'. Van Warmelo translates this as 'A girl goes to the water to be soaked... when she goes for the second time they say "she has cast midday from her, she has got up"'. However, in the context of the Tshivenda narrative this could more accurately be translated as 'A girl goes to the water to be cleansed/purified by the removal of menstrual blood (*u tamba* – to wash; *u tambiswa* – to be cleansed of). When she goes for the second time they say "the pollution has been removed (*o lata matavha*), it has stopped (*o ima*)"'.[21] This is not to suggest that van

[21] Van Warmelo's translation is fascinating in that it plays on the ambiguity of a Tshivenda term for a woman's period. The next phrase in the Tshivenda account is given as '*Ha tsha maduvha a dzheni madini*', which he translates as 'she does not go into the water again', and which he incorporates into the previous explanation that 'she has cast midday from her'. However this phrase could also be translated in this context as 'if she is not bleeding, she does not enter the water'. A woman's period is often referred to as '*o vhonna maduvha*' (she has seen the days) but *duvha* also translates directly as 'day' or 'the sun'. Also '*ima*' translates directly as 'stand up' or 'come to a halt'. He thus maintains a degree of linguistic integrity by translating literally what was clearly intended in a figurative, metaphorical sense. I must credit Noriah (who found van Warmelo's sanitised version highly amusing) with noticing these transgressions. She suggested that it was possibly narrated to him in these terms as there were uninitiated women present at the time, or that the narrator did not want to divulge the 'whole story' to him in the interests of preserving ritual knowledge.

Warmelo was in any way ignorant of the actual meaning here (given that his ability to converse in Tshivenda was legendary), but rather that, as a conservative, Christian commentator of the time, he would have been uncomfortable publishing the intimate details of Venda girls' menstrual ablutions. Nonetheless, such menstrual ablutions are key to understanding this aspect of *vhusha*, and the removal of menstrual blood from the female body is fundamental to Venda aetiology of sexual health through which HIV/AIDS has been widely interpreted by local men and women alike.

Blacking's accounts of female initiation, on the other hand, are less coy. In his agglomeration of *vhusha* songs, he relates a rendition that 'refer[s] to the onset of a girl's menses':

Wele Wele phosho vhasidzana!	What a noise there is, girls!
Wele wele phoso ndi ya'ni?	What is causing all this noise?
Hu na dinnyo lo mpha vhuyada.	My monstrous fanny has given me filth.

(Blacking 1969a: 21)

The theme of pollution is extended in other songs, in which notions of morality and respect for conservative norms, namely fidelity and deference, are counterposed against the dangers of pollution. During the first stage of a *domba* at Tsianda village in April 2004 (which I witnessed again in 2009), the ritual mother (*Mme a Domba*) decided to recap the central themes the girls 'learned' in *vhusha*. Her summary covered three thematic areas of respect (*u thonifha*), work (*u shuma*), and health (*mutakalo*). Each was given a résumé by means of a riddle, a narrative with clay figures, and a song. Regarding health, the narrative told of 'Nya Vhasedza', a woman whose husband passed her a sexually transmitted illness after he slept with a beer hall prostitute, because his wife did not care for him adequately. She was sent to Ha-Makuya in search of a cure, but was unsuccessful in her quest. The song reinforced the story like this:[22]

Nya Vhasedza u a lwalwa, u na thusula.	Vhasedza's mother is sick with syphilis.
O ya wana ha munna wawe.	She got it from her husband.
Vha muise hanengei Ha-Makuya	They took her to Ha-Makuya
Vha do vhuya ngauri thusula a fheli	They will return because syphilis isn't finished (not cured).[23]

[22] You can hear this song, as recorded during the Tsianda *domba*, at http://www.cambridge.org/us/9781107009912.

[23] Ha-Makuya is a remote region of Venda, in the extreme north-east corner on the border with the Kruger National Park and Zimbabwe (see Map 2). It is a very dry area. Trees that grow there are believed to yield concentrated bark and roots, and are thus associated with powerful herbal medicines. It is also mentioned in Solomon Mathase's *Zwidzumbe* in his search for a traditional cure for AIDS (see Appendix B, line 51).

Venda aetiology of sexual health, then, is enshrined in female initiation. Sexual health, in this context, is intimately related to menstrual blood, and is achieved through the cleansing and purging of the perceived source of pollution. This is also central to male circumcision rites, and it forms the basis upon which traditional healers such as Noriah diagnose and treat problems of a sexual nature. This aetiology constitutes the building blocks for the ancestral knowledge of sexual health, expressed through a 'folk model' of illness representation (Good 1994: 37; Liddell et al. 2005) through which HIV/AIDS has been interpreted by many men and older (initiated) women in Venda. This line of thought will be taken up again in Chapter 6 through the analysis of male guitar songs. For now, the point to remember is that sex education in Venda has its culturally appropriate home within the ritual confines of initiation schools.[24]

Ritual Knowledge and Experience

During *ludodo*, the breaching of strict taboos with reference to adultery, bestiality, witchcraft, death, illness, and accusations clearly placed the initiates in an awkward position, but this was encouraged by the elders and was an expected part of the ritual. As an initiate told me weeks later, 'We were *told* to be rude and insult people!' For the initiates, the elders' complacency legitimised the unnerving boundlessness of their permitted actions, and most of them – eventually – revelled in the moment. And yet it was this very complacency of the elders which imposed new boundaries in place of those that had been removed.

From the examples outlined above, it is clear that authority in the *vhusha* is based on elders' monopoly, and gradual release, of esoteric knowledge. This, in turn, engenders a broader consensus of 'knowing' through experience. Indeed, it could be argued that the logic of experience is fundamental to the creation and legitimation of ritual knowledge (or, at least that which is differentiated from common sense) throughout Southern Africa.[25] This is evident not only in processes of male and female initiation but to various degrees in *ngoma* cults of affliction, in which the experience of illness legitimises possession and the ability to heal; in traditional healers' training rites, where dreams lead to the identification of herbal remedies; in the proliferation of Christian prophets through epiphanies which augment the 'live and direct' contact with God (even in the absence of scripture; Engelke 2007); and at the very heart of

---

[24] See Kotanyi and Krings-Neg (2009) for an ethnographic outline of female initiation and sex education in Mozambique.

[25] A close reading of ethnographic descriptions of ritual practice in Papua New Guinea and Bali (Barth 1975; 2002) and Mayotte (Lambek 1993) suggests a strong connection between ritual knowledge and experience beyond Southern Africa. See Chapter 6.

occult discourses when misfortune opens the door to authoritative accusation. In these examples, all of which are perceived (albeit with very diverse capacities) as central to securing healthy social and sexual reproduction in Southern Africa, it is primarily through lived and/or embodied experience that claims to legitimate knowledge are made.

At the *vhusha* in Dopeni, the connection between ritual knowledge and experience was self-evident; those with more experience of the ritual process had a more legitimate claim to authoritative knowledge. But the logic of experience created spaces in which *vhusha* knowledge was regularly contested in heated debates between previously initiated women of all ages as to what the 'correct' order of things should be. Issues such as the specific sequence and content of the rites, words, and actions in songs, or the detail of *milayo* and *ndayo* dances, were all, in this way, 'up for grabs'. The ritual experts joined these debates but were often overruled by older and more senior women who thus directly influenced the instruction of the initiates. The end product, the accumulative process of initiation, was a *bricolage* (cf. Hebdige 1979: 103-4) of contributions from all the initiated women based upon widely accepted principles and patterns they had experienced when, as girls, they were themselves 'sung for'. For the initiates at Dopeni, *ludodo* appeared to offer a break from this structural position in which they were powerless to influence proceedings. Ultimately, however, the improvisation of obscene insults and death threats took place within a strictly controlled ritual context and should never have threatened the stratification of authority within the *tshivhambo* ritual hut in any way.

Up to the point at which a biomedical interpretation of AIDS infection became a threat to health and life, the imagined scenarios were controversial and provocative, but nonetheless plausible and quite within the accepted boundaries of what experience and knowledge the girls, ideally, should have had at that stage of initiation. The only knowledge which was acceptable was that which was shared by the older women – all of whom could conceive the possibilities of (but would not necessarily discuss openly) poison, bestiality, and promiscuity. What did not constitute plausible courses of social action, however, for the senior elderly women who were most dismissive of the girls' references to AIDS, were antiretroviral therapy and the use of condoms. Whilst undoubtedly such things were known to these women, their material existence and physical usage fell outside the core of a lived experience and social milieu shared by old women in rural Venda.

The initiates' introduction of biomedical discourse through singing about AIDS and its attempted prevention/treatment thus quite unintentionally posed a genuine threat to the monopoly of knowledge held by initiated women. This, in turn, put into potential jeopardy the hierarchical structure of authority, recently bolstered by King Tshivhase's public support of the project. In this way, the words 'AIDS', '*khondomisa*', and 'antiretroviral therapy' appeared to the elders through *ludodo* as a subversive esoteric code which clearly had been internalised by the young girls, but from which they remained largely excluded. The hostile reaction to the introduction of biomedical discourse was thus instigated not by the mention of AIDS per se but by the suggestive manner in which the initiates introduced a separate sphere of understanding that fell beyond the broad consensus of acceptable ritual knowledge or experience in the *tshivhambo*. In this way, the biomedical model appeared to be outside of the elders' control. For them, it was in direct contradiction to the *milayo* based on colour symbolism through which supposedly the *vhatei* had learned about sexual illness and morality in terms of blood taboos, the build-up of pollution, and conservative, appropriate sexual behaviour for young girls and in their future role as wives.[26]

A central reason for this clash of sexual cosmologies lay in the advocated use of condoms. The mention of condoms took on a multitude of unacceptable meanings for the initiated women. In a ceremony largely concerned with preparing girls with the moral and physical education to enter and endure marriage, condoms represented a serious threat to fertility and rendered the *ndayo* outlined above potentially obsolete. Despite the incorporation of masturbation into the rites, the *ndayo* associated sex not primarily with pleasure but rather with procreativity, within which barrier methods of contraception have no place. Fhatuwani's final attempt to lead the *ludodo* by singing about AIDS infection thus brought the biomedical model into direct conflict with Venda aetiology. However, condoms are tolerated in very specific social situations. Conversations with initiated women after the *vhusha* indicated, for example, that they were closely associated with extra-marital affairs, secret lovers (*mafarakano*; singular, *mufarakano*), and liaisons between men and commercial sex workers. All of these contrast with the 'ideal' behaviour of a good wife in South Africa (cf. Campbell 2003; Hunter 2002; Wojkicki 2002), and they speak instead of how men may avoid the pollution from dirty blood (see Chapter 6).

Thus, in emphasising the rites designed to teach sexual positions, Noriah actively drew my attention to the *ndayo* of what we both agreed – although on somewhat different grounds – was a dangerous locus of disease transmission: sexual intercourse. She did not suggest that they were more important per se than other lessons of the *vhusha*; it was more that she thought they were what I – as a researcher interested in AIDS – was really there to see.

---

[26] Recent research in Mozambique strongly suggests that training ritual experts in the nuances of the biomedical approach to AIDS may facilitate the incorporation of scientific AIDS education into female initiation rites. See Kotanyi and Krings-Neg (2009).

There was a further way in which the specific aesthetics of this *ludodo* performance blurred the familiar hierarchy of initiates. It spoke of a new youth solidarity that transgressed the particularities of initiation hierarchy. Girls from stages one, two, and three were all, in a seemingly united group, implicated in constructing the new narrative. To some extent, this collapsed the established status groups between stage one and ritual leader (see Figure 3.1), yielding a provocative 'us against them' scenario. The way in which this appeared to the initiated women can be explained by referring beyond the ritual context to the realm of secular life – and particularly to the recent history of youth uprisings in Venda and neighbouring areas. Much of this (extensively documented) unrest was hostile to structures of traditional and generational authority and directly aimed at significant numbers of elderly people who were accused of practising witchcraft or committing '*muti* murder' for body parts (Delius 1996; Bozzoli 2004; Niehaus 2000; 2001a; and Ralushai 1996). Typically, these outbreaks have been associated with wider political changes in which groups of young people have formed new identities outside of chiefly or generational authority. The initiated women at Dopeni, having had direct experiences of similar insurrections, were thus aware of the potential danger inherent in youth rebellion. However, although the introduction of AIDS into *vhusha* might have been vaguely reminiscent of recent activist disturbances, it was by no means intended to be a challenge to the status quo; the initiates were merely following orders. This reflects a (broadly Marxist) argument that initiates would not challenge the authority of the elders as, by enduring the ritual, they too would eventually inherit positions of authority (cf. Bloch 1992).

Nonetheless, in other rural regions of South Africa, processes of initiation have been transformed along such generational divisions. In Cancele, Transkei, Ngwane has traced the changing symbolic significance and structural articulation, in the context of rising unemployment, between formal (state) education and male initiation, both of which brand young men with the 'marks of home' (2004: 184). The state school, no longer the domain of white missionaries, is now just one of a number of local institutions orientated towards Xhosa social reproduction. Ngwane demonstrates the ways in which young, schoolgoing men, through the partial incorporation of the Sotho-Tswana initiation system, eventually appropriated the ritual process at the expense of older men's authority:

For older men the [initiation] school, juxtaposed with incomplete manhood, referenced a perceived threat to their control of the means of social reproduction while for younger men the school, juxtaposed with proper manhood, referenced an alternative site for, and mode of, producing social subjectivity... which ameliorated... their politically infantilised relation to older men. (Ngwane 2004: 191)

For the older men in question, the loss of ritual authority, on top of the widespread erosion of employment opportunities, represented a new low point in an ongoing, and seemingly collective, crisis of masculinity. For the younger men, the appropriation of ritual authority was partly a way of dealing with their oppression by older men and the 'impossibility' of their becoming prosperous household heads in the current economic climate. The result of this, in the initiation, was a shift from disciplining of bodies to articulating rhetorical conversational processes (2004: 189). Ngwane accounts for this in terms of different 'local' and 'Sotho-Tswana' traditions of knowledge. To some extent, however, given the apparent shortage of older men with appropriate ritual knowledge, the young local initiation leaders had little choice but to 'construct speaking subjects' as opposed to the older generation's concern with 'listening'. The ritual knowledge had vanished along with the elders. There was thus little to listen to.

This is a revealing comparison. In some ways, this may be precisely the scenario of 'intergenerational disarticulation' (Comaroff and Comaroff 2004: 337) that Noriah and the ritual experts in Venda were keen to avoid. Such an analogy underplays, however, the extent to which *vhusha* initiates were motivated by deferential attitudes towards their ritual elders. The relative ease with which the Xhosa elders relinquished their ritual duties contrasts with the Venda case. In the latter, recent chiefly politics have bolstered ritual hierarchies, making it practically unfeasible for younger generations to trump elders' ritual authority.

But the Transkei example also raises the important issue of how formal state education figures in the relationship between sexual health, knowledge, and experience. AIDS awareness is the subject of a 'life orientation' course in the national schools curriculum. From 2005, all high school children have been taught about the immune system, the possibility of infection with a virus, and the role of killer T cells in the blood (Coetzee et al. 2004). Literature on this subject has questioned, however, the extent to which school teachers can discuss issues such as contraception and sexuality effectively in rural African contexts (Gallant and Maticka-Tyndale 2004). Moreover, such governmental attempts at AIDS education are largely presented with a strong urban bias and against the backdrop of the government's previously confusing and contradictory public statements on AIDS, to which I turn in the following chapter. On the whole, these depersonalised government information campaigns have been received with a mixture of embarrassment, confusion, and scepticism (cf. Leclerc-Madlala 2005), leaving young female volunteers, in the guise of HIV/AIDS peer educators, to become the public face of AIDS education.

Young women in Venda have been forced to carry a disproportionate burden: it is they alone who are charged with conveying this biomedical information to the general public. Indeed, the uneven, and unevenly targeted, character of AIDS education in South Africa can perhaps help to explain, at least partially, why the biomedical model appeared as an esoteric code, threatening to elderly women. Government and NGO intervention strategies such as Love Life, Soul City, Khomanani, and the Limpopo-based Forum for AIDS Prevention target predominantly younger people to the exclusion of older generations. Aiming educational campaigns at poor, young, females carries the danger, however, of disregarding those presumed to be at low risk (Stadler 2003: 138–9). Although Stadler's comments highlight the absence of affluent men in HIV/AIDS awareness programmes, they hold equally true for the situation regarding old rural women. As an elderly passer-by at a peer education performance told me, 'This AIDS talk sounds like Chinese (*Tshitshainna*) to us'.

Assuming, then, that intervention strategies and the national school curriculum have at least partial success in raising awareness of AIDS, it is hardly surprising that the initiates had a better grasp of scientific explanations than did their elders. In this sense, the drama played out at *ludodo* was reflective of connections between 'closed' female hierarchies of ritual authority and national policy priorities. It provided a succinct demonstration of what happens when elderly people are excluded from the experience of AIDS education, and the ways in which this can impinge on – and stymie – innovative approaches to prevention.

And yet national education policies alone cannot explain adequately the elders' rejection of the girls' innovation. As several authors have shown, scientific explanations – even if they are part of a comprehensive educational programme – are easily reinterpreted and incorporated within non-scientific systems of belief (Ashforth 2005; Campbell 2003: 167; Stadler 2003; Walker et al. 2004; Farmer 2006). For Noriah, and most of the ritual experts at Dopeni, the very term AIDS was problematic and biomedical explanations posed more questions than the solutions they proposed. She had heard accurate versions of the biomedical model from her eldest daughter, the peer educator and ritual expert, who had convinced her to attend a workshop facilitated by the Department of Health in which traditional healers were trained to deal with symptomatic ailments of AIDS-related illness. Nonetheless, Noriah remained wholly unconvinced by the scientific explanation.

Like many middle-aged rural people in Venda and throughout Southern Africa,[27] Noriah acknowledges the accuracy of the biomedical model inasmuch as it maintains that AIDS is part of a complex of sexual illness, transmitted through blood (see Chapter 6). But she also shares with them a strong suspicion that it is part of a longer trajectory through

---

[27] See Ingstad (1990); Heald (1995); de Bruyn (1992); McDonald and Schatz (2006).

which such illnesses have evolved over time, whose explanation lies in neglect of moral considerations rather than in biomedicine. For Noriah and her ilk, the current surge of illness and death – the perceived crisis of reproduction – is attributable to a wider neglect of spiritual responsibilities and generational respect. She argues that this has heralded a rise in immoral sexual behaviour by youth who have 'become lost' (*ono xela*) and are more influenced by 'modern ways' (*misalaino*) than by *mvelele* (culture) (see Bujra 2000a and Baylies 2000 for an account of this in Tanzania; and Kotanyi and Krings-Ney 2009 for Mozambique).

While the cause of this broader malaise might lie beyond the remit of medicine of any kind, Noriah maintains that the symptomatic cure for what doctors are calling AIDS lies in treatment with *mushonga* (herbal medicine), which as an experienced traditional healer she can provide. Antiretroviral therapy, like a course of antibiotics or the contraceptive pill, therefore constitutes a distinctly alien method of dealing with illness, which by ignoring the Venda aetiology of sexual illness renders itself unable to 'cure' – and may even exacerbate – ill health. I will return to this theme in Chapter 6 in relation to musical interpretations of HIV/AIDS, when I look in more detail at the ways in which AIDS has been incorporated into the folk model.

Conclusion

This chapter has demonstrated the dynamics of traditionalism and generational conflict in post-apartheid Venda through an historical and ethnographic analysis of the *vhusha* initiation. The resurgence of traditional leadership and fortification of custom in Venda, however, displays quite different dynamics to similar concurrent revivals in KwaZulu-Natal described by Scorgie (2002) and Leclerc-Madlala (2001; 2005). Such accounts depict groups of women actively engaging with the biomedical model to reinvent virginity testing as a modern and relevant, if ethically questionable, means of promoting chastity in the name of HIV prevention. In Venda, the ritual experts at Dopeni forcefully excluded this model in the belief that it contradicted their pre-existing strategies to avoid sexual illness, and as such challenged their authority. It would appear, then, that retraditionalisation in Venda has bolstered structures that are based on ritual knowledge, whilst in KwaZulu-Natal similar processes have promoted biomedical understandings of the virus.

However, this apparent dichotomy cannot be explained by recourse to the differing structures of chieftainship in the two regions alone. It also sheds light on the supposed distinction between the two bodies of knowledge. To be sure, ancestral knowledge and biomedicine are distinct in important ways, and, as the account presented above suggests, their coexistence can be antagonistic. However, there is also a sense in which they partially complement each other. Both are mobilised in everyday life, in a pragmatic manner, to similar ends. They are both considered powerful and potentially beneficial to humanity; they use similar symbols and the boundary between them often blurs in the search for ways to recapture lost capacities to act meaningfully in the world. Thus we see in following chapters that aspects of the peer educators' biomedical model have been incorporated into, and are regarded as part of, ritual knowledge.

However, if chiefly power in Venda – buttressed by the state – has largely supported ritual authority, the evidence in this chapter suggests that monarchs hold little influence over the female hierarchies in control of ritual knowledge. Indeed, the official promotion of initiation, despite its new streamlined and bureaucratised form, has reinforced this internal stratification and, crucially, further entrenched the body of ritual knowledge and experience upon which that authority structure is based. Paradoxically, this process has rendered the *vhusha* even less amenable to change. Thus, although female initiation may appear to be a viable site for innovative AIDS education among young women, it is in fact highly unlikely that the biomedical model will be incorporated into the ritual curriculum as it is currently beyond the boundaries of what should be known and what can be controlled by the ritual experts. It is not part of a shared experience to which the elders could relate and, in Long's terms (1992), on the 'battlefield of knowledge' – at least in the ritual context – biomedicine stood no chance of victory.

The initiated women were motivated largely by a concern for their own positions of privilege, but this speaks to wider regional trends of generational conflict and a perception of widespread concern with the nature of social reproduction. Contemporary Southern Africa, it has been noted recently, appears to be 'mired in a crisis of generation and regeneration... a crisis of an increasing cleavage between the "young" and the "old"' (Comaroff and Comaroff 2004: 329). Whilst generational conflicts are by no means new phenomena, the dynamics of *vhusha* in Venda provide a specific example of the nature of this conflict in terms of a post-apartheid discourse and practice of traditionalism, articulated through the connections between knowledge and experience in a ritual context. The elders' rejection of biomedicine, and the subsequent upholding of the hierarchy, were thus motivated by a sense of losing control not only over ritual knowledge, but over the very means of social reproduction itself. For King Tshivhase, *vhusha* may have represented a political opportunity to invoke the African renaissance in his failed quest to have the legitimacy of his kingship recognised officially, but for the ritual elders it is fundamental to the production of personhood, and their actions demonstrated the concern that its 'protracted failure, real or imagined, carries with it the spectre of *de*generation: of the future as stillborn, an impossibility, as a telos-in-retreat' (ibid.: 329, 336).

In a context of widespread death caused by AIDS-related illness, the 'future as stillborn' is a reality of everyday life in South Africa. Whilst this chapter has been concerned with attempts to rectify this perceived crisis through recourse to tradition, the following one looks at the official government response and the role of NGOs in more conventional attempts to fix the social problems that have accompanied the epidemic.

4 'We Want a Job in the Government'

Motivation and Mobility in HIV/AIDS Peer Education

The eighth birthday party of the Ha-Rabali HIV/AIDS peer education project was well under way as I crept into the large tent through the back entrance. Some volunteers squeezed up on the benches to give me a seat, and I got out my notebook and pen to make a record of proceedings. The tent was full of young women dressed in their best finery of colourful *minwenda* cloth, and, as usual, I felt completely underdressed. It was unbearably hot, and the photocopied order of proceedings was being used by guests as a makeshift fan. At the top table, the project coordinator sat in a line of distinguished dignitaries including the local traditional leader, the ANC ward councillor, a pastor, the director of a local NGO, and a policewoman. In due course, they rose to give lengthy contributions concerning the work of the project, pausing occasionally to sip water and wipe sweat from their brows. They were met with polite applause from the crowd. A car drew up outside and four women in very expensive *minwenda* dresses and headscarves walked into the front of the tent, accompanied by ululations that drowned out the policewoman's speech. I recognised them as peer educators from the very start of the project in 1998, whom I had not seen for years. They were now working for the government, in the Department of Public Works, as AIDS counsellors and trainers. When the dignitaries had completed their speeches, the four ex-educators rose to give a brief presentation – more like a motivational speech – on their humble beginnings and their new-found status. As they received rapturous applause at the end of their contribution, a current volunteer leaned over to me and pointed at my notebook. 'Write this down', she said. 'These women are the *real* peer educators.'

Over the past decade, most people in Venda have been exposed to biomedical ideas about AIDS through voluntary, exclusively female, peer group education. In this chapter, I begin a critical evaluation of these peer education projects based on an analysis of the contradictions between the intentions of project designers, on the one hand, and the motivational incentives of peer educators on the other. Subsequent chapters build on this: developing the analysis to consider the ways in which volunteers use music in an attempt to transfer biomedical knowledge; showing that volunteer efforts are at best partially successful and at worst counterproductive; and then arguing that the very process of peer education frames the volunteers – and condoms as their most widely recognised symbol of prevention – as vectors of the virus. The overall picture that emerges is an unsettling one. HIV/AIDS peer education has become part of the problem, as opposed to part of the solution.

But it is not completely worthless. On the contrary – for the women involved – peer education presents a significant window of opportunity. The nature of divergent status groups in Venda, as demonstrated by the *vhusha* initiation in the previous chapter, leads to individuals joining highly differentiated social groups at various stages of their life cycles. Whilst ascribed status may seem immutable, there is some room for bettering one's position over the life course. Thus, although male authority trumps that of females, as royal status trumps that of commoners, it is possible for young girls with no chiefly connections to enter initiation schools and gradually achieve positions of status by progressing over the course of several years to the position of initiated woman or ritual expert through the accumulation of knowledge, age, and experience.

The HIV/AIDS peer educators who form the central focus of this chapter are involved in analogous attempts to achieve status and authority through a gradual accumulation of knowledge and experience. Theirs is realised, however, by progressing not through a ritual hierarchy, but through the networks of health-related NGOs, with the ultimate aim of securing employment somewhere 'in the government'. In doing so, they seek to professionalise what remains a largely voluntary vocation – capitalising on years of informal experience in the health industry, and on the government's desperate need for health/social workers 'on the ground'. The blurred boundary between health-related NGOs and government service provision creates a space in which this profound transition in social and economic status is sought after by many, but achieved by few. The desire for social and economic mobility directly affects the efficacy of peer education: the educators' desire to change the social/sexual health environment is matched by their aspirations to transcend and move away from it.

This chapter has three sections. First, it outlines the South African government's response to the AIDS epidemic and the ways in which this created spaces for the participation of NGOs in grassroots AIDS interventions. Second, in an analysis of 'participatory approaches' and an ethnographic account of peer education in a local NGO, I elucidate some of the ways in which prevention programmes in Venda have attempted to change health-related behaviour and encourage safer sex. Last, I draw on data taken from other projects at the same non-governmental organisation to consider the experiences and motivations of peer educators. This demonstrates fundamental contradictions between the aims and objectives stated by project designers – quasi-state proponents of 'participatory' approaches – and the everyday experience of being a voluntary peer educator.

Thabo Mbeki and the End of a Dark Era?

Mbeki's legacy is a South Africa filled with AIDS orphans, child-headed households, grandparents forced to parent their dead children's children, poor women having to home-nurse the sick and dying without remuneration, and a phalanx of businesses selling untested remedies to desperately ill people with promises of healing and cure. (Cullinan and Thom 2009: xv)

The South African government's infamous response to the HIV epidemic has been well documented in literature on the subject.[1] From the late 1990s to his downfall in 2008, ex-President Mbeki courted unorthodox scientists such as David Rasnick and Peter Doesberg, who in turn draw on critics of 'premature consensus' (see Root-Bernstein 1993) in their challenge to conventional biomedical approaches to HIV and AIDS. Mbeki chose to share his dissident sympathies with the world at the International AIDS Conference in Durban in 2000, where he informed a bemused audience that 'not everything could be blamed on a single virus' and that poverty, not sex, was fuelling the nation's epidemic (Mbali 2004: 105; cf. Fassin 2007). In the same year, he convened the Presidential Advisory Panel on AIDS to which dissident scientists were invited, and although the resultant statement from the panel said nothing new, it cemented the relationship between Mbeki and the international community of unorthodox AIDS pseudo-scientists.[2]

In 2002, amid widespread outrage at his seemingly negligent stance, and possibly out of concern that it might be damaging international confidence in the country's currency and economy, Mbeki withdrew from public debate on AIDS. Health Minister Dr Manto Tshabalala Msimang took up where Mbeki left off. Msimang made no secret of her belief that antiretroviral drugs (ARVs) are poisonous and that the consumption of

---

[1] See inter alia Nattrass (2004; 2008), Gevisser (2007), Whiteside and Suntner (2000), Schneider (2002), Schneider and Stein (2001), Quinlan and Willan (2005), van der Vliet (2004), Walker et al. (2004), Mbali (2004), Achmat (2004), Robins (2004), McGregor (2005), Leclerc-Madlala (2005), Fassin (2007), Thornton (2008), and Cullinan and Thom (2009).

[2] This international community of dissident journalists, scientists, People Living With HIV and AIDS (PLWHA), and others is not insignificant. It contains several high-profile individuals such as Nobel Prize winner for Chemistry Karry Mullise and Harim Caton, a retired professor of politics and history, and a fellow of the Australian Institute for Biology. They are joined by numerous eminent professors of biology and virology who all question the scientific AIDS orthodoxy. Such 'communities' have, along with other conspiracy theorists, flourished on the internet, and through websites such as <www.aidsmyth.addr.com> and <www.virusmyth.net> they have established networks, email lists, and petitions through which they lobby policy makers. These websites support Mbeki explicitly, and promote him as a champion of their cause.

raw garlic, lemon juice, the African potato (*hypoxis rooperi*), beetroot, and multi-vitamin supplements are more beneficial to patients with immunodeficiency than ARVs (cf. Cullinan and Thom 2009).

Two explanations have been proposed for Mbeki's controversial stance on AIDS. One is rooted in economic policy and the other can be traced to 'Africanist' interpretations of the African renaissance, outlined in the introductory chapter. The first possibility, according to Mbali (2004), is that the turn to conservative macro-economic policy in the form of the Growth, Employment, and Redistribution Strategy (GEAR) in the latter half of the 1990s repositioned AIDS as primarily a fiscal problem. Following this line of thought, Mbali suggests that Mbeki's denial of HIV/AIDS acted as a convenient clause to avoid the drastic public spending that a full acceptance of the problem would entail. This argument lacks evidence, and has been refuted, at least partially, by Nattrass (2007); she highlights the substantial amount of state welfare that is in fact available for people who are infected and affected by the virus. The economic explanation also underestimates the extent of funding that flows into South Africa from international charitable organisations such as Oxfam or Save the Children, and foreign government development agencies such as the UK's Department for International Development (DfID), the US Agency for International Development (USAID), or the American President's Emergency Plan for AIDS Relief (PEPFAR).

A more convincing explanation for the 'state of denial', as Elaine Epstein dubbed it in her 1999 documentary, may be that it is 'a response to the history of racist colonial and apartheid discourses of African sexuality' (Mbali 2004: 111). In this reading, Mbeki's refusal to accept scientific orthodoxy should be seen in the context of his wider rejection of notions that he believes underpin science as a vehicle for neo-imperialism:

[W]e [black people] are germ carriers, and human beings of a lower order [who] cannot subject... passion to reason... we are but natural born promiscuous carriers of germs... they [scientists] proclaim that our continent is doomed to an inevitable mortal end because of our devotion to the sin of lust. (Mbeki, *Mail and Guardian*, 26 October 2001, in Mbali 2004: 111)

To be sure, the colonial construction of African sexuality did indeed frame Africans as inter alia rampantly promiscuous, with endemic immorality and barbaric, animalistic qualities. Whether this was as a result of the colonists' construction of 'the other' in such as way as to free themselves of any vestiges of barbarism and clear the path for their own psychological and material development (McGrane 1989), or whether it reflected simply the fear of difference, was not of central concern to Mbeki. In it, he read the tendency to stereotype African sexuality as a means to dehumanise and discriminate against black Africans.

In this context, then, Mbeki's controversial response to AIDS was a call for 'African solutions to African problems' à la the African renaissance. It was an attempt at the decolonisation of consciousness; an endeavour to foreground African-initiated science and question convention. For Mbeki and his ilk, the imposition of orthodox science as a compulsory explanatory paradigm through which they must *think* and engage in debates about AIDS was unacceptable. Essentially, this constituted a critique of the political economy of biomedical research (Schneider 2002). However, as Mbali points out (2004), from the late 1980s the dominant discourse around AIDS in development and interventionist circles was framed in rights-based terms that actively avoided potentially racist stereotypes.

However, whilst Mbeki's hawkish questioning of AIDS orthodoxy and Tshabalala-Msimang's promotion of lemon juice and garlic over ARV drugs clearly underpinned the Department of Health's sluggish response to the epidemic, policy on the ground has been framed in conventional scientific terms. Anomalously, at the same time that Tshabalala-Msimang was advocating the nutritional benefits of garlic and beetroot, she was signing national health policy documents rooted in conventional scientific understanding. Paradoxically, then, despite the very public support for pseudo-scientists, there has been consistency at the national level in developing AIDS policy that has promoted scientific orthodoxy as opposed to dissident points of view. The support for AIDS denialists did not materialise in policy. Rather, it was manifest in the continual stalling of policies that could have saved hundreds of thousands of lives, and the victimisation of anyone who dared to depart from the party line (cf. Cullinan and Thom 2009).

In 1997, the same year as Mbeki declared an African renaissance, the government unveiled Virodene: its miracle cure for the looming epidemic. To deep embarrassment, upon testing by conventional scientific means, Virodene turned out to be a commonly used industrial solvent and was scrapped. At the same time, *Sarafina 2*, a musical drama intended to promote safer sex among young people, became embroiled in allegations of corruption as the total cost escalated to over R14 million. Both the Virodene and the *Sarafina 2* debacles put the government on the defensive, and President Mbeki in particular began his descent into 'an obsession with AIDS "denialism" and the "demon" of white racism' (Myburgh 2009: 8). The highly critical responses from civil society in opposition to its early interventions set the government on a path to which participation with groups representing civil structures became increasingly marginal. From this early stage, non-governmental groups were largely excluded from AIDS policy making, but they were becoming increasingly responsible for the implementation of foreign-funded prevention projects on the ground.

The failure of the first National AIDS Plan, and the combined embarrassments of Virodene and *Sarafina 2*, set the tone for state responses to follow. The Treatment Action Campaign (TAC), which has become a perennial thorn in government's side, was established in 1998 on a tide of anger and frustration flowing from the Department of Health's refusal to provide the antiretroviral drug AZT. AZT, and later Nevirapine, had been widely proven to reduce mother-to-child transmission of HIV, but Mbeki had read on the internet that they were poisonous and so pregnant South African women were denied access to them. In 2001, the TAC and other AIDS-related pressure groups began constitutional court proceedings against the government in an attempt to force it to provide the drugs. 'One year and about 100,000 infant infections later' (Coovadia 2009: 73), the Minister of Health was ordered 'without delay' to lift restrictions on Nevirapine, and the slow process of initiating pilot projects for its distribution began.[3] Reflecting and exacerbating the government's uneasy relationship with AIDS activists, when the South African National AIDS Council (SANAC)[4] was established in 2000, prominent pressure groups such as the TAC and the AIDS consortium were excluded from it.[5]

Simultaneously, the 'Comprehensive National HIV/AIDS and STI Strategic Plan for 2000–2005' (South African Government 2000) was released. A largely non-committal statement of intention, the plan reads more like a PowerPoint presentation that a policy document – although it did recognise and encourage NGOs in various partnership roles with the state to provide preventative and antiretroviral treatment. This effectively legitimised NGOs as parastatal groups, incepted as local-level initiatives but with remits to fulfil national and regional policy priorities. As James has noted, 'in the wake of initial state indifference about AIDS in South Africa, early non-governmental initiatives seemed to promise the best that civil society could offer' (2002: 176). Thus state provision of AIDS prevention initiatives, especially in rural areas lacking infrastructure such as Venda, was effectively outsourced to NGOs who received overseas subsidy and followed a hodgepodge of directives from both their funding bodies and regional or local government representatives.

---

[3] The TAC won on the basis that concurrent trials in Thailand had demonstrated that AZT (the ARV in question) can help prevent mother-to-child transmission of the virus by up to 50 per cent during childbirth. AZT was later to be replaced by a similar ARV known as Nevirapine (Coovadia 2009).

[4] The South African National AIDS Council (SANAC) is always headed by the Deputy President of the country. SANAC is composed of up to 30 individuals from across a broad spectrum of government departments, faith-based groups, private enterprise, and civil society.

[5] Johnson (2009: 207) argues that the government began to finance its own organisation, the National Association for People Living with AIDS (NAPWA), as an NGO designed to harass and counteract the TAC and other AIDS-related NGOs.

Away from the rural peripheries and towards more urbanised centres, events took a quite different turn. Most civil society organisations concerned with AIDS in Gauteng, KwaZulu-Natal, and Western Cape provinces seem to have remained relatively separate from government structures, taking a proactive role in advocacy, and only supporting the government on rare occasions. This was the case in 2001 when the TAC joined the Congress of South African Trade Unions (COSATU) in supporting the government during a court hearing brought by pharmaceutical multinationals to 'prevent regulatory measures to reduce the cost of AIDS drugs' (Schneider 2002: 149). The pharmaceutical companies lost their case, and the government won the right to import generic drugs – mostly from Brazil – and to produce the drugs in South Africa. This cooperation, however, was short-lived. Even after the dramatic fall in price of ARVs, the government continued to insist that provision by the public sector was financially unviable.[6] The TAC and associated bodies again threatened to take Tshabalala-Msimang to court, on the grounds of her continual reluctance to facilitate the provision of treatment which had been agreed to in yet another HIV/AIDS Operational Plan in September 2003. She subsequently capitulated to their demands, giving assurance that the Department of Health would meet its targets. By the end of December 2005, in the midst of the 'denialism debacle', UNAIDS (2007) estimated that over 111,000 South Africans were accessing free antiretroviral treatment in 200 public health sector facilities, while an additional 60,000 were receiving care through the private sector. This provision was inadequate to cover even half of those who were in need of, and entitled to, treatment.

Moreover, provision has been unequal regionally. Provincial governments in Gauteng and especially the Western Cape led the way, often acting independently of national-level guidance, notably in defiance of Mbeki's instruction to withhold AZT and later Nevirapine medication for the prevention of mother-to-child transmission. Conversely, the provision of ARV therapy in Limpopo Province has been seriously hampered by a lack of political will both at regional and local levels of government. Limpopo remains an ANC stronghold, and dissent from the party line has rarely been rewarded.

Whilst potentially the removal of Thabo Mbeki in 2008 may have signalled the end of a dark era for AIDS activists in the country, President Zuma's track record of prophylactic showering has been less

---

[6] See Nattrass (2004) for a comprehensive critique of the government's calculations on this. The argument that AIDS drugs were too expensive was thrown into further contestation in 2004/5 when the Clinton Foundation negotiated a deal that gave South Africa access to the cheapest antiretroviral drugs in the world (Johnson 2009: 206).

than inspirational.[7] Still, Zuma's government pledged to implement yet another 'strategic plan', with the aim of halving new HIV infections by 2011 (South African Government 2007). In doing so, the Department of Health at last seemed to be sincere about tackling its own statistical estimations that national HIV prevalence among antenatal clinic attendees rose from 7.6 per cent in 1994 to 30.2 per cent in 2005 (South African Government 2006), and continues to rise (cf. Thornton 2008). However, current targets are unlikely to be realised without a profound change in approaches to HIV prevention. The strategic plan for reducing infection rates by 2011 clearly outlines the government's continued priority: '[to] implement [preventative] interventions targeted at reducing HIV infection in young people, *focusing on young women*' (South African Government 2007: 11, my italics). As the previous chapter demonstrated, targeting high-risk groups such as young women is in itself a risky strategy; the uneven distribution of biomedical knowledge in rural areas such as Venda can have serious unintended consequences.

Nonetheless, there is scope for optimism. In the aftermath of Mbeki's denialism, Zuma's new Minister of Health, Dr Aaron Motsoaledi, and his deputy, (the late) Dr Molefi Sefularo, have openly accepted that HIV causes AIDS, and implemented a progressive campaign encouraging high-profile South Africans to be tested. Whilst Minister Motsoaledi stopped short of revealing his own status, he did openly admit to being tested. President Zuma himself later announced his HIV-negative status. This sent out profoundly mixed messages: on the one hand, he had tested and openly disclosed – ostensibly in the name of reducing AIDS-related stigma. And yet, at the same time, against the background of his recently publicised reluctance to use condoms, the President's announcement suggested that unprotected sex may not be that risky after all.

In a bid to test up to 15 million people, in 2010 the Department of Health announced that everyone attending a public heath facility would be tested for HIV and encouraged to ask for the results. This aggressive approach to righting previous wrongs has seen the Department pledging to provide ARVs to all those in need. Until recently, a person living with HIV in South Africa was eligible for free treatment only when their CD4 count fell to 200, thus nearing full blown AIDS. In early 2010, President Zuma announced that ARVs will be provided when a patient's CD4

---

[7] Jacob Zuma revealed in a 2006 court appearance on charges of rape (of which he was acquitted) that he knowingly had unprotected sex with an HIV-positive family friend and used a post-coital shower as his only means of protecting himself – and his three wives – against contracting the virus. Later, in early 2010, revelations of a love child he fathered out of wedlock with a prominent politician's daughter again reminded the nation that President Zuma himself does not practise safe sex. The sex scandals, and his insistence on living a very public polygamy, have provoked both impassioned criticism of, and support for, the President into his second term in office.

count falls to 350, meaning that people will get treatment earlier. However, demand continues to outweigh provision. In 2007 almost 900,000 South Africans needed ARVs, but just over 350,000 were actually receiving them through the public sector (South African Government 2008c; cf. McNeill and Niehaus 2010).

But figures can be misleading. A serious shortcoming of data that measure the uptake of ARVs in public health facilities is the assumption that if medication is offered, it will be accepted. Low numbers of patients on ARV regimens are taken to represent inadequate standards of service provision. However, having had regular access to a project at which ARVs have been distributed through a rural hospital since 2005, it is apparent to me that many patients have refused and continue to refuse treatment. This is either because they are suspicious of the efficacy of ARVs, or because of the perverse economic incentive to stay sick: the monthly disability grant of R800 (in 2010) is removed when a person starts to become healthy. Alternatively, the requirement that they will be accepted onto a treatment programme only if they disclose their status to a friend or family member has encouraged many people to suffer in silence.

In Venda, the socio-cultural environment is not yet conducive to full, public disclosure (see McNeill 2009). This is borne out by the fact that people do not 'live openly' with HIV in Venda. In 2010, there was not one openly HIV-positive individual in the region. Unlike much of South Africa – especially in parts of Gauteng, KwaZulu-Natal, and the Western Cape – there is no recent history of AIDS activism in Venda. HIV/AIDS NGOs in the region, like the one I describe below, are partisan and follow instructions rather than engaging in advocacy. The Treatment Action Campaign, Médecins Sans Frontières (MSF) and the National Association for People Living with HIV-AIDS (NAPWA) have yet to establish offices there, and have no presence in or around Venda. The concept of an openly 'positive identity', in the absence of support networks or local precedent, is yet to emerge. Stigma is king, and positive people live a public life of secrets.

And yet those who develop full-blown AIDS are effectively forced to disclose their HIV-positive status to at least one person before they can enrol on an ARV programme.[8] In the Venda context described above, the recipient of disclosure is generally not a friend or family member, but another HIV-positive stranger – contacted through nursing networks – who understands the necessity for secrecy. This has had far-reaching, unintended consequences: by encouraging secretive social clusters of

---

[8] There is evidence that disclosure helps HIV-positive clients adhere to their medical regimens, and that the psychological burden of relief is in and of its self conducive to attaining and maintaining mental and physical health. Whilst national guidelines 'strongly recommend' that a client discloses before being enrolled on a programme, it has, in effect, become a prerequisite for accessing treatment.

AIDS patients, forced disclosure has contributed directly to the construction of stigma (McNeill and Niehaus 2010). Thus, whilst it was widely believed, and indeed hoped, that increasing access to ARV therapy would help to mitigate AIDS-related stigma through more people being open about their status (Norman et al. 2005; Eba 2007), in this case medical provision has actually exacerbated the stigmatisation of people living with AIDS. As I demonstrate in the following chapter, HIV/AIDS peer group educators in Venda are subject to stigmatisation of a different, although not unrelated, kind.

As this brief sketch of AIDS policy in South Africa has shown, the relationship between government and NGOs in the provision of prevention and treatment programmes has often been a tense one. Connections between the two have developed along pragmatic lines, and a lack of high-level political leadership has led to pervasive confusion and uncertainty in public reception of treatment interventions. Whilst many critics have blamed this lack of political direction for the extent of the AIDS crisis in South Africa, it cannot be held solely responsible for the mixed fortunes that NGO-led interventions have encountered. A closer look at the micro-dynamics of AIDS programmes is required to ascertain exactly what form these mixed fortunes have taken, and what their implications may be.

The Forum for AIDS Prevention[9]

The Forum for AIDS Prevention (FAP) is the brainchild of Harold Lemke, an American Buddhist monk who lived in Venda between 1980 and 1998. In 1993, after nursing a close friend who died of an AIDS-related illness, Harold became a self-styled, completely untrained, AIDS educator, holding public meetings and distributing the few condoms with which he was provided by the Department of Health and Welfare. I was with him at many of the early meetings, during which his eloquent but apocalyptic talks were met with a combination of suspicion and dread, creating a state of fear that he hoped would induce the practice of safer sex.

By 1997 Harold had procured the voluntary services of two Venda co-workers, a man and a woman. Munaki, the woman, worked at the local hotel, whilst Rudzani had been a commander in the ANC's military wing, *UmKhonto weSizwe* (MK). They registered the Forum for AIDS Prevention with the Department of Social Development as an NGO in 1997 and secured a start-up grant from the Department of Health for

---

[9] As mentioned earlier, the title of the organisation has been changed. All the names of people working for it, with the exception of the founder who has granted permission for his name to be used, are pseudonyms.

R80,000. This paid rent for their first single-room office in down-town Thohoyandou and provided a small stipend for the two volunteers.

Rudzani's high-profile ANC contacts were to prove invaluable in future dealings with the government, especially in securing funding. Since 1994, it has been official procedure for all foreign donations to NGOs in South Africa to be diverted to a central fund, and the government has initiated a centralised system of tendering intended to systematise the unprecedented level of aid and promote competition amongst 'service providers' (James 2002: 176). James has noted that this manner of funding generated confusion in many 'formalised anti-AIDS education initiatives' (ibid.) – but for the FAP, at least in its early format, it was a blessing. Still, not all funding comes via state regulators. Excessive bureaucratic procedures have driven many funders to bypass the central pot and deposit money directly into the FAP bank account. Given its regularly maintained connections to government and the distinct lack of advocacy work in its activities, it may be misleading to think of the FAP as non-governmental. Indeed, as Ferguson argues, 'local voluntary organisations... very often, on inspection, turn out to be integrally linked with national- and transnational-level entities' (2006: 101). In a wider commentary on the ways in which such organisations have often 'taken over the most basic functions and powers of the state [in post-colonial African countries]', he argues that '[some] NGOs are not as NG as they might wish us to believe' (ibid.). NGOs often turn out to be BONGOs (bank-organised NGOs) and GONGOs (government-organised NGOs). In this context, perhaps the FAP could best be referred to as a non-profit organisation (NPO), or even as a community-based initiative (CBI). Both terms are common in South Africa's burgeoning lexicon of development jargon. However, simply changing the acronym does not change the inherently ambiguous status of voluntary organisations. They are neither 'governmental' nor 'non-governmental'. As I demonstrate below, they are commonly used – at least in the Venda region – as a stepping-stone between voluntary and state employment. In this context they may also be thought of as 'quasi-governmental' (Ferguson 1994: 6; cf. Fisher 1997; James 2002). In the knowledge, then, that there is an intrinsic tension in these organisations' allegedly non-governmental character, I shall continue to use the term NGO when referring to the FAP.

Having secured tenders from the government for the provision of home-based care (HBC) and voluntary counselling and testing (VCT) in the Vhembe District, the FAP has become an important service provider for out-sourced government initiatives. As the director of the organisation explained to me:

We don't really have a 'good' relationship with the government – most of it is just forced... people in government positions are always changing and we cannot waste time by trying to become friends with them... we have jobs to do and people are dying. But we do not own these people [the volunteers], we do not own the projects, we are just an extended hand of what the government is supposed to do, but it can't – so you see we can assist in that. (Interview, 4 February 2005)

Thus, although the close relationship between the FAP and government was born out of necessity (to access funds), it later became a virtue, allowing the remit of the organisation to mushroom rapidly. In addition to this, it has maintained very strong connections with a number of national and international development organisations and faith-based groups such as the Evangelical Lutheran Church of South Africa (ELCSA), Lawyers for Human Rights (LHR), and Voluntary Services Overseas (VSO, UK). An important exemption from this list is the TAC, whose presence is yet to be felt in the region but is widely influential in other regions of South Africa.

Moreover, whilst much funding is secured via government bodies, a significant number of FAP projects are sponsored directly by national and international donors.[10] From most of these organisations donations are deposited directly into the FAP account, avoiding the extra bureaucracy of going through national or provincial government offices. This does not, however, guarantee that funding will reach the intended projects. Missing cash is often blamed on complications such as the international currency exchange rate or exorbitant bank fees.

Highly critical of international patterns of development in which NGOs often become dependent on foreign support for daily survival and accountability, and having trained the two volunteers in basic administration and proposal writing, Harold Lemke decided to leave in 1998. Besides his disaffection with these patterns of dependency, his departure was also prompted by his astute observation that for the FAP to achieve its objectives and survive in post-apartheid South Africa it would have to be run 'by Vendas for Vendas'. By 1999 the organisation had received a second supplementary grant of R50,000 from the Department of Health and Welfare that enabled it to take on three more volunteers. The new recruits, all young men, played pivotal roles in developing the HBC and 'youth in school' awareness programmes.

As the result of a chance encounter with the head of the Department of Psychology at the University of Zimbabwe in 1998, Munaki and Rudzani travelled to Harare for training that would equip them with the skills to

---

[10] In May 2005 these included AusAID (Australian government), USAID (United States), Bristol-Myers Squibb Foundation – Secure the Future (BMS-STF), Christian Aid, Family Health International (FHI), National Development Agency (NDA), Nelson Mandela Children's Fund (NMCF), OXFAM Australia (joint HIV/AIDS programme – JOHAP), Reggio nel Mondo, and Save the Children (UK and Sweden).

establish peer group education and HBC projects in Venda. These programmes were designed in Zimbabwe in collaboration with the Project Support Group (PSG), an organisation funded largely by the Norwegian, Netherlands, and Swedish governments, that has assisted in setting up and funding many AIDS interventions in Southern Africa (cf. Campbell 2003).[11] Establishing a partnership with PSG was a significant turning point in the development of the FAP: it initiated the now-ingrained emphasis on participatory approaches and offered models for the means by which these could be established, coordinated, and evaluated.

Today, the FAP has grown into a major player in the provision of health care in Limpopo Province and acts in its own capacity as a mentor and reference point for emerging NGOs in the area. It 'facilitates' peer education, HBC, VCT, and projects for orphans and vulnerable children (OVC) throughout the province and in neighbouring Botswana. Munaki, the first volunteer, is now the director of the organisation, and in 2002 Rudzani secured a managerial position at the regional level in the Department of Health and Welfare. Such examples of upward mobility into the echelons of government are important and I will return to them in due course.

However, in order to consider the ways in which the FAP exemplifies broader trends in NGO-organised peer education, I must look at the spread of participatory approaches to public health, and examine the theory of effective learning which underpins these approaches.

The Knowledge Politics of Planned AIDS Intervention

Manifesting a very different understanding of the relationship between knowledge and experience from that illustrated in the *vhusha* initiation, health policies reveal the conviction that a deliberate change in the former will alter the latter. The process whereby planned interventions are designed to change behaviour through education is neatly conceptualised in the acronym KAP: 'Knowledge, Attitudes and Practice'. The extent to which the process is ineffectual, constrained by economic, social, and 'cultural' factors, has been theorised as the 'KAP gap' (cf. Mathews et al. 1995). Whilst it is widely acknowledged that KAP approaches are inadequate, the reasons for their failure are not well understood. And yet they remain popular in health intervention models (cf. Turner and Shepherd 1999; Campbell 2003).

Based on the premise of knowledge transfer, KAP can be conceptualised fundamentally as the attempt to draw together separate 'traditions' or corpuses of knowledge (cf. Lambek 1993). Instead of thinking of knowledge transfer from experts to initiates in a controlled ritual

---

[11] For more details about PSG, see <www.psgsa.org.za>.

environment, this points the way to the distribution of knowledge through public programmes such as peer group education. In AIDS interventions, the biomedical tradition is clearly the most powerful in terms of international support and access to resources, but, through the agency of the actors involved, local understandings can and do usurp this power in a variety of ways. Long has termed these contestations 'battlefields of knowledge' (Long 1992; Cernea 1991; 1995).[12]

Concepts of intervention have changed over time. The dominant theoretical paradigms of the 1960s and 1970s offered a mechanical model of the relationship between policy, implementation, and outcomes that relied on a linear progression from policy formulation, through outcomes, to evaluation (Long 2001: 31). This has been criticised on several grounds, and contemporary approaches are more likely to factor in the transformation and 'evaluation' of policy during implementation and the 'external' influence of factors such as 'culture'. In the development of HIV/AIDS interventions, this has led to the promotion of 'finding ways of negotiating social hierarchies, or [culturally appropriate] methods of communicating creatively' (Healthlink 2007: 6). Although interventions remain mostly diagnostic and prescriptive, the linear model has been displaced by 'actor-centred' approaches that seek to construct 'bottom-up' interventions as opposed to the previously dominant 'top-down' approach, and thus need to:

understand the processes by which interventions enter the lifeworlds of the individuals and groups affected and thus come to form part of the resources and constraints of the social strategies they develop... the concept of intervention [is] an ongoing, socially constructed and negotiated progress, not simply the execution of an already-specified plan of action with expected outcomes. (Long 2001: 31)

Commentators have argued, however, that actor-centred approaches overemphasise individual behaviour. It is far more likely that AIDS intervention projects fail, they argue, because of social factors (poverty, patriarchy, et cetera) and 'cultural' understandings that impinge upon people's abilities to change behaviour.[13] Writers such as McDonald (1996) and Campbell (2002; 2003) thus demonstrate that the failure to induce change in sexual behaviour reflects a lack of sensitivity to local cultural norms as well as socio-economic circumstances that might make such

---

[12] Cernea identifies two categories: knowledge for understanding and knowledge for action (1995: 343). The two categories are distinct, but have a symbiotic relationship. Knowledge for action is valid, according to Cernea, only if it increases knowledge for understanding, whilst knowledge for understanding on its own can be 'pedestrian and deceptive' (ibid.)

[13] See Packard and Epstein (1991), Parker (1996), Campbell and Williams (1998; 1999), Barnett and Whiteside (2002), Delius and Walker (2002), and Kalipeni et al. (2004). See Waterston (1997) for an example of this kind of critique based on ethnographic research among homeless women in New York.

behaviour change impossible. For example, highlighting the role of 'cultural attitudes to fertility', McDonald (1996: 1325) has shown the ways in which condoms impinge on the desire for a large family in Botswana (cf. Heald 2006). But such studies have inevitably raised more questions than they have answered, providing cursory and often utilitarian explanations as to why interventions do not always achieve their intentions and avoiding the issue of how they might be more successful in achieving their objectives.

Such studies, by de-emphasising the strategies and intentions of actors and stressing the intractabililty of 'culture', also run the risk of ignoring how individuals may contest and transform meanings. The female HIV/AIDS peer group educators in Venda, as mostly young, unmarried, and unemployed women, embrace their new-found identity as (quasi) social workers and, ultimately, aim for employment in the government health sector. In part, this identity is predicated upon their promotion of biomedical understandings of the virus. As the following chapter demonstrates, music – some of it sanctioned by 'tradition' – is fundamental to these educators' enterprise, but they use it to sing about new things: things they 'cannot talk about'. Sanctioned by international funding agencies, the peer educators' account of AIDS is centred on the promotion of prevention and treatment. Their approach thus represents a complex hybrid in which pre-existing culture intersects with international development discourse.

If anthropologists have been slow to consider the knowledge politics of AIDS intervention, they have not ignored it completely. A small but relevant body of research, situated at the interface of anthropology and development, has initiated the task of making connections between the biomedical model of AIDS and representations of sickness and health in 'folk models' or, as they are also known in the inevitable development jargon, indigenous knowledge systems (IKS).[14] As I describe in more detail in Chapter 6, these studies have made important connections between the centrality of (certain) women, (menstrual) blood, and (inappropriate) sex in IKS. They demonstrate that high levels of cross-over between the arenas of biomedical and indigenous knowledge have occurred since AIDS education projects began to be pursued in earnest.

The precise nature of this 'marginal change' (Barth 2002) in a body of knowledge is difficult but not impossible to map out, as I show in Chapter 8. These authors have made significant headway in understanding the interdependence and commensurability of biomedical science and IKS in the context of the AIDS pandemic. Whilst drawing on these ideas, I want to develop an argument based on the ways in which folk

---

[14] Foremost in this vein have been Green (1994), Liddell et al. (2005), de Bruyn (1992), Heald (1995; 2006), Ingstad (1990), Leclerc-Madlala (2002), and McDonald and Schatz (2006).

models are rooted, essentially, in contemporary political processes, such as the recent battle for paramount chieftaincy discussed in Chapter 2. By interpreting the commensurability of the folk and biomedical models through the relationship between knowledge and experience, it is possible to see biomedicine – as it is often understood in Venda – as a form of ritual knowledge. This has profound implications for the processes of knowledge transfer that have been widely adopted by policy planners who design AIDS interventions.

The 'Participatory' Approach to Peer Education

The current dominance of peer group education as a method of HIV/AIDS prevention can be traced to the emergence of participatory approaches to development in the 1980s and early 1990s. Seminal texts such as those by Chambers (1983; 1994) and Cernea (1991) paved the way for a plethora of literature devoted to the promotion of 'participation' where previously top-down, state-centred approaches had prevailed. This literature was both influenced by and had influence on the strategic planning of institutions such as the World Bank, which began to support 'greater involvement of "local" people's perspectives, knowledge, priorities and skills... [as an alternative to] ... outsider-led development' (Cooke and Kothari 2001: 5).

The surge in the popularity of 'participation' in development projects has reflected the increasing concern that citizens ought to participate fully in the processes of democracy. To this end, the African Union (AU) made a constitutional undertaking in favour of 'democratic principles (and) *popular participation*' (Lodge 2002: 233, my italics). The broad aim of this participatory development is to 'increase the involvement of socially and economically marginalised peoples in decision making over their own lives' (Parker 1996). Baylies has captured the essence of this by arguing that a participatory, 'bottom-up approach' acknowledges the 'legitimacy of local knowledge and the ability of individuals to know and verbalise their needs' (2000: 133).

In development projects devoted to the promotion of public health, this also reflected and was influenced by a general acceptance that wellbeing should not be considered the end result of an individual's life choices, but rather a social phenomenon played out among historically and culturally constituted class and status groups with distinct life chances. This heralded a paradigm shift in models for the promotion of public health in developed and developing countries. 'Behavioural' interventions, common before this shift, had been influenced heavily by European and US experiences of HIV among groups of gay men and injecting drug users, and had sought to provide knowledge and encourage individual action from the top down. Largely because it was promoted effectively by organisational structures developed by groups of gay men, this strategy was reasonably successful (Watney 1989) – and policy makers assumed its universality. In Africa, this translated into models that assumed people practised risky sex because they lacked adequate information, and the overwhelming early focus on KAP was implemented in this context (cf. Heald 2006).

However, public health policy makers soon realised that education alone was insufficient as a motivational factor for the instigation of behavioural change. As HIV began to have more substantial impacts on heterosexual populations in Europe and elsewhere, models in Africa for the promotion of public health moved towards 'community'-based strategies that were intended to promote collective responses, from the 'grassroots'. Following this logic, the reason why education alone had failed to induce safer sex was to be found in the often ill-defined concept of power. Specific groups such as 'youth' and 'women' came to be – and still are – defined as characteristically in a state of disempowerment, and thus in need of empowerment – which, in reality, translated into the provision of employment, more education, or both. Moreover, for this process to be successful, it would have to be participatory, and as this logic has been adapted more recently to HIV/AIDS peer education, the notions of empowerment and participation have become central tenets of project designs (cf. Kalipeni et al. 2007).

This is reflected in development/social psychology approaches that emphasise the key role of participation in health-related behaviours and in the reconstruction of sexual identities. In this process, Campbell has suggested, people are motivated by a 'fundamental human need for positive self-esteem, self-efficacy or empowerment' (1998: 57). For Campbell, HIV/AIDS peer education thus seeks to empower educators by:

> transferring health-related knowledge from the hands of outside experts to the hands of ordinary people, increasing their sense of perceived control over their health... [and]... deriving respect and recognition for their role in promoting health. (Campbell 2000: 492)

Although these theoretical assumptions will be criticised later in more detail, it must be noted here that they continue to employ overtly Eurocentric notions pertaining to the bounded, objectified self, albeit in a group context. For several generations now, a fundamental contribution of anthropology to intellectual debates has been to demonstrate that such a 'self' cannot be assumed to exist in an apolitical or non-historical vacuum – or, more generally, as a desirable construction of identity across cultures (cf., for example, Chabal and Daloz 1999: 52–3; Erikson 1995; Keesing and Strathern 1998). Indeed, if it is to be of use in determining the efficacy of peer education projects, any 'fundamental human need for... empowerment' must be qualified strictly in terms of culturally and historically constituted understandings of the self and sexualities which may or may not reflect post-enlightenment conceptions. Without such qualification, authors and project designers may be in danger of imposing etic, authoritative notions of human nature which are as likely to impede our understanding of the potential of participatory efforts to promote safer sex as they are to complement or assist them.[15]

Failing to recognise this, HIV/AIDS peer education has been deemed successful by project designers if, encompassing the prospects for self-directed change, it instigates the collective renegotiation of social and sexual roles among target groups. In South Africa, these are generally young women, commercial sex workers, compound-dwelling migrant labourers, and 'youth', all of whom are held to be disempowered and to experience low levels of control over the construction of their sexual identities. In its ideal context and under ideal conditions, peer education is thus based on the premise that

People evaluate changes not on the basis of scientific evidence or authoritative testimony, but by subjective judgements of close, trusted peers who have adopted changes and provide persuasive role models for change. (Wilson 2000)

For example, current projects aimed at young people in South Africa, such as Love Life, train a core of individuals known as 'groundbreakers' from schools and youth centres in participatory teaching methods.[16] These include interactive dramas, role plays, songs, and public performances in which groundbreakers are intended to transmit their newly acquired life skills and health-related knowledge to their contemporaries. In theory, the peer groups in these projects are made critically conscious (Freire 1972) of the potentially dangerous impact that socially and historically constructed gender roles such as 'macho-style' masculinity in boys and passiveness in girls can have on their sexual health. They are then made aware of the effect that poverty and unemployment can have in structuring and reinforcing these identities. On this basis, with the peer educators as positive role models who are intended to lead by example, it is hoped that others will follow their lead and renegotiate health-enhancing behaviour.

---

[15] By 'sexual identities', authors seem to be referring to the ways in which people have sex, and power relationships that mould this. There is scope here for a wider engagement with criticisms of identity as an analytical term (Cooper 2005). It is not clear, for example, why such a fluid, contested, and consistently reconstructed concept should be labelled a (sexual) identity, nor if we can really ascribe such a category to groups of people who are unaware that they ought to have one.

[16] Love Life was initially established by the Department of Health and Welfare with funding from the Kaiser Foundation, and is now well funded by the Bill and Melinda Gates Foundation, which works in partnership with the Department on several HIV/AIDS projects.

With such financial and institutional support, and with backing from academics concerned with development, participation, and empowerment, peer education has become 'one of the most commonly used strategies of health promotion in the world' (Campbell 2003: 42). The proliferation of the strategy in South Africa is thus reflective of trends throughout the continent[17] and beyond.[18]

However, although considerable resources have been channelled into peer education, there is a distinct absence of research on or knowledge of 'the means by which, and the effectiveness with which the programmes change sexual behaviour' (James 2002: 180; cf. Turner and Shepherd 1999; Campbell 2003). Our understanding of the social processes underlying the alleged efficacy of so-called participatory approaches to health promotion thus remains in its infancy, and the faith with which donors continue to fund programmes seems increasingly problematic given the possibility that they are 'costing lives as well as funds' (Kalipeni et al. 2007).[19]

Peer Education in Venda

The Forum for AIDS Prevention has been facilitating peer education projects among groups of young women in Venda since 1998. The rationale for its intervention is the finding that young women in Southern Africa are the demographic category most susceptible to HIV infection.[20] Since 1998, the FAP has expanded from two projects to 24, covering Limpopo Province from Doreen farm project in the north to Ha-Muila in the south. In February 2009 there were over 600 peer educators, the vast majority of whom were young (18–30) unmarried women. The bulk of my data is drawn from four peer education projects comprising an average of 25 volunteers each at Tshikombani (which included my host village Fondwe), Ha-Matsa (towards the N1 motorway to Zimbabwe), Ha-Rabali (in the central Nzhelele region), and Tshakhuma (to the south: see Map 4).[21]

---

[17] See Hope (2003), Basset (1998), Leonard et al. (2000), Wolf et al. (2000).

[18] Fernandes et al. (1999); Lamptey and Gayle (2001); Barnett and Whiteside (2002); Campbell and MacPhail (2002).

[19] Current strategies for prevention are not limited to peer education. For example, a great deal of research is currently under way to assess the efficacy of microbicides, the female diaphragm, and male circumcision. See the 2006 UNAIDS report, <http://data.unaids.org/pub/GlobalReport/2006/2006_GR_CH06_en.pdf>.

[20] See Oppong (1998), MacDonald (1996), Baylies (2000), Bujra and Baylies (2000), Bujra (2000a), Craddock (2000; 2007), Kalipeni (2000), Sikwibele et al. (2000), and Kalipeni et al. (2004).

[21] The Tshakhuma project is an integrated prevention and HBC programme. The FAP has recently established three such integrated projects, where the volunteers have responsibility for home-based care and peer education.

The recruitment process for peer educators is intended to follow a conventional structure designed by the Project Support Group (Wilson 2000). According to this model, an initial baseline survey is conducted in which FAP staff request permission first from local traditional leaders (*Vhamusanda/Magota:* see Chapter 2) to start work in the area. Permission has never been withheld, and in general peer education projects have a good working relationship with traditional authorities. Indeed, traditional leaders are encouraged to send young women from their homesteads to join projects. This is done in the knowledge that such women will report back to royal circles; they thus fulfil a dual role as project members and royal spies. This is advantageous to project leaders in that it maintains corridors of communication with traditional leaders, although the recent rise in numbers of headmen has created some confusion: with whom, exactly, should they be in communication?

At the same time, FAP staff frequent beer halls, cafes, and night spots, and initiate dialogue with working girls in an attempt to recruit them. Potential volunteers are always told up-front that their time will be offered on a voluntary basis, but that eventually they will receive a small stipend. In reality a monthly stipend of R250 (in September 2005) is given to the volunteers from their first meeting. The strategy of misleading them about the regularity of payment is intended to dissuade transient, migrating women, often encountered in the border areas, who may be tempted to take the first payment and leave the area.

The social origins and modes of livelihood of the educators themselves are significant. Some were recruited from beer halls where they engaged in sex work; others heard of the projects through friends. In addition to the small monthly stipend, volunteers are encouraged by the FAP to initiate income-generating activities, some of which have been relatively successful. Cooperative efforts farming chickens, making bricks, or organising *stokvels* (rotating credit schemes)[22] have generally suffered, however, from a chronic lack of sustainable funding. Thus, whilst some peer educators climb the ladder of promotion into the role of 'coordinator', and possibly beyond to employment, most of them remain dependent on either state welfare or their families for an income. It is hardly surprising, then, that many continue to earn a living through sex work in its loose definition – exchanging sex for food, money, clothes, and phones with multiple concurrent partners, with whom they often maintain long-term transactional relationships (Hunter 2002; Bähre 2002). Clearly, then, the safe-sex message is contextualised by the limited extent

---

[22] Individual members receive a lump sum of cash at the end of the month. In other parts of South Africa, women *stokvel* members wear uniforms and sing initiation songs and church hymns during monthly meetings (Lukhele 1990), in a manner similar to groups of peer educators.

to which educators can 'practise what they preach' under the conditions imposed on them through such unequal power relations.

In accordance with the PSG model, the projects are intended to consist mostly of commercial sex workers. As a 'peer group', they should encourage and support each other (and their clients) to adopt safer sexual behaviour.[23] With the exception of a few projects on the borders, however, the recruitment process has failed to attract enough sex workers (or women who would admit to selling sex) and thus other women have been asked to join. Local church groups, civic associations, and burial societies are all targeted in an attempt to make up the numbers. Women also volunteer after hearing of a project through word of mouth or 'pavement radio' (Ellis 1989). The resultant mixed bag of motivations, aspirations, and expectations of such different groups of women throws the very notion of 'peer' education into question.

Volunteers are introduced to their project coordinator at the first meeting. Coordinators are chosen from established projects for their ability to communicate information and to impart participatory methods clearly to new recruits. They must, for example, have a vast repertoire of songs and drama topics from which to draw during their training. The coordinators and volunteers are frequently 'workshopped' by representatives from the Department of Health to ensure that their knowledge – their biomedical knowledge – is up-to-date. Thus the content of peer education programmes has changed markedly with the provision of government-funded ARV medication and VCT. This is reflected in the songs analysed in the next chapter. The lyrical content, dramas, and role-plays have changed significantly over time in line with government and international funding priorities. Thus the early emphasis on AIDS-related information, condoms, and prevention has been replaced to a large extent by an emphasis on the prominence of HIV testing and the provision of ARVs and other treatment in support of the national roll-out. In this context, the role of peer education can be seen not just as a means of attempting to enable health-enhancing social situations, but also as a peripatetic advertisement for the various services provided by the FAP and the state at hospitals, clinics, and health centres.

As the weekly ongoing training continues, the coordinator gives out bright red uniforms and explains about their R250 monthly stipend (the coordinators themselves receive around R1,000 per month). The volunteers learn that this is in return for a minimum of 27 hours a week, divided between training (six to seven hours), house meetings (six meetings of three hours each), and a Friday public performance (two to three

---

[23] Hunter (2002) and Wojcicki (2005) have problematised the notion of 'sex worker' with a discussion on wider transactional relationships through which trust and obligation often develop. The term 'sex worker' is used here with reference to women who sell sex at beer halls or on main roads – but any precise definition of the term remains problematic.

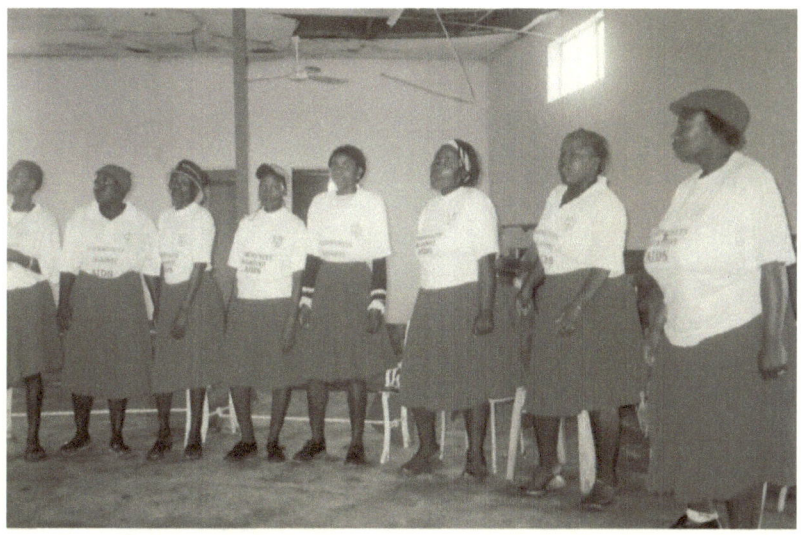

Figure 4.1. Peer educators at the Tshikombani project rehearsing songs during their weekly ongoing training in 2004.

hours). They are then divided into three or four geographical 'zones' in which they conduct house-to-house meetings, and each zone nominates a leader. This system also helps to organise the pragmatics of project management: a rota system dictates which zone will have certain responsibilities each week, such as cooking at the training sessions or organising and facilitating the Friday public performance. The first task of each zone is to draw a map of its area – indicating such features as roads, houses, farms, beer halls, churches, and clinics – onto which they record their activities and plan future outings.

During training, peer educators are taught biomedical HIV/AIDS information within a broader context of general health and life skills such as hygiene, basic dietetics, and methods of family planning. Armed with – and in theory empowered by – this knowledge, and wielding the equipment necessary to demonstrate the use of a condom, peer educators are then sent into the surrounding villages to visit homes in their respective zones on Monday and Wednesday mornings. The home visits are not usually prearranged, and, although they should last up to three hours, in fact they generally occupy no more than half an hour.

Dressed in their bright red uniforms (see Figure 4.1), they approach homesteads in which they can see people are present. If they are permitted to enter, they are seated (like all visitors) outside the main room of the kraal. As the reason for their visit has been disclosed by their uniform, pleasantries are kept to a minimum and the zone leader initiates a conversation about general health and wellbeing in the homestead. The hosts

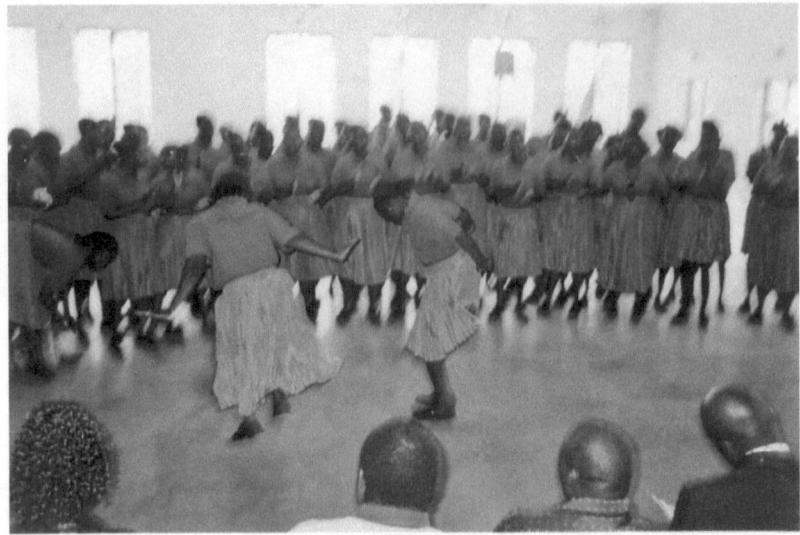

Figure 4.2. Peer educators at the Ha-Dumasi project perform a *malende* traditional dance (from stage five of the public performance) for a visiting delegation from the Project Support Group (PSG) and the South African Department of Health.

are encouraged to be open with any questions they may have regarding HIV/AIDS; the peer educators answer them as best they can, often using diagrams and pictures. If they come across any house-bound people, they are reported to the nearest HBC project, which will then make follow-up visits. When they leave, they offer condoms and government leaflets, and provide a contact number for any questions that may arise in the future. As I show in the following chapters, however, it is common for people to hide inside their homes when they see the red uniforms approaching, and the educators are often refused entry to a homestead. The houses to which visits are paid, then, are often the default ones of a relative or sympathetic friend. Alternatively, educators target people who are walking around, trying to instigate conversations with them as they walk. A strict record of the proceedings is kept and presented to the group at the next ongoing training meeting.

This weekly pattern of activity has resulted in a staggering volume of statistics that record 'facts' and figures such as 'clients served', 'females/males reached', and 'condoms distributed'. These figures are reproduced in donor reports and made into PowerPoint presentations for visiting 'experts' from overseas funding groups and government departments (see Figure 4.2).[24] They create a sense of efficacy and are ultimately manufactured into documents that encourage the continuation

---

[24] See Huges-d'Aeth (2002); Lindegger and Maxwell (2005); Raman (2005).

of funding. This set of procedures has contributed to a lack of critical appraisal in programme design and evaluation: the FAP has modified the structure of its peer education projects hardly at all since their original implementation in 1998.

One significant exception to this was the recent attempt to incorporate men into several peer education projects. Although 'targeting men' has received some attention in the literature, the incorporation of men into pre-existing female projects has not been studied.[25] Following instructions from several funders to extend peer education projects beyond their exclusively female focus, from 2003 the FAP attempted to recruit males. This was, without exception, a resounding failure. Most of the women resented the few men who did get involved, as they dominated any discussion while refusing to take part in what they perceived to be women's songs. This led to a recruitment drive for younger men, aged 18–23, who in turn were bullied by many of the women and looked ridiculous impersonating female dances. A few who joined did so with the ulterior motive of forming intimate relationships with peer educators, citing this advantage in their defence when they were ridiculed by other men at public performances. The current FAP policy on male peer educators is unclear. It raises issues, to which I shall return shortly, of how pragmatic experience may undermine funding priorities. Nonetheless, the exclusively female quality of projects reflects a broader trait, whereby it is women who tend to interact more with health services, as is evidenced by their attendance at antenatal clinics and the subsequent visits they make with their children.

A central tenet of the peer education programme, as designed by PSG, is the Friday afternoon public performance. This mostly takes place in beer halls, but also at market places, taxi ranks, clinics, or other such public arenas, and it involves a progression through six distinct stages:

Stage 1: Introduction by means of a variation of the *domba* initiation python dance or a popular song in which the lyrical content has been changed to include information on the FAP. They gather about 200 metres from the 'stage', which can be anything from a dancing arena in a beer hall to an open space in a market place, then move towards it slowly and loudly.

---

[25] Although their contributions have yet to match the volumes on women, authors such as Kaler (2004), Niehaus and Jonnson (2005), Simpson (2005; 2007), and Hunter (2005) have made important improvements to our understanding of the ways in which men in a variety of social and economic contexts have adapted and reacted to the virus. Niehaus (2002) has pointed to the complexities of male–male sex in migrant labour compounds and prisons. MacPhail (2003) and Wood et al. (1998) emphasise the manner in which heterosexual men are defined through acquisition of multiple partners, through 'macho' masculinities, exercising power over women, and espousing negative attitudes towards condoms, although MacPhail indicates that this can often be in conflict with the 'true' emotional vulnerabilities of young men. See also Stadler (2003).

Stage 2: Once the stage has been taken, two or three popular songs fused with HIV/AIDS information are sung *a capella* to draw and entertain a crowd.

Stage 3: Drama/role-plays – inspired by life experience and introducing themes such as polygamy, rape, domestic violence, alcoholism, commercial sexual encounters, sexual health, family relations, HIV transmission, and AIDS-related illness. These provide amusement to some and discomfort to others. The discomfort is usually manifest in men leaving the space created for peer education, heckling, or attempting to hinder proceedings.

Stage 4: A facilitated question-and-answer session, developing issues emerging from or emotions generated by the previous section. The zone leader asks such questions as: 'What did you see there?' 'Does this happen in your community?' 'How do you respond when this happens?' 'Do you think this behaviour is acceptable?' This stage usually involves the circulation of a phallic prop in the form of a large wooden penis, onto which individuals are encouraged to roll a condom. This potentially chaotic section is thought of as the climax of the performance, during which peer educators stand in a two-deep solid line of red, behind the leader who is responsible for coordinating the discussion and circulating the prop. If the conversation is slow to develop, some peer educators may stand amongst the crowd and ask provocative questions to stimulate discussion (see Figure 4.3).

Stage 5: *U tamba ngoma!* (To play the drums!) This section, which is often the most lengthy and exuberant, involves performances adapted from the repertoire of 'traditional' Venda music. This can include *malende* beer songs, *tshifhase* adolescent dances, songs from girls' initiation schools, and the female *tshigombela*. Like the gospel songs adapted in the earlier stages, the 'traditional' renditions are fused with biomedical HIV/AIDS information (see the next chapter). The 'traditional' dancing involves solo performances in which peer educators compete with each other in technique and innovation. This can get overtly sexual and provocative as buttocks are shaken towards the crowd.

Stage 6: The distribution of condoms. The entire performance hinges on condoms being free and plentiful. The Department of Health and Welfare has vastly improved the previously inconsistent supply of condoms. They are now freely available – although it is not clear what percentage of those taken as 'freebies' are actually used in the desired manner.[26]

---

[26] There are two types of government condoms in South Africa: the 'old' ones that come in a silver packaging; and the newer 'trust condoms', that come in a fashionable 8-pack with blue plastic wrapping and a recognisable trade mark on the front. Although 'trust'

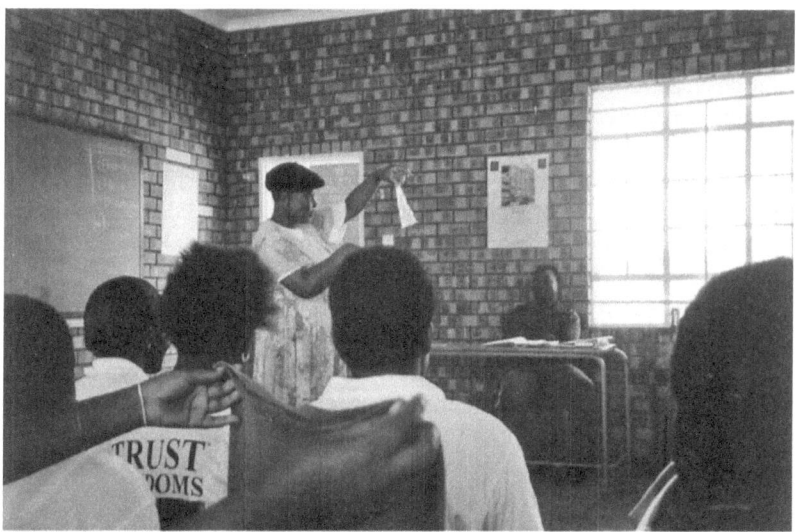

Figure 4.3. Facilitated 'question and answer' session (stage four of the public performance) by educators at the Tshikombani project, at a meeting held for teachers and learners in a local school. The educator holds up a female condom and asks the headteacher (at the desk): 'What is this?'

The way in which different song types, acting, performance, and AIDS-related information are strung together in the FAP formula for peer education bears distinct resemblance to 'cultural productions' by Mayibuye and the Amandla Cultural Ensemble by ANC members in exile during the struggle (Gilbert 2007). Such productions were used to raise support for the anti-apartheid movement outside South Africa. The symbolic resonance between the two, especially with regard to the use of freedom songs to convey a radical message, is another theme of the next chapter – where I will also discuss the extent to which peer educators' actions can be interpreted as resistance.

Each FAP performance, apparently a mere repetition of previous meetings, involves what performance theorists have termed 'critical difference' (Drewal 1991). Each is newly created in every new setting. For example, depending on where a performance is held, the composition of the audience can vary dramatically. Men in beer halls, women at clinics, and combined audiences at taxi ranks react very differently to similar performances. The peer educators often persuade friends and family to come

condoms enjoy greater popularity, due to the marketing that has been invested in them, they are smaller, thinner, and much more likely to break during intercourse than the old silver brand, known in Venda beer halls as *masokisi* (socks). The female condom is popular among sex workers as it can be used without a man's knowledge, but demand regularly outstrips supply.

along for moral support, and their presence significantly changes the dynamics of a performance. Often, the only people in the audience are friends and family, who help the educators through the familiar motions of their performance, but at other times a small crowd gathers to watch the proceedings.

Moreover, the weekly content varies according to which zone leader has organised the performance. Some are known to be humorous, others to be serious, and one in particular excels in overtly sexual innuendo. She encourages the educators to attract the attention of men by exaggerating their own sexuality to encourage male participation in the performance. Under such guidance, songs such as 'Jojo Tshilangano' (see next chapter) can take on overtly sexual characteristics. However, the extent to which this participation encourages men to accept the biomedical model of AIDS is unclear. Given that the package in which this model is wrapped is often one of titillation, they are often disappointed to discover that the educators were merely teasing them.

Or were they? Recent research has drawn attention to women's motivations for extra-marital or casual sexual relationships, showing that the construction of women as victims of their own need for survival (cf. Wojcicki 2002), or as merely in pursuit of economic or emotional security, is often inaccurate. Tawfik and Watkins (2007) offer a timely reminder that women, even in circumstances of extreme poverty, are often active agents in defining their own sexuality, and can be motivated by an array of incitements from passion to revenge for a partner's infidelity. Whilst the structural determinants of gender construction are important, it is equally important not to lose sight of the potential for agency in social and sexual encounters.

Although performance may incorporate critical difference as mentioned above, the mode of delivery of these NGO-initiated sessions has become somewhat formulaic. Over time, both performers and audience have begun to experience fatigue. The audience can easily anticipate the familiar pattern of delivery, and the educators get bored in delivering it. Although volunteers have suggested significant changes to the running order of public performances, these have not been permitted by FAP office staff, as they claim to have a legally binding contractual agreement with funders to provide a specific form of participatory AIDS education.

Furthermore, generational authority and gender become salient markers of divergent group identity during the public performances. These markers distinguish the volunteers from their beer hall audiences (mostly older men). To have a group of (ex)-commercial sex workers performing AIDS education in beer halls where they previously operated certainly makes some sense from the point of view of transforming sexual practice through peer example. In practice, however, volunteers with a history of beer hall sex work are a minority. Most sex workers do not frequent beer halls until they are hidden by the darkness of night. The peer educators, by contrast, perform very early in the evening, as most of them must return home by sunset to perform household chores. The result is that a group of young women often perform to groups of older men who, in Venda, could not possibly be defined as their peers. For this reason, performers are often verbally abused and occasionally ejected from the performance arena. On the other hand, when the public performances are held at clinics or market places, the balance between the educators and the audience is often more conducive to creating an 'enabling' environment, in that more young women are likely to be present in the crowd. Nonetheless, funding priorities stipulate that beer halls – as sites for illicit sexual encounters – should be 'targeted', and the volunteers are powerless to modify this to any significant extent.

As I suggested above, this may be related to a dependence on internally produced documents for the evaluation of projects, but it also points to a situation where a supposedly 'bottom-up' project is, in practice, orchestrated by the needs and expectations of donors and government agencies. The same argument can be made with regard to the confusion over recruitment of educators and the experimental inclusion of men. In this regard, funding priorities consistently take precedence over the content or efficacy of actual projects, and while the FAP office staff ensure their own regular salary, the volunteers 'on the ground' are often left frustrated and experience a distinct lack of participation in project design or management. Indeed, as I now go on to explain, the experience of being a peer educator generally contradicts what project designers expect.

Peer Education and Religious Affiliation

The term 'peer' in peer education projects can be misleading in a variety of ways. It is a highly ambiguous term, imposed by project designers who associate it with equality and high levels of social capital among trusted cohorts (cf. Campbell 2003: 51). However, with reference to an alternative usage of the term, James discusses peer pressure among Zulu adolescents around the time of sexual debut, arguing that 'the egalitarian cosiness associated with peer education in an ideal context must surely be more frequently experienced as the duress of peer pressure in a less-than-ideal context' (2002: 172; cf. Wood et al. 1998). If notions of peer pressure speak to inequalities of power in the gendered construction of sexual identities, then we must pay due attention to the nature of the groups from which the peers are drawn. The evidence presented above demonstrates that the processes of volunteer recruitment in Venda have led to peer education being conducted by a conglomerate of different groups of women from various sections of society.

As the vast majority of young women's time outside of working hours is spent either performing domestic chores or at religious gatherings, Christian denomination is central to the construction of group identities both in Venda and throughout South Africa. With over half of South Africans attending worship once a week or more, it is 'one of the most "churchy" countries in the world' (Garner 2000: 46). Because of this, the church an educator attends is likely to furnish her most important peer group on a day-to-day basis.

This is apparent during the leisure time at weekly training sessions. For example, without coercion by the coordinator to remain in their 'working zones', volunteers consistently sit down to eat in little cliques. The gossiping, eating, laughing, plaiting hair, and resting on each other – in a way that was quite different to the formalised behaviour of the 'zone group' – was suggestive of more genuine friendship networks from which the volunteers at each project were recruited. Those who ate together generally spent more leisure time together outside of working hours, and were members of the same social groups and religious networks. This was evidenced at family funerals every weekend. While the entire group was regularly called upon by the coordinator to assist with cooking and other tasks, those who actually turned up to assist were generally members of the same church-based cliques.

In reality, then, the alleged 'peer group' of AIDS educators in Venda was strongly undermined by separations wrought through religious affiliation. In one project alone, there were several clearly identifiable groups made up of members from the local Apostolic, Zion Christian Church (ZCC), and Lutheran congregations. In other projects there were small groups who did not attend any church. Moreover, whilst groups of royal women from the traditional leader's kraal maintained a certain superiority, their royal status was subsumed under church affiliation. At all projects, there were some women who mostly sat alone and did not seem to be part of any clique. They had been full-time sex workers or had engaged intermittently in 'survival sex' (Wojcicki 2002) before joining the projects. They were stigmatised by the others for having engaged in the open sale of sex in beer halls as a subsistence measure. However, this was never discussed openly, at least not in my presence. Conversely, it was this latter group that received preferential treatment from FAP office staff, especially during visits from funders who were keen to see 'real prostitutes' in their projects.[27]

---

[27] It is very important to note here that different projects have very different group dynamics. At projects towards the Musina border, for example, the majority of educators are engaged in full-time sex work in beer halls, and the recruits from Christian groups are in the minority. I only spent a few weeks at these projects and my data are drawn from projects deeper inside Venda that are not in such proximity to commercial centres or migration highways like the N1.

Religious affiliation is a good indicator of an educator's previous lived experience. It emerged from my collection of life histories that most peer educators who had been through stages of female initiation as they grew up were members of African Independent Churches (AICs) such as the ZCC or Apostolic churches. These denominations of Christianity are highly syncretic, permitting members to participate in symbolic acts of initiation (*vhusha ya vhatendi* – '*vhusha* of the believers'; see Chapter 3). Some peer educators explained during interviews that their attendance at these churches was prompted in part by their wish to worship with other initiated women as well as by their provision of the possibility for their own daughters to 'be sung for' (*u imbelwa*). By becoming initiated women in the church, they take an active part in the initiation of young girls. Through this they create and sustain hierarchies of authority within the wider church community. Although the secretive nature of initiation prevents them from discussing many details openly, they clearly take pride in their associations with and exhaustive knowledge of *mvelele* (culture):

We, at the project [traditional dancing project], understand our responsibilities and respect our ancestors when they come to us to help. These days most people have forgotten these things, and you see now we have no jobs, and people are getting sick. (Interview, F. R., 2 April 2004)

Most of the several non-Christian cohorts were recruited from networks associated with 'culture industry' projects that promote traditional practices, such as the one at Dopeni. These women are well known to be specialists not only in the arts of initiation and ancestral worship but also the *malombo* possession ritual (*ngoma dza vhadzimu*). During *malombo*, ancestral spirits (*Vhadzimu* or *Midzimu*) communicate with their living relatives during all-night dancing sessions through which therapeutic mediation of affliction is achieved (cf. van Warmelo 1932: 141; Jansen 1992: 108; Blacking 1995a). Like the girls undergoing the *vhusha* ceremony described in the previous chapter, the position of such peer educators is perhaps similar to that of the 'salempore girls' described by Blacking. They are drawn from the significant minority of traditionalists who reject Christianity despite, or perhaps even in reaction against, the influence of the Christian majority.

In the peer education projects I worked with, these traditionalists made up about 10 per cent of the volunteers, while members of AICs were in the majority (roughly 60 per cent), followed by those who attended mission/mainline churches (roughly 30 per cent).[28] The mission Christians,

---

[28] See Chapter 3 for a definition of this taxonomy of Christian churches. These figures are taken from in-depth interviews with 96 peer educators between April and July 2004, and from 60 questionnaires distributed at different projects in 2003. Of course, at different projects some denominations are more common than others. The percentages are rounded off and should be used as a rough guide only, as volunteer turnover in projects is significant.

in line with established literature on the subject, placed more importance on formal education and their fathers generally belonged to an established middle class of relatively wealthy migrant labourers, successful local farmers, teachers, or civil servants (Cochrane 1986; de Gruchy and de Gruchy 2004; Egan 2007). The members of ZCC or Apostolic churches, on the other hand, exhibited markedly lower standards of educational achievement and had annual household incomes that reflected their lower economic status. Nonetheless, in terms of time and money, they donated more on a weekly basis to their churches than members of mission or mainline denominations.

Zionist and Apostolic congregations believe that possession can be the work of the Holy Spirit or the ancestors, and it is generally accepted that their convention of nocturnal dancing sessions (*mkuku* – to stamp the Devil back into the ground) is associated with possession by denizens of the wider spirit world (Comaroff 1985; Naude 1995; Anderson 1999). The doctrine of mission denominations (mostly Lutheran), on the other hand, remains heavily influenced by the teachings of German missionaries: they have long defined traditional activities such as initiation and *malombo* as constituting unacceptable acts of pagan worship (Kirkaldy 2005: 182). Peer educators from mission denominations are thus prone to seeing their relationship with those in the African Independent Churches in judgemental and hierarchical terms. They represent their own lifestyles as modern and progressive in contrast to the backward, less Christian practices of others:

At church last Sunday we were addressed by a pastor from Pretoria. He was fantastic! He told us that we should only praise one God, and that he knows many people here in Venda continue to praise the dead. He read to us from the Bible that this is a great sin... and it is true, even the girls at the [peer education] project are doing it.... They say they even make money from it [here she is referring to the commoditisation/rationalisation of ritual described in the previous chapter]. (G. R., Diary 13: p. 44, translated from Tshivenda)

Whilst these religious divisions derive from events in individual life histories, they also influence directly the ways in which peer education is practised on a daily basis. At the weekly training session, for example, important decisions about the Friday public performance must be made. These include choosing who will lead a melody, change a song lyric, or correct a dance routine. As arguments are usually settled through recourse to previous experience, those affiliated with AICs (and thus with more experience of traditional activities) take more responsibility for stage five's traditional drumming session; likewise, those from mission churches, with more experience of gospel and choral songs, tend to take charge of organising stage two's choral arrangements. Religious divisions that were formed outside of peer education thus provide the basis for a pragmatic division of musical labour within the projects.

However, at the same time, members of these different groups harbour grudges, jealousies, and suspicions about each other. Although these feelings do not often come to the fore, their 'backstage' presence is unstintingly acknowledged. At one project, during the weekly training session a Roman Catholic group openly accused members of the Apostolic Faith Mission church of poisoning them. Despite interventions from several office staff (and me) the matter was never fully resolved, and the volunteers remained suspicious of each other. Several of them left the project. Seen in this light, claims by advocates of peer education in Venda to have achieved behaviour change through the 'subjective judgements of close, trusted peers' (Wilson 2000) can seem rather hollow. If such change has occurred, it has happened only at the micro-level of religious cliques, and not within the group as a whole.

In this section I have argued that, in peer educator projects in Venda, the notion of 'peer' embodies considerable ambiguity and is even misleading. The implications of this are not necessarily such as to induce pessimism. As Mosse has suggested, the relative success or failure of such projects depends upon having groups of people buy into them on whatever seem to be the most appropriate terms (Mosse 2004). Peer education has brought together divergent groups: the continued distinction between them is productive in that it provides for a division of labour in the projects. Nonetheless, this has created volatile cliques which, based on religious affiliation, represent peer groups in a more accurate sense. The divisiveness of religious separation potentially inhibits the overall efficacy of the project, and calls into question the notion of a uniform and homogeneous group of peers. Instead of conducting peer education within previously existing social networks, the FAP has attempted to smooth over differences between divergent social groups by creating a 'one size fits all' scheme that leaves the 'peer' in peer education a potentially misleading term. The pressure to produce funder-friendly statistics indicating how many males have been reached, condoms distributed and the like, forces the FAP to maintain its rigid format for peer education, and impinges on the extent to which educators can actually 'participate' in the processes of project design and implementation.

As I now go on to demonstrate, however, religious divisions – whilst important for understanding the group dynamics of peer education projects – should be seen in relation to wider affiliation with the NGO and, by extension, aspired-to association with the government. Becoming a peer educator presents the potential to create a new, upwardly mobile 'self' in which religious affiliation does not play a defining role. In this context, we must re-evaluate the extent to which membership of mission or African Independent Churches – originally influential in the creation of class identities – continue to be divisive in the post-apartheid dispensation. Instead, I now go on to consider the role of NGOs (especially the least 'non-governmental' among them) in providing new opportunities for class mobility.

Peer Educators' Motivations

Altruism and empowerment are only part of the motivation for joining a peer education project. To shed some light on the peer educator experience, I start this section with two condensed career histories.

Career History One

Tshifhiwa became a volunteer at the Ha-Rabali peer education project in 1998. She had been out of school and not working for some time, and heard about people doing voluntary work through a friend at the Lutheran church. She went along and became a volunteer on the same day. Her favourite aspect of it at that time was the gospel singing and dancing as practice for public performances. In 2000 she was promoted to 'field support coordinator' and given responsibility for supervising several new projects – some of which were over 40 miles away. In late 2000 she was 'contracted' by a health promotion and research organisation to be the 'outreach officer' for their farm worker intervention project on the Zimbabwe border. In 2002, having seen out the contract, she moved back to the FAP to become the 'peer education outreach officer'. This put her in charge of coordinating and supervising all of the organisation's prevention programmes – where she remains today.

Career History Two

Mavhungu also joined the Ha-Rabali peer education project in 1998. Like Tshifhiwa, she had heard about it through word of mouth and was already volunteering in several church-based groups in her local branch of the ZCC. She had a real desire to make living conditions in Venda better in the post-apartheid era, and joined in all the peer education activities with a passion. In 1999 she became a zone leader and then, in 2000, coordinator of the project. With the award of a government lay counselling tender to the FAP, she successfully applied for one of the positions. She was instrumental in setting up the first support group for people living with AIDS at Siloam hospital in 2003 and then in 2005 she got a permanent position in the public sector as part of the management team in the AIDS clinic at the same hospital.

The career histories above represent a well-established pattern of employment opportunities for volunteers within the FAP. The first case of which I became aware in Venda was that of Munaki, the original volunteer at the project, who now travels the world to give presentations at AIDS conferences as the organisation's director. That a similar process of graduation through the ranks is aspired to by peer educators was demonstrated in the opening story of this chapter, which describes a group's birthday party. Of the many dignitaries and keynote speakers invited to attend that function, the premier slot (just before lunch) was given to a small group of ex-volunteers who had progressed into fulltime positions working as HIV/AIDS trainers in the local government municipality's Department of Public Works. Their presentation evoked rapturous applause, and they spoke explicitly about how the FAP had been a 'stepping stone' for them from poverty, through security, and into relative prosperity. In the eyes of current volunteers, these were classic examples of *real* peer educators since their positions had led them to find stable employment. This important pattern must be explained through other programmes coordinated by the FAP, such as voluntary counselling and testing and home-based care. A brief outline of their activities will serve to make the point.

Voluntary counselling and testing (VCT)

The FAP was awarded a highly sought-after government tender (partly funded by Oxfam Australia) in late 2004 to provide VCT and facilitate support groups for people living with AIDS in the Vhembe District.[29] This was part of a wider national government agenda to make HIV testing and ARV medication more accessible in rural areas, and also to provide more accurate HIV prevalence statistics, which had previously been formulated only on the basis of pregnant women attending antenatal clinics. The lay counsellors, as they are known, receive a relatively substantial monthly wage of R2,500, for which they work as quasi-nursing assistants on a nine-to-five, Monday-to-Friday basis. They undergo several weeks of government training and examination, after which they receive official certificates and are given the title of lay counsellor. As experienced volunteers, skilled in confidentiality and AIDS-related knowledge, they are responsible for pre- and post-test counselling, performing HIV antibody tests, administering Nevirapine for the prevention of mother-to-child transmission (PMTCT), and running the support groups for people with AIDS at rural clinics and health centres. They cannot, however, administer antiretroviral medication, a role confined to selected larger hospitals and official projects in the region.

Of the 56 lay counsellors employed at over 30 rural clinics and health centres in May 2005, all but six had been recruited directly from peer education programmes.

---

[29] The other two organisations in the district to be awarded the tender were the Planned Parenthood Association of South Africa (PPASA) and Takalani Nama, an NGO for people living with AIDS in the Polokwane area.

Home-based care (HBC)

The section of the FAP responsible for providing HBC works in partnership with the provincial government, church groups, and the PSG. The volunteers (almost 500 in May 2006, working with over 6,000 patients in 24 project sites) attend a comprehensive 'minimum standards' training course provided by provincial government, and are subject to annual assessment in which their knowledge and skills are evaluated.[30] With few exceptions, HBC volunteers are women, with an average age of 38 (in 2005); they receive a stipend of R1,000 per month (cf. Raman 2005 for an account of how men have been integrated into HBC activities).

There is a strong emphasis on 'spiritual counselling' within HBC and almost all of the volunteers are recruited through a broad spectrum of local church networks. This reflects the existence of substantial pastoral care programmes undertaken by many churches throughout the Venda region. HBC volunteers work closely with their respective churches, and generally conduct their daily business within these existing social groupings. For example, the project at Tshakhuma (see maps) has a strong connection with the local Catholic mission clinic and many of the volunteers are members of the congregation there. Indeed, Catholic churches have been pioneers in cooperative palliative care projects in much of rural South Africa (Egan 2007). At other projects, based on both mission and AIC churches, the same kind of relationship between church membership and volunteer recruitment applies. Volunteers often use church meetings to request information about house-bound friends or relatives who are then visited by the HBC volunteers in the congregation. In an attempt to reduce the stigma attached to their actions, and in line with PSG instruction, HBC volunteers treat and care for *any* house-bound individuals, regardless of their affliction.

A trained HBC volunteer is qualified to prescribe and administer simple medication such as antibiotics and TB drugs, and in two pilot projects they work with Family Health International (FHI) to provide palliative care and assistance in the distribution of ARV drugs to patients who have full-blown AIDS. They are trained in pre- and post-test counselling but cannot perform the HIV antibody test except in the presence of a qualified nurse. Daily activities include praying with and washing clients, most of whom are bed-bound with open sores, and delivering food and clothes parcels donated by various local and national charities.

---

[30] The content of national government minimum standards workshops for VCT and HBC was drawn up in close collaboration with the FAP project coordinators.

> HBC groups provide another important example of career opportunities from within the ranks of peer education. As HBC was established from 1999/2000, the most promising and committed peer educators (who had often developed 'close' relationships with various office staff) were selected as candidates for the positions: they already had basic HIV/AIDS training and were acquainted with the bureaucratic procedures of the FAP office. Of the 24 projects that were functional in 2005, *every* HBC project coordinator had a career history of peer education.

In terms of the argument being made here, there was no recognisable pattern of religious affiliation amongst the educators who became lay counsellors or HBC coordinators. Neither did earlier promotions to the position of zone leader demonstrate any religious bias. These decisions were made by office staff (on a panel that included two board members) on the basis of career history, reliability, and 'potential to develop a career in public health'. Of the 74 appointees (50 lay counsellors and 24 HBC coordinators), 29 were from mainline churches and 40 from AIC denominations. The remaining five were either Pentecostal or non-Christian. Although this appears unbalanced, it is quite consistent with the general pattern of religious affiliation within peer education projects (roughly 30 per cent mainline and 60 per cent AIC), and from this cursory use of statistics – with an accepted margin of error – it would appear that Christian denomination, previously so determinant of or associated with socio-economic class division, no longer affects a young woman's chances of progressing towards full-time, stable employment.

This pattern of social mobility can be mapped onto wider trends of class formation in post-apartheid South Africa. Seekings and Nattrass (2005: 247) have suggested that we can stratify class position in South Africa into five broad categories: upper class (managers, professionals); semi-professional class (teachers, nurses); intermediate class (white collar, skilled, supervisory); core working class (semi- and unskilled workers); and marginal working class (farm and domestic workers). Whilst they demonstrate that in the post-apartheid era there has been a rise in very visible African 'middle' classes[31] that have benefited inter alia from governmental policies of Black Economic Empowerment, they also show that the main economic change since the 1990s has been a fall in formal employment (ibid.: 314).

It is difficult to fit peer education into this schema with any accuracy, but attempting to do so puts the data presented in this chapter into a wider context. Given that an overall trend in the post-apartheid

---

[31] They suggest that, relatively, these were a very privileged upper class, but that models of class analysis are incapable of contextualising this adequately.

era has been a marked rise in levels of unemployment (Daniel et al. 2005; Southall 2007) and that the few jobs that have become available have largely gone to the previously privileged (Seekings and Nattrass 2006: 336), it is hardly surprising that unemployed, rural women such as peer educators are keen to grasp the opportunity for employment when it arises. Peer education would appear to provide a significant opportunity for 'intragenerational' upward class mobility – a rise in status occurring within the course of an individual's lifetime (ibid.: 261). But from what, and to what?

Given that the starting point is one of extremely low status, the aspired-to position promises a considerable leap up the ladder of social mobility. However, voluntary work is not included in the stratification suggested by Seekings and Nattrass. This omission may yield an inaccurate picture, given that peer educators receive a monthly stipend of between R500 and R1,000. Domestic workers in rural South Africa (part of the 'marginal working class') do not receive much more than this. The full-time positions that peer educators have achieved in government programmes for voluntary counselling and testing, however, fall between semi-professional and intermediate classes. Acquiring such a position represents a significant leap in socio-economic status, and a class mobility that is all the more remarkable given the general context of endemic unemployment within which it is occurring.

This may help to contextualise the excerpts from peer educator diaries below, in which this upward mobility (whether experienced or aspirational) is consistently expressed in terms of government, not NGO, employment (*muvhusoni* – 'in the government'):

When I came here [to the project] I thought it would be good to help other people because I was just lying around all day. My mother always told me to keep busy, but as we all know there are no jobs here in Venda these days. Still, it is good to help other people. In church and in town people now look at me and think that I am working for the government. (Book D/4: 33. This and the following excerpts translated from Tshivenda)

Before [I joined the project] I was drinking and just making money through men. It was not a good life before, but I hope that being at the project can help change that. Men can be so cruel, but when we love them [have sex] it is still nice. Things will be better when I get a real job [*mushumu vhukhuma*] ... we want a job in the government. (Book T/20: 2)

I was really happy today to find people at my home waiting for condoms. They addressed me just like a nurse working at the hospital, and I gave them some and showed them how to use them. (Book T/7: 4)

I really wanted to make a change, to help people here in Venda. I want to be a nurse, and marry a doctor [she was joking here] maybe, and travel abroad... being a peer educator is good for us, but the money is not enough. How can I feed my children? It is just not enough. (Book T/16: 22–3)

Really, we were just selling our bodies, me and the others... we enjoyed it at times, getting gifts and going to the hotel... we all miss that but now we are trying to change it... these things are painful [to talk about]. (Book D/15: 10)

Clearly, such sentiments indicate that altruism and the desire to modify lifestyles are significant motivational incentives for some to volunteer. However, they also reflect the powerful desire to get onto a rung of the ladder of employment outlined in the career histories and through the examples of VCT and HBC. These two incentives are not mutually exclusive. Rather, when experienced together, they vigorously propel young women into positions as peer educators.

This is expressed by the volunteer whose ambition is to change her lifestyle in order to 'get a real job'. For this woman the crucial factor, the ultimate destination, in becoming a volunteer is the ambition to progress through the ranks and find alternative, stable employment. 'Real' peer educators, if they are successful, should get real jobs, and such opportunities exist in the public health sector. It is expected that this progression will be gradual, with incremental promotions from volunteer to zone leader, to coordinator, then to lay counsellor or other such positions. This upward social mobility is associated with a substantial increase in remuneration and elevation in status and authority. In other words, a central intention in becoming a peer educator is to leave the group in which they are deemed peers – to rise above it and '[to] acquire distance from, rather than being embedded more deeply in, an undifferentiated "community"' (James 2002: 183).

As James goes on to suggest, peer educators often feel more attached to the NGO they are working for than to any peer group. The evidence presented here indicates that this can be explained, at least partially, by the perception that volunteering is the first step to public sector employment. In the current economic climate, where a small but rapidly rising and highly visible middle class – known cynically as 'tenderpreneurs' – is funded largely by the award of government contracts to its members, it is hardly surprising that peer educators express a desire for government employment. The flattery of being recognised as a government employee, as a nurse or a quasi-social worker, is thus welcomed and appreciated by peer educators. Given the recent history of successful FAP government tenders, they have every reason to believe that their ambitions may one day be fulfilled. With a relatively high labour turnover brought on by the regular opportunities for promotion, peer education can be a competitive enterprise, and the stakes are high.

This state of affairs exposes a fundamental contradiction. The desire of programme designers for long-term, sustainable, and efficacious projects clashes with the pragmatic ways in which the ANC-led government – through NGOs – has sought to train and employ as many rural unemployed people as possible. The government has been expected not only to create jobs, but also to provide training for the rural poor who were marginalised under apartheid. Black Economic Empowerment has created small, mostly urban, elites – many of whom had their roots in the black middle class created under apartheid. But it has done little to address the concerns of those on the periphery. In this wider context, then, government may claim that the frequent and expensive 'workshops' through which HBC volunteers and lay counsellors are trained and assessed on an annual basis are long-term investments in the rural poor. It is hoped that the Department of Health will receive returns from this if, and when, volunteers progress into the public health care sector as nurses, counsellors, trainers, or HIV support workers. As an FAP project coordinator told me: 'the government wants our volunteers to be career-minded! In fact, it needs them to be so'.

This throws significant doubt on the implicit assumption made by project designers that most peer educators will (want to) remain in the voluntary sector long enough to assist in the creation of 'enabling contexts' for the promotion of health-enhancing behaviour. It further suggests that, for peer educators in Venda, the notion of empowerment is understood more in terms of the individual social and financial benefits of getting a 'real job' in the public sector than it is in deriving 'respect and recognition' for a voluntary role in promoting health (cf. Campbell 2000: 492), although the two are not unrelated. In practice, peer education projects are more successful at improving the life chances of the few volunteers who join them than benefiting the 'peers' with whom they attempt to renegotiate sexual identities.[32]

Conclusion

Religious divisions that form genuine 'peer' groups in the projects, then, are mediated rather than exacerbated by new opportunities for upward social mobility through affiliation with an NGO. In an overall context of rising unemployment, joining the peer educators offers a potential route into employment and out of the overwhelming perception of a crisis in social reproduction. Ironically, while the AIDS pandemic has contributed significantly to the perception of emergency, it has also provoked a catalyst through which these young, poor, women seek upward mobility in the hope of mediating their own personal crises.

---

[32] I have evidence to suggest that many peer educators have not led by example in using condoms, which has broad implications for the 'creation of an enabling context'. The evidence includes secrets told to me by men who have had illicit relationships with peer educators and is reflected in high rates of pregnancy among unmarried educators. Also, not one peer educator has become open about her HIV status. This hardly creates an enabling context for others.

I shall end by underscoring the themes to be picked up in the following chapter. Clearly, the recruitment process of peer education has led to a situation that is far from ideal for a collective renegotiation of sexual behaviour. The projects' division into zones cross-cut rather than reflect pre-existing social networks based on religious affiliation. This forms a barrier to group cohesion and to the kind of effective 'community contact' that might be based upon pre-existing connections. HBC volunteers, in contrast, work more closely within their religious groups and use the networks of sociality that surround church life to their advantage. Thus, as peer education projects attempt unsuccessfully to traverse the boundaries between historically divergent social and economic groups, HBC projects work within religious and domestic arrangements that make their programmes more likely to succeed.

The importance of secrecy employed by the HBC volunteers should not be underestimated. HBC is relatively successful precisely because of its discretion and use of existing networks and, as we shall see in Chapter 7, the lack of these qualities in peer education contributes greatly to the difficulties experienced by the volunteers. By avoiding open, public conversation about AIDS, by treating house-bound clients regardless of their affliction, and by working under the guise of relatives, home-based carers are able to avoid the suspicions of the wider public. This is part of a process through which they construct 'degrees of separation' in the negotiation of limited responsibility for deaths perceived to be unnatural. In stark contrast to this, peer educators regularly exhibit their expert knowledge of HIV/AIDS in public, drawing attention to their fluency in biomedical discourse. This is largely expressed through musical performance, and it is to the music incorporated into public performances that I now turn.

5 'We Sing about What We Cannot Talk About'

Biomedical Knowledge in Stanza

In Venda – and throughout Southern Africa – knowledge can be dangerous. Potentially hazardous information, such as that pertaining to sexual health or death, is conventionally transferred through the lyrics of songs in highly prescribed ritual contexts, under the protection of an ancestral hierarchy or a Christian God. In this way, the bearers of dangerous knowledge in Venda negotiate limited responsibility for what they know. With the accumulation of such knowledge comes a responsibility to manage the associated risks. Most peer educators have direct experience of this through their attendance at female initiation, where girls become women by entering into the stratified structures of ritual knowledge, and where they graduate with the socially recognised ability to manage monthly ablutions and maintain fertility. In this controlled ritual context, stratified by hierarchies of ritual knowledge, the ancestors (through the authority of ritual elders) actively facilitate healthy reproduction – mostly through the didactic performance of initiation songs and the learning of 'laws' (*milayo*). Music, in this context, acts as a medium for the complete and safe transference of ritual knowledge whilst the songs, dances, and *milayo* of initiation represent the desire for continuity in healthy social and sexual reproduction (cf. Blacking 1969a–1969e; 1973; La Fontaine 1985).

Peer educators use music in a broadly similar manner. In one sense – and in the eyes of project designers – songs and dances are a cheap and readily available medium through which educators can pursue their goal of knowledge transfer during public performances. But their use of music is multifaceted, and must be understood on different levels. They intentionally select specific songs within certain genres through which they construct a complex group identity by association with their chosen performances. In addition to this, by framing AIDS education through music, peer educators seek – but do not necessarily achieve – the relative protection which these genres afford in different contexts. In this way they pursue new ends by old means.

In the previous chapter I analysed the ways in which peer education has been adapted to HIV prevention in South Africa and the fluctuating social and economic dynamics to which this has given rise. I now want to focus on the songs used in this enterprise before turning, in the following chapter, to the male-dominated *zwilombe* guitar songs with which I will compare them. This approach will allow me to assess the extent to which the biomedical model has interacted with alternative understandings of the HI virus, and the implications of this for people's understandings of the epidemic. My specific focus on songs is not arbitrary; nor is it simply a result of the widespread use of musical performance in Venda peer education. Rather, it reflects explicit concerns of the peer educators who regularly claim to 'sing about what [they] cannot talk about' (McNeill 2008).

Peer educators group the songs they perform into specific categories.[1] To some extent, this categorisation is the result of the training received by representatives of the Forum for AIDS Prevention (FAP) who learned peer education techniques from psychologists at the University of Zimbabwe. They were taught that using locally recognised songs would increase the impact of their performances. Educators in Venda decided to have four categories of music, which they defined as 'church', 'struggle', 'traditional', and 'original'. Public performances are structured around different mini-performances in each of these genres.

The imposition of boundaries between musical genres is clearly problematic. In the South African context, for example, where Christian hymns were regularly adapted into anthems for the anti-apartheid movement, when does a 'church' song transform to become a 'struggle' song? South Africa's national anthem, *Nkosi Sikelele Afrika* (God Bless Africa), is a case in point. In religious groups such as the Zion Christian Church (ZCC), in which the synchronistic blending of pre- and post-missionary elements takes on new meanings, when does a 'traditional' drumbeat become a 'church' one? One might argue that in any specific historical and social context, the extent of borrowing between musical genres as they develop over time erodes the extent to which any form of musical expression can be deemed truly 'original'.

But the peer educators are not exercised by matters of academic abstraction. They are well aware that the categories into which they group songs are fluid. It is this very fluidity that they seek to manipulate in redefining the songs as vehicles for AIDS education. By categorising their repertoire, they are laying claim to meanings that are very much 'up for grabs', and their sense of ownership over the songs comes from their creative engagement with them. Most of the songs looked at in this chapter could be defined in at least two of the educators' categories. But through this categorisation they seek to achieve symbolic associations with different forms of power and authority by blending political, church, and traditional elements into their public performances. In doing

[1] I have recorded over 200 of these songs since 1999.

so, they hope to legitimate their enterprise and to garner public support through regular demonstrations of their creativity.

When looked at in isolation as a group of 'peer educator songs', these forms of cultural expression reflect the new-found optimism of quasi-social workers, fluent in the nuances of biomedical discourse and well-acquainted with the subtle fluctuations in government policy that we saw in the previous chapter. The combination of politically motivated songs of struggle, church, and tradition serves, in culturally appropriate ways, to laminate this new content together with existing melodic and dance patterns familiar to the general public.

Without any convincing evidence, project designers, funders, and NGO 'experts' have assumed that this hybridising strategy will contribute to behavioural change in the target population. By the end of this book, serious questions will have arisen as to the validity of this assumption. Foremost among these is the extent to which songs about AIDS can really be a powerful force for change in an environment where open conversation – and the public display of knowledge – about death and illness can have far-reaching and potentially counter-productive consequences.

Both the peer educators and the male *zwilombe* musicians with whom I compare them in Chapter 6 represent distinctly marginal social groups. Both propagate distinct, and partly conflicting, forms of knowledge with the hope of consolidating their prospects of social advancement. Creative musicality is the central process through which this knowledge is transferred to the wider public. These two bodies of somewhat distinct yet partially converging knowledge represent attempts to secure productive and reproductive capacities to act on the world; but they lead to very different conclusions about how best to avoid disease. Thus peer educators employ music and fluency in biomedicine as a means of asserting new individualised and entrepreneurial strategies of self-advancement, with the aim of full-time government employment. As I show in the following chapter, *zwilombe* musicians – in contrast – mobilise their musicality as a means of reacting against new, imposed, and fragmentary forms of (re)production, exchange, and consciousness in favour of the older identities which they reassert. In doing so, they enunciate a rather different political alignment. Symbolic references to post-apartheid traditionalism are woven into guitar songs designed to restore, and show their singer/composer's allegiance to, collective patriarchal/ancestral authority in preference to the perceived rise of fragmented individualism.

Performance as the 'Tip of an Iceberg'

Ethnomusicologists and anthropologists of Southern and South Africa have long argued that the composition and performance of songs and dances is integral to the affirming or creating of identities. Early research, with an apparently more conservative emphasis, highlighted the role of musical performance in the configuring of fixed social contexts, delineating life-cycle stages, political allegiances, or gender positions. A subsequent generation of scholars, with a more transformative focus, has embraced social theories which account for the emergence of popular forms in the wake of capitalism and industrialisation, examining how musical performance can transcend social positioning to create new practices and ideas of society and selfhood (Erlmann 1991; 1996; Coplan 1994; James 1999; 2006).

The peer educators' claim that they sing about what they cannot talk about struck me as familiar. It resonates with anthropological approaches that suggest performance may allow people to say things they would not otherwise be able to articulate and thus provide access to what Vail and White have called ethnography from 'within' and history 'from below' (1983: 887; cf. Vail and White 1990). Thus the analysis of musical performance can grant the anthropologist 'privileged access to layers of consciousness that are normally not available to scholarly examination' (Erlmann 1991: 12). In this vein, Fabian (1990: 12–13) has suggested that performance is 'the tip of the iceberg of culture floating in a sea of history and consciousness'.[2] Fabian's analysis of Shaba-Swahili performing arts was inspired by Victor Turner's earlier theoretical concern with plays, ritual, and festivals. These, he argued, must be read not as mere enactment but as the regeneration of symbols and meanings that constantly change (1982). Fabian builds on this to construct a notion of 'performative ethnography' through which anthropologists can understand culture not only through interpretation of a set of symbols but also through enactment and performance. Such an approach is intended to facilitate the reading of forms of knowledge that are not expressed in discursive statements, but which find their way into the public domain through alternative action, such as plays, poems, and songs (1990: 6).

In the South African context, Erlmann (1996) and Coplan (1994) have provided accounts of how anthropological analysis of performance can reveal more than meets the eye. Their studies validate the later claim that the performance of popular culture 'enable[s] people to engage with present difficulties in a creative manner' (Kaarsholm and James 2000: 198). Coplan's analysis, for example, does this by looking at sung and spoken poetry (*sefela*). The active role of writing and performing *sefela* in the construction of working-class Basotho migrant consciousness shapes the agency through which a migrant makes life choices in the face of the structural constraints and expectations he encounters. The historically salient transition from herd boy to heroic male through the course of

---

[2] Fabian and Erlmann here use 'consciousness' to refer to the active process in which human actors deploy historically salient cultural categories to construct their self-awareness (Comaroff and Comaroff 1987).

one's travels is at once remembered and reconstructed by the active, and apparently simultaneous, process of *sefela* composition and performance.

Erlmann's account of *isicathamiya* demonstrates migrant Zulu males' musical performance as resistance: an ongoing 'form of struggle' (Erlmann 1996: xix). Challenging the dominant power relations of social and political oppression under apartheid, the performers propose an alternative ideal social order. They attempt to fuse the negative structural relationships of their immediate environment with positive meaning by replicating its competitive logic on a smaller and more manageable scale in *isicathamiya* performances and competitions. Exponents of the genre thus attempt to return coherence into a world shattered beyond their control by singing critically about the alienation of migrant life. Their concerns over the loss of domestic cohesion and the loosening of patriarchal authority are contained in musical and choreographic arrangements which as performers they do control. Erlmann suggests that performance is thus not merely a response to or reflection of social relationships, but 'in itself a form of realistic praxis that asks questions about society' (1996: 242).

Performance thus constitutes the search for an autonomous social and political sphere, a created space able to connect notions of the past and the present, and through which new ideas are spun and contested.[3] The songs and social processes involved in singing about AIDS in Venda reveal the interconnections between gendered and generational ways of understanding sex, health, and death. Whilst these dovetailing relationships are historically constituted, they have been recast in the face of the AIDS pandemic, breathing new life into old songs and bringing hopes of social advancement to the young women who sing them.

The pervasive culture of performance in Venda has been exceptionally well documented and analysed. Primarily through John Blacking's work, the region became famous in ethnomusicological circles with seminars, conferences, and edited volumes making consistent reference to the area and to his work there (cf. Byron 1995; Reily 2006). Blacking's research, as I suggested in the introductory chapter, covered almost every social, political, and aesthetic aspect of musical performance in Venda. He mapped the many different genres onto specific stages in the progression of a calendar year, such as the performance of *malende* party songs after harvest and working songs (*dzinyimbo dza davhani*) during the sowing season (1965: 30). Blacking's work also stressed the connections between musical repertoire and an individual's life cycle, such as the songs of children (1967) or female initiates (1969a–1969e), or the *tshikona* dance in relation to traditional political power in the region

---

[3] See Meintjes (2003; 2004), James (1999), Muller (1999), and Gunner (1991) for further examples of musical performance in South Africa as historically constituted social practice, and Vail and White (1983) for an example of this in Mozambique.

(1965: 37). In this way, he demonstrated that the performance of specific genres plays a central role in the designation of fixed social positions, and that musical recital is central to the ways in which people in Venda recognise and maintain social difference and deference to the hierarchical order upon which political power and ritual authority is based.

But Blacking's Venda material also revealed his view that music has the potential to radically alter the world in which it is a part. It is this aspect of his work, the conviction that music can embody 'resilience in the face of oppression', that has made a lasting impact on ethnomusicology in the region and beyond, and is now akin to conventional wisdom (James 2006: 74). Blacking mostly developed this theoretical angle in *How Musical Is Man?* (1973) – his most widely read and influential work – in which he argued for the innate musical capacity of humans and the mystical potential of that music to effect positive changes among those who perform it. In the analysis of songs that follows, I draw on this theoretical legacy. Between music's role as a conservative force for equilibrium and a radical force for change can be found the clues to understanding the lyrical content of contemporary music performances.

The Songs of HIV/AIDS Peer Educators[4]

The Tshikombani peer educators hold a weekly training session in the disused hall behind Ha-Netisa Restaurant.[5] In the evenings, the hall is frequented by local drinkers seeking moments of solitude with their lovers. Over the years, the empty beer crates and broken bottles left behind by the revellers have been a constant annoyance to the educators, most of whom do not drink alcohol. I joined the educators on a warm, rainy morning in 2005, and they had come prepared – after the previous day's rehearsal – to have some of their songs recorded for my research. As usual, they set about sweeping the floor with grass brooms (*luswielo*) before rearranging the beer crates into small clusters, one in each corner for each zone group.

I was standing outside waiting for my assistant when I heard Mme a Mapule, the group coordinator, open the session with a well-known Lutheran church hymn. 'Jesus, Jesus, Jesus is number one! No matter what the people say, but Jesus is number one!' Clapping hands provided percussion. Two latecomers, dressed in their bright red skirts, began to sing along as they idled slowly up the track towards the hall. One of them stopped. A slither of glass from the broken bottles that had been swept

---

[4] With the exceptions of 'Condom is Number One!', '*I Ya Vhulaya*', and '*Lele*', the peer educator songs discussed in this chapter can be heard on the accompanying website at http://www.cambridge.org/us/9781107009912, along with renditions of *tshikona* and *domba* music. See Appendix A for details.

[5] Not the real name.

out of the hall was now lodged in her foot. She cursed as she picked it out.

Then she burst out laughing, distracting the assembled educators much to Mme a Mapule's frustration. Under a trashed cardboard box next to the broken glass, the latecomer had spotted the bright silver corner of an empty 'government issue' condom wrapper. '*Ro winna!*' she shouted, '*Zwidakwa zwi khou shumisa dzikhondomu dzashu!*' (We have won! The drunkards are using our condoms!) Holding the empty wrapper aloft, she entered the sparse hall in a shuffle that picked up the time of clapping hands. Taking the next verse before anyone else had a chance and pitching it high, she declared that condoms, not Jesus, were now number one: 'Condom, condom, condom is number one, no matter what the people say, but condom is number one!'

Not everyone approved. A few educators who attend the local Lutheran church told her to stop, as Jesus could never be compared to a condom. They argued that people would be offended by the lyrics, and that the educator in question (a prominent member of the local Zionist church) had the intention of degrading 'real' Christian beliefs. Her Zionist friends came to her defence, shouting in response that the Lutherans were 'lost' (*no xela*) and that many ZCC songs had been made into AIDS slogans. After the dust had settled, they took a vote. It was decided that 'Condom is number one!' would indeed be adopted as part of the group repertoire. Whilst some educators remained uncomfortable with the decision, they were swayed by the group coordinator's argument that 'shock tactics' might convince people to take more notice of their public performances and that, ultimately, it was worth the gamble.

As this narrative demonstrates, peer educators change the lyrics to well-known songs, but they try to keep any modifications as simple as possible. They practise cyclical repetition of 'call' (*u sima* – to plant) and 'response' (*u bvumela* – to thunder) vocal parts, broken down into arrangements of rhythm and harmony which reflect their varied music backgrounds. Religious affiliation is an important characteristic, and hence indicator, of the socially embedded groups from which peer educators are constituted, and church songs are used throughout their weekly training sessions for opening and closing prayers, and for the blessing of food. As the example above demonstrates, different groups bring songs and melodies from their Sunday worship into the peer education arena. The hymns used in this way thus combine elements of 'mission' with African Independent Christianity, and in different areas they fluctuate in popularity to reflect the demographic dynamics of divergent projects. Sometimes an adaptation is spontaneous, but they usually present a previously written piece, or work within their zone group to find alternative lyrics that can encapsulate succinctly biomedical notions of HIV, AIDS, treatment, and prevention. As we have seen, the micro-politics of these sessions can reveal tensions and alliances that are concealed beneath the peer educators' wider, collective identity.

In keeping with a general principle of all peer education music, programme designers hope that a receptive audience will learn the simple lyrical adaptations and participate in the singing through prior knowledge of the melodic shifts. This tactic enjoys some success, especially when a weekly performance is held in a clinic or other female space. But the public response to peer education songs does not always end in participation. Audience reactions range from shock or amusement to discomfort and, occasionally, outright anger.

For example, when 'Condom is number one!' was performed in public, it was met – as the Lutheran educators had predicted – by varying degrees of discomfort and disdain. Many people in the audience associated church songs with sacred spaces, and regarded their secularisation as blasphemous. The group coordinator was acutely aware of this, even regarding it as a point in the songs' didactic favour:

When we are busy singing these songs from church, some people [laughing], they can get very cross with us. Even my auntie, she told me she was not happy about us doing it like this. It's like we are stealing from them, or laughing at Jesus, but we say 'No!' They should be blessing us because isn't it that the Bible says 'God is Love'? And how can you love if there is no life? Really, if people are getting shocked then we think that is good! They must just get tested and use condoms. (Interview in Tshivenda)

At the same time, however, the Tshikombani educators were mindful of the need to 'cushion' their potentially controversial songs by slotting them in between more conservative offerings in the performance. One such song is known as '*Vho i vhonna naa?*' (Did you see it?), which is usually performed before or after 'Condom is number one!':

<u>*Vho i vhonna naa?* – Did you see it?</u>

Leader:	*Ahee, Vho i vhonna naa?*	Hey! Did you see it?
	Ahee, Vho i, Nevirapini a vhonna naa?	Hey! Did you see Nevirapine?
Chorus:	*Ahee, Vho i vhonna naa?*	Hey, did you see it? (Repeated)
Leader:	*I thusa nwana wa vhone*	It helps your child
	Uri a bebwi a si na tshitshili.	That it is born without the virus.

'*Vho i vhonna naa?*', I was told, is an adaptation of a ZCC song, prevalent in much of eastern Venda. A church version is known as '*Vhavhonna Murena naa?*' (Do you see the Lord?) and is performed by peer educators with the characteristic 'stamp dancing' that accompanies much of the ZCC musical repertoire (cf. Comaroff 1985: 244–5). However, the melody is also sung in times of protest, for example by a group of villagers demonstrating against police inefficiency in a ritual murder trial in 2000, which suggests that it may also be associated with the struggle.[6] So, whilst the peer educators place this performance squarely in their list of 'church songs', we can take it as an example of 'genre blurring' in which the boundary between 'church' music and songs of the 'struggle' is not clearly defined.

Nonetheless, peer educators appeal directly through the song to pregnant women (*vhaimana*; singular, *muimana*), informing them that Nevirapine is freely available at clinics, and that it can help prevent mother-to-child transmission (PMTCT) of HIV. At the time I recorded this track, in May 2004, the government had recently made a commitment to the provision of PMTCT medication to all HIV-positive pregnant women and rape survivors (see Chapter 4). Department of Health representatives and non-governmental actors at the regional and local levels often demonstrated significant independence from the ex-President's dissidence, and they did not always share the eccentric ideas of the former Minister of Health. Over the years, the information passed down to peer educators has thus consisted of conventional biomedical knowledge. In the song above, we see the signs of a relatively progressive (if poorly implemented) government policy that allowed for free provision of antiretroviral drugs (ARVs) to every HIV-positive person whose CD4 count was low enough.[7]

The song below demonstrates recent modifications in government policy. '*I ya vhulaya*' (It kills) was recorded in 1998 before the 2003 AIDS policy shift, and the lyrics proclaim that 'there is no medicine'. Previous to government provision of antiretrovirals, the FAP chose not to assume a role in advocacy or lobbying for treatment. Project coordinators were advised in their weekly meetings with FAP management as to what their songs should, and should not, promote. Whilst many educators privately advocated a more critical approach, they were prevented from taking it. Some often spoke of their frustration that pressure groups such as the Treatment Action Campaign (TAC) had very limited impact in the Venda region. In 2010 a peer educator at the Ha-Rabali project made this clear: 'The TAC don't have offices here. Everything

---

[6] This demonstration was in the Mukumbani area of Venda. King Kennedy Tshivhase made an appearance on the front line of the protest when police threatened to shoot at the crowd. He exclaimed that the police should 'Rather shoot the king of Tshivhase than any of his subjects!' Again, this was a shrewd publicity stunt in the strategy to gain legitimacy with sections of the citizenry in his quest to have his kingship recognised officially, and it was widely covered in the press.

[7] Until recently a person living with AIDS had to wait until their CD4 count fell below 200 before they could receive treatment. In 2010 this was changed to a CD4 count of 350. See Chapter 4.

'We Sing about What We Cannot Talk About' 163

for them [TAC] stops at Polokwane. If they were here we would leave FAP and join them... but they are not [here] so as educators we have no choice but to support our government and try to put food on the table.'

The songs of the peer educators have thus been reflective of existing government policy rather than attempting to influence it: they have advertised services and medicine as these gradually became available through the national roll-out of AIDS treatment. FAP's slowness to speak out and its tendency to endorse existing policy must be understood in the context of the comfortable relationship between regional government and the FAP office staff discussed in the previous chapter, and the necessity to maintain this for the continuation of funding. From the mid to late 1990s to the early years of the new millennium, the focus of peer educator songs has thus shifted in line with government policy: from prevention to the promotion of voluntary counselling, testing, and treatment.

I ya vhulaya – It Kills

Leader (one line, then echo by chorus)
Ndi tshitshili tshi no fhirela   It is a virus that goes through/past you
Kha muthu a renatsho   And goes from and to another
Are natsho, na a renatsho   One to another, one to another,
A huna mushonga   There is no medicine
U bva kha tshikhuwa kana wa tshirema   From white or black medicine
Mushonga ndi lufu   The only cure is death
Mufumakhadzi wa muimana   The pregnant woman
A nga pfukisela kha nwana   Will pass it to her child
A ro vha na AIDS   And the child gets AIDS

Chorus (echo throughout):
HIV, AIDSE, i ya vhulaya, i ya vhulaya HIV, AIDS, it kills, it kills.

Another song recorded in mid-2004, '*Diraga*' (Drugs), demonstrates the stance taken by the FAP to endorse the government's shifting approach to HIV and AIDS: from 'There is no medicine' to 'We use drugs, these days'. '*Diraga*' is an adaptation of another very popular choral song used by several church groups throughout Venda. It is usually performed in Shangaan, and most versions of it are reportedly sung to celebrate changes in the seasons, or at christenings or weddings when a significant life-cycle rite of passage is being undergone by members of the congregation. In the peer education version available on the website,[8] it was being rehearsed for a public performance, and the leader changes in the middle of the rendition.

[8] http://www.cambridge.org/us/9781107009912.

Diraga (Drugs – ARV)

Leader:	Hu shuma diraga maduvha ano,	We use drugs (ARV), these days,
	Hu shuma diraga maduvha Ee, Ahh!	We use drugs, these days, oh!
Chorus:	Diraga maduvha ano, iyo! weah! (x3)	Drugs, these days, oh!
	Hu shuma diraga maduvha ano	We use drugs, these days
Leader:	Vha tshi ya Vhufuli[9] vha do i wana	You will get it at Lufule [clinic]
	Vha tshi ya Siloam vha do i wana.	You will get it at Siloam [hospital].[10]

Whilst the songs above show the ways in which FAP's closeness to the government has influenced the content of peer educators' songs, they also represent, at least for the educators, a quest for legitimacy. The desire to shroud their particular brand of AIDS education in songs that are usually about God may have been born – at least partly – out of familiarity with them. But their attempt at association with the sacred is intended to bolster their anti-AIDS message and thus, ultimately, to lend authority to the educators' actions.

Songs from the Apartheid Era

Their association with God is one part of a wider plan to secure symbolic alignment with other sources of legitimacy. The appropriation of songs associated with the anti-apartheid struggle is also central to this strategy.[11] Struggle or freedom songs have been described as:

[S]hort slogans... set to simple melodic phrases, sung *a cappella* (unaccompanied) and repeated over and over in a call and response style. They are created and sung collectively, and frequently modified as politics, attitudes and circumstances change, and are almost exclusively non-commercial. (Gilbert 2007: 426)

Although reference to these songs is scarce in the existing literature on South African music, they are clearly related to the Zulu *isicathamiya* genre (Erlmann 1996) and, like it, are descended from pre-struggle church music. They are also strongly derivative of, and arguably an example of, the *makwaya* (choir) genre (James 1999; 2006: 155) that has stylistic origins in the combination of 'Southern African singing traditions with Christian hymnody' (Gilbert 2007: 426).

Moreover, they are 'ubiquitous but largely informal and un-professionalised' (ibid.: 423) and currently constitute a dominant medium of

---

[9] Vhufuli here refers to Donald Fraser Hospital, close to King Kennedy's palace in Mukumbani.

[10] See Map 4 for Lufule and Siloam; at the time the clinics in these areas were participating in pilot studies for the ARV roll-out.

[11] The role that music played in the struggle was commemorated in the excellent SABC documentary 'Amandla! – A revolution in four-part harmony' (BMG South Africa 79102-21510-2).

popular political expression throughout the country. This was especially so just after the April 2009 general election during which Jacob Zuma seduced ANC rally goers across the land with renditions of his trademark struggle song, *'Umshini wami'* (Bring me my machine gun). Following Zuma's lead, the president of the ANC Youth League, Julius Malema, caused considerable controversy in early 2010 by repeatedly performing another struggle song, 'Kill the Boer'. In the context of racial tensions in the wake of the murder of Eugene Terreblanche (Afrikaner white-supremacist leader and iconic latter-day 'Boer hero'), and a concern for international perceptions of South Africa in the run-up to the 2010 World Cup, a court hearing ruled that the song constituted 'hate speech' and the ANC's most senior body – the National Executive Committee – instructed Malema to refrain from singing it. The song was effectively banned. Malema reportedly responded by changing the lyrics at political rallies from 'Kill the Boer' to 'Kiss the Boer', but clearly the underlying sentiment of redress for historical injustice remained prominent in the performance.

In part, struggle songs remain hugely popular in South Africa because of their great adaptability. Gilbert points to their historical significance in the construction of ANC propaganda outside the country during the fight against apartheid. At this time, music, literature, graphic art, dance, and theatre were 'actively recruited to promote the anti-apartheid struggle internationally' (ibid.: 422). These songs, and the culture of which they were a part, grew to be central to ANC policy during the struggle. An official project (Amandla Cultural Ensemble) was established, and soldiers who were talented singers, actors, and performers were deployed there to be 'cultural workers'. A considerable number of their songs made reference to ANC leaders like Albert Luthuli, Oliver Thambo, Walter Sisulu, and especially Nelson Mandela, 'honouring their leadership and calling for political guidance' (ibid.: 435).

The primary purpose of this was to send out a political message and encourage collective political action (Nolwin 1996). Given the historical context and explicit political critique inherent in this music, it is perhaps not surprising that until the unbanning of the ANC in 1990 they remained illegal, were primarily an oral form, and were only (officially) recorded outside South Africa. Some recordings, such as *'Hey, Wena Gatsha!'*, are kept in the archives of Radio Freedom – the name of the ANC station when it was still underground and broadcasting from Ethiopia, Zambia, Angola, Tanzania, and Madagascar. The music of many other black and coloured South African artists who recorded on record deals outside the country reached black listeners in South Africa in a similar fashion over the airwaves of Radio Freedom or through a bustling trade in contraband.

Although the purveyors of many genres such as jazz, reggae, gospel, choral, and some traditional music were actively engaged in challenging the policies of segregation, the struggle songs in question were distinct in several ways. Chief among these was the accompanying *toyi toyi* dance that grew to symbolise the preparation for warfare (McGregor 2005). During the apartheid era, the lyrical content of struggle songs was highly politicised. '*Hey, Wena Gatsha!*' has a threatening message for the political leaders of the apartheid-era homelands. The chanting comrades exchange Mangosuthu ('Gatsha') Buthelezi, previous head of the KwaZulu homeland, for other leaders of the puppet regimes such as (Patrick) Mphephu in Venda and (Lennox) Sebe in Ciskei, and prophesy their rendez-vous thus:

Hey, wena Gatsha! (Hey you, Gatsha!)[12]

Hey, wena Gatsha!	Hey you, Gatsha!
Amasi abekwe elangeni	It's only a matter of time
Sodibanda	We shall meet
Ngebazuka.	With a bazooka.

As if to exemplify Blacking's claims about the dual capacity of music, however, official productions at the same time by the South African Broadcasting Corporation (SABC), ideologically driven and even propagandistic in intention, promoted racial segregation and depicted black people as country dwellers rather than townsmen (James 1997), thus supporting the apartheid status quo. Through stations on the state-controlled broadcasting network such as Radio Thohoyandou in Venda, local artists (largely motivated by instant cash payments for which they relinquished copyright) recorded in the SABC studios and tailored their lyrical content to banal love songs with essentialist, nationalist sentiments such as that expressed in Tshigwada tsha Toronto's hit song '*Ndi a tuwa*', in a genre that became known as 'radio jive'.

Ndi a tuwa (I am going)[13]

Thi dzuli Makhuwani,	I don't live in Johannesburg
Ndo da fhano nga mushumo	I just came here to work
Ndo da u shumela musadziwanga	I came to work for my wife
Ri a tuwa, hayani Venda.	We go, home to Venda.

A vast and previously unreleased collection of these recordings was recently released as the *African Renaissance* series – showcasing the ways

---

[12] The version was recorded by Canadian journalists at ANC headquarters in Lusaka, Zambia, in 1985 and later appeared on the commemorative Radio Freedom CD (Rounder Records USA 11661–4019–2).

[13] Performed by Tshigwada Tsha Toronto. Recorded at the Radio Venda studio in Thohoyandou, and later included in *African Renaissance*, Vol. 2: Venda (Eagle Records SABC002 GAS 0000002 SAB).

in which government propaganda at the time combined the recording of popular music with traditional pieces that were designed to create a longing for 'home'. As Hamm (1987) has argued, however, radio jive had genuine popular support amongst urban-based Africans who reinterpreted its intended propagandistic agenda. To some extent this section of the populace thus dictated the choice of music broadcast by the SABC and reinterpreted it in their own terms (James 1997). Songs of the struggle, then, existed illegally in relation to strict state regulations over what could, and could not, become popular music – whilst state-sanctioned genres such as radio jive were reconstrued along political lines.

During apartheid, struggle songs accompanied illegal political rallies and demonstrations. The recognised experts in leading them were groups of ANC members, especially the Youth League and the military wing of the ANC, *Umkhonto we Sizwe* (MK) soldiers in training, or their commanders such as the late Peter Mokaba who championed the 'one settler, one bullet' slogan through the genre. Thus struggle songs were both illegal and hugely popular. However, as a result of the lack of recordings, they circulated largely in formats that were not standardised, and the lyrics changed depending on the leader. The versions aired on Radio Freedom would be reinvented in different languages throughout the country. After 1990, with the unbanning of the ANC, this began to change. Record companies such as BMG started making commercial recordings and artists such as Amaqabane, Blondie Makhene and various African church choirs began to produce standardised versions with synthesised backing instrumentation.

Given that contemporary Venda remains an ANC stronghold, songs of the struggle regularly become part of the entertainment at public gatherings during and after local ANC ward meetings when they are sung in praise of old and new comrades. They often form part of beer-drinking/meat-eating repertoires through which men remember the past and comment on the present. They are also widely associated today with general protests, and have been performed by groups of women presenting a petition to Parliament in anger at the extent of sexual violence or by people protesting against alleged police involvement in the sale of human body parts. During their 2009 election campaigns, supporters of both the ANC and the newly formed Congress of the People (COPE) often engaged in musical battle, attempting to out-sing each other in crowded beer halls and on the way to and from election rallies in overloaded pick-up trucks. The songs they sang were contemporary interpretations of older struggle songs, and they changed the lyrics to suit political causes in much the same way as peer educators manipulate well-known songs to promote safer sex.

The considerable influence that struggle songs had in the past has thus been brought into the post-apartheid political arena. They are used by politicians such as President Jacob Zuma and Julius Malema, in pursuit of popular support. At the same time, they are sung by the electorate both in praise of and in anger against the ANC-led government. It is in this context that peer educators attempt to harness the power associated with them by utilising the genre in public performances:

[T]he struggle is not yet over. We are still struggling, can't you see? It is not enough that we can vote, but voting is important. My house remains without water and I still cook on a fire at night. Anyway, now AIDS is the enemy, it kills us secretly just like the Boer used to, and we should fight it [AIDS] as we did before with the Boer. (Interview in Tshivenda)

The song below is an adaptation of a very famous struggle song in praise of ANC comrade Joe '*Ntate*' (Father) Modise and other heroes of the struggle. A standardised recording was released in 1990 by the band Amaqabane. In the peer education version, the four syllables of the opening line 'Nta/te/ Mod/ise/' are replaced with the four syllables in '/Khondomu/ndi /bosso/'. It is performed with variations on these themes, in verses, with the call and response differing depending on the leader. In 2005, peer educators were unaware of the recorded version but were encouraged to modify the song initially by Rudzani, the original volunteer (now government employee) and a previous commander in the ANC's military wing.

'*Khondomu ndi bosso!*' (Condom is the boss!)

Leader:	*Khondomu ndi bosso!*	Condom is the boss!
Chorus:	*Ndi bo...*	It is...
	Ndi bosso	It is the boss
	Ndi bosso, Khondom ndi bosso.	The boss, condom is the boss.
(x2)		
Leader:	*I thivhela malwadze.*	It prevents sickness.
Chorus:	*Malwa...*	Sick...
	Malwadze...	Sickness...
	Malwadze a vhudzekani.	Sexually transmitted sickness.
Leader:	*Khondomu nga i shume!*	Use condoms!
Chorus:	*Nga i shu...*	To be...
	Nga i shume...	To be used...
	Nga i shume....Khondom nga i shume!	To be used....Use condoms!
Leader:	*Khondomu ndi ngwena.*	Condoms are crocodiles.[14]

[14] The crocodile is a symbol of chieftainship, and of incontestable strength. But the literal meaning here is misleading. It is used in this context to symbolise a hero. It is usually used in this manner after a fight to show victory, such as the winner of a Venda boxing contest (*musangwe*), who is referred to as *ngwena*.

Chorus: *Ndi ngwe...*	It's a croc...
Ndi ngwena...	It's a crocodile...
Ndi ngwena, khondom ndi ngwena.	A crocodile, condoms are crocodiles.

The emotion with which peer educators perform struggle songs is a stark reminder that freedom is a recent acquisition and that AIDS threatens to destroy it. Sometimes they are overcome with sentiment, such as during the rendition of '*Aidse*', below. The woman leading it had to wipe tears from her tightly closed eyes as she recited the melody, supported by the backing harmonies of her fellow educators. Many had their right fists raised, swaying and shuffling gently to the rhythm, creating percussive brushes by scuffing the soles of their shoes in unison against the ground.

<u>Aidse (AIDS)</u>

Leader:	*Aidse!*(x3)	AIDS!
Chorus:	*I ya vhulaya* (x2)	It is killing
	I ya vhulaya, Aidse	It is killing, this AIDS
Leader:	*Kha ri luge*	Let's get ready
Chorus:	*Kha ri luge Afurika,*	Let's get ready, Africa
	Ri thivhele, Aidse.	To prevent this AIDS.
Leader:	*ARV!* (x3)	Antiretrovirals
Chorus:	*I ya dzidzivha...* (x2)	It knocks out[15]...
	I ya dzidzivhadza tshitshili.	It knocks out the virus.

Struck by the emotional response to her own performance, I later asked the lead singer on '*Aidse*' if that song was of particular significance to her. 'No', she replied. 'Not just "*Aidse*", but all songs of the struggle remind us of the past, and we have all lost loved ones to this [AIDS].' She continued: 'I remember my brother who died last year, and we still miss him at home.' I later learned that '*Aidse*', like most of the songs discussed here, has had multiple reincarnations, and is associated with different activities by various groups throughout Venda. The peer educators recalled it as a funeral song performed by women during the Bantustan era. Others contradicted this and argued that it was a military song of *Umkhonto we Sizwe* sung by soldiers asking God to bless them and their families, who were left behind in South Africa while the comrades underwent training in neighbouring countries. Given the adaptability of struggle songs, the two explanations are not necessarily mutually exclusive.

[15] *U dzidzivhala* literally means to be unconscious. In this context it could be translated as 'it does not cure, but it minimises the pain'.

The association between peer educators and the struggle, like the sought-after connection with God, is achieved – at least partially – by their recasting of music associated with that era. In a similar manner, songs that are popularly known as 'traditional' present another opportunity for peer educators to secure legitimacy for their actions.

'Traditional' Songs in Peer Education

The concept of 'tradition' is as contested as it is frequently invoked. The word *sialala* is used by peer educators, for example, to describe that moment in a public performance when they use a *murumba* drum.[16] Performing traditional songs at weekly public performances provides the occasion for audience participation with impromptu solo dances (*maluselo*) that go on until the dancer has outshone the previous soloist or accepted defeat in the competition.

The potential repertoire of traditional songs is connected to and restricted by the classification of communal Venda music into genres performed by men, women, adults, and children (see Chapter 1 in this book; also Stayt 1931; Blacking 1965). As mostly young to middle–aged women, peer educators use a combination of *malende* (sung by men and women at beer drinks, and for general entertainment at various occasions), *vhusha*, *domba* (from the female initiation schools – see Chapter 3), *tshifhase* (a courting dance for teenagers), and *tshigombela* (young girls/women's entertainment; cf. Kruger 1999).

Malende: 'Zwonaka' (It's Beautiful) and 'Khondomisa!'
(Condomise!)

Of all these genres, *malende* is the most popular among both peer educators and the wider public. Songs such as *'Zwonaka'* (It's beautiful) and *'Khondomisa!'* (Condomise!) are the educators' interpretation of widely performed *malende* tunes. Their inclusion in public performances regularly results in some form of audience participation, although this could perhaps more often be described as drunken interference. The educators have discovered the difficulties of performing *malende* and other 'traditional' songs 'out of context'. For the public performance to 'work', according to the educators' criteria, the inclusion of two or three traditional songs should last no more than 15–20 minutes in the public performance. In a 'non-peer education' context, however, each individual song can last up to half an hour, and beyond. During a performance in Feburary 2010, a group of drunken men refused to stop singing

---

[16] The *murumba* drum is used as it is symbolic of female initiation, and is used in the rites of *vhusha* and *domba*, as described in Chapter 3.

'Zwonaka' after the educators had moved onto the next part of the programme. The men reverted to the 'original' lyrics and the echos of their deep baritone and bass harmonies slapping against the cold, sparsely decorated concrete walls of the beer hall drowned out the rest of the peer educators' show.

<u>Zwonaka (It's Beautiful) (Commonly used lyrics)</u>

Chorus:	(opens the song and then becomes the response throughout)	
	Zwonaka, zwonaka, zwonakela	It's beautiful, so beautiful, to become beautiful
	Zwonaka u tshila na vhathu zwavhudi	It's beautiful to live nicely with others
Leader:[17]	(a sample of the 'call' throughout)	
	U dzula na vhatu, zwo nakelela	Living with others, having parties, it's nice.
	Na vhana vhavhudi vha do aluwa ngauralo	And good children will come of it.

<u>Zwonaka (It's Beautiful) (Peer education lyrics)</u>

Chorus:	*Zwonaka, zwonaka, zwonakela*	It's beautiful, so beautiful to become beautiful
	Zwonaka u shumisa khondomu zwonakalela	It's nice, so nice to use a condom.
Leader:	*U shumisa khondom zwi a tsireledza*	Using a condom will prevent disease.
	Na thusula i a tsireledzwa	And it will prevent Syphilis
	Na AIDS i a tsireledzwa	And it will prevent AIDS.

<u>Khondomisa! (Condomise!): Peer education lyrics</u>

Chorus:	*Khondomiza!*	Condomise!
Leader:	*Nda lila iyo wee! Mara ngoho ndi tshi shumisa khondomu*	I am crying oh! but really, I am using condoms
	Khondomu yanga, mara ngoho nne ndo I sia gai naa?	My condom, but really, where did I leave it?
	Nne ndi shumisa yone	I work with it
	Nne ndi tshimbilonayo	I travel around, walk with it.

The original version of *'Khondomisa!'* is the extremely popular *'Syendekela'*. It is intended to mock, in a jovial way, the husband of a wife when he visits his mother-in-law. She claims that the children he has given her daughter are ugly, lazy, stupid, with big heads and small ears, and that they are not beautiful enough to be born of her daughter. The song is reflective of the joking relationship that exists between a man and his wives' matrilineal relatives, but is also extended to make general mocking statements about anyone who happens to be present, if the leader is so inclined at the time of performance.

---

[17] In representing 'traditional' songs, I have used a sample selection of the possible lyrics that are all variations on the same theme of biomedical AIDS-related information. However these songs are rarely performed with the same lyrics twice and the textual content of these songs varies significantly depending on the performer and the region. This applies for both the 'commonly occurring' and the peer education versions. The general themes, however, remain consistent. In the 'original' version from which the educators took *'Khondomisa!'*, for example, the chorus remains consistent – '*nwana si wanga*' – (the child is not mine). This is also the case for *'Zwonaka'*, in which the chorus reminds listeners of the need to live peacefully with their neighbours.

In the context of peer education, the joking relationship expressed in '*Syendekela*' can be extrapolated in several ways: it facilitates the airing of latent tensions between sub-groups of educators and between the educators and the audience. For example, in the dispute I mentioned in the previous chapter between two religious cliques who suspected each other of poisonous activity at ongoing training, accusations were made initially through the performance of this song – as were various attempts at mediation some months later.

Female Initiation Songs

In addition to *malende*, peer educators furnish their performances with 'traditional' elements from female initiation and a genre known as *tshifhase*. For example, '*Lele*' is sung, according to the peer educators, in the *musivheto* initiation school prior to *vhusha* (see Chapter 3), urging young girls to ignore the advances of boys. Blacking, however, has recorded a version of it as part of the *ndayo* sessions of the *vhusha* female initiation ceremony (1969a).

Lele (Be patient) (Initiation lyrics)

Chorus:	*Iyo lele, lele, lele*	Be patient, be patient, be patient
Leader:	*Vhatukana havha vha mmbondolola mmawe*	These boys are looking at me
	U vhonna a thina khaladzi	They see I don't have a brother
	Thi malli khaladzi nnduni mmawe	I don't marry my brother/sister.

In the song, the initiates are reminded that their brothers have a duty to protect them against any unwanted attention. But the girls' predicament is also important; they may marry a young suitor, but could never marry an over-protective brother. The message to girls here is that there comes a time when you will be in a position to be married and relinquish your brothers' protection, but until then you must refrain from intercourse. In the peer educators' version, the social context is transformed and the sexual instruction manipulated to suit the new content. First, the song has moved from a relatively closed, quasi-sacred female initiation ceremony into a male-dominated public arena. Second, the lyrical content is transformed from a sympathetic riddle promoting abstinence to a direct confession of an STI, in which the condom is an unambiguously advantageous addition to the average girl's handbag (*phesini* – literally, 'in the purse').

Lele (Be patient) (Peer education lyrics)

Chorus:	*Iyo lele, lele lele...*	
Leader:	*Dorobo yo thoma nga nne mmawe*	The drop (gonorrhoea) started with me
	Ngauri a tho ngo ita nga khondomu mmawe	Because I didn't do it with a condom
	Zwino khondomu i phesini mmawe	Now the condom is in my handbag.

Tshifhase, Malombo, and Other Traditional Genres

Whilst the songs from female initiation are intended, in their ritual context, to impose rules and regulations on the sexuality and productivity of young women, songs in the *tshifhase* genre are set in opposition to this, giving light relief in the form of flirtatious dances. In *tshifhase* the sexual and social tensions between young men and young women are brought into the open and, at least theoretically, resolved. For van Warmelo (1989: 397) *tshifhase* is:

[S]ong and dance of young folk... a diversion for moonlit evenings. Boys and girls stand in two groups apart, singing. A girl comes across to the boys, hooks her choice by the arm and leads him to her own group. A lad now does likewise, and so on until the groups are sorted out again.

Although the only lyric in '*Jojo Tshilangano*' is a repetition of the song title, the young performers are made aware of a story behind it. Jojo is said to be a migrant labourer (*mugaraba*) who has returned from the Reef in characteristic style with money to spend, and is in demand with the local girls.[18] As performed outside of the peer education context, the girls stage a competition to impress Jojo and he subsequently chooses the best dancer. Jojo and his new girlfriend then meet in the middle of the two groups, until another young man is chosen to play Jojo, and so it continues.

The dramatic presentation of '*Jojo Tshilangano*', and others like it, places it stylistically between song and drama in the peer education repertoire. In the version they stage, one of the women dresses in drag as Jojo – donning dungarees, a hat, boots, and whatever else she can find. In an elaborate and exaggerated mime, (s)he approaches a girl in the other group and tempts her to dance in a sexually explicit, but comical, routine. With the rest of the peer educators now forming a circle around the pair, she accepts his proposition and they frolic in the middle, until eventually he offers her money for sex. She is tempted, but refuses. Dramatically, Jojo then produces a condom, thrusts it high into the air as the peer educators ululate and the girl falls into his arms – generally to the great amusement of the audience.

But not all 'traditional' songs performed by women have made it into the peer educator catalogue. Although several educators dance *malombo*, also known as *ngoma dza vhadzimu* (literally, the drum of the ancestors – a ritual of affliction), at fairly regular intervals in their private lives, no songs from this genre appear in the FAP repertoire. Given that *malombo* is

---

[18] The term *mugaraba* is derived from the verb *u garaba* – to skin/scrape a slaughtered pig. Upon their return, migrant labourers are expected to hold a party, for which they purchase and slaughter a pig. They have been named colloquially after this practice, although the extent to which it actually happens is highly variable.

explicitly concerned with the social, personal, and metaphysical processes of healing (Blacking 1995a), this absence is perhaps puzzling. It is part of the complex of healing/possession rites that occur throughout Central and Southern Africa known as *ngoma*, documented by Janzen (1992), van Dijk et al. (2000), and more recently West and Luedke (2005). Drews (2000) provides an analysis focusing on gender dynamics in *ngoma* to demonstrate that, like peer education, *ngoma* rites are often dominated by female participants. And yet despite this historical female dominance and an association with healing, *malombo* music does not feature in FAP AIDS education.

The absence of *malombo* music has a simple explanation, however, which lies in its ritually separate, taboo, and group-specific character. Although there is considerable evidence of hybridisation between traditional and Christian religious practices, especially in African Independent Churches as discussed previously, *malombo* remains taboo even for most Zionist or Apostolic Christians in Venda. Those who perform it are members of a very specific social and spiritual group, inclusion in which is achieved only through experience of possession and thus being healed of a specific affliction. Only once a person has been possessed (*o wa* – literally, to have fallen) will she (or, increasingly, he – see Rezacova 2007) be called upon to assist in the next *malombo*?[19]

The taboo attached to *malombo* and those who perform it, usually identifiable by a copper bracelet (*mulinga*) around a wrist, has prevented it being used in AIDS education: the Christian majority of peer educators simply would not be associated with it in public or private form. Moreover, the few educators who do take an active role in possession dances recognised its role in healing, but would not perform it 'out of context'. The ritual arena in which *malombo* is danced must be carefully prepared and adequately protected with *mushonga* (medicine), and to invoke possession without this would quite literally risk the wrath of the ancestors. In this way, the non-optative nature of *malombo* music renders it unsuitable for the objectives of peer education. For the peer educators, this is self-evident: as a form of treatment for affliction, its worth is measured by its efficacy rather than its aesthetic appeal, and of all the genres

---

[19] Over the years I have been lucky enough to attend many *malombo* dances under the instruction of Noriah at Dopeni (see Chapter 3). She went to great pains to ensure that I had accurate data on the various stages, costumes, and objects used throughout the possession. She talked me through the three stages (*tshele, malombo, u kwasha tshele mavhidani*) several times, and permitted my access to the 'spirit house', place of mysterious noises where the shadows of the ancestors rest and eat during the period of their brief incarnation in human bodies. Late in the evening during a *malombo* in June 2004 a spirit, who was known to be partial to the traditional beer from a specific *shebeen* in a neighbouring village, stole the drum stick (*tshiombo*) and ran off into the night to drink there. Only at 6.30 the next morning did he return, drunk, for the rites to be completed.

mentioned here it is the least likely to transcend its context and be used for anything else besides its original purpose.

The same cannot be said, however, for songs from the various stages of female initiation. Although they are intimately associated with ancestors (*vhadzimu*) in many ways, this is to some extent countered by the ways in which they constitute the more neutral (and recently fashionable) notions of *mvelele* (culture) and *sialala* (tradition). As we have seen in previous chapters, many peer educators have 'been sung for' (initiated), either through the Christian or royal *vhusha*, and this entails the accumulation of esoteric knowledge. This information is not divulged through peer education songs, however: neither do peer educators perform the *ndayo* described in Chapter 3. Rather, mindful of the need to avoid betraying ritual knowledge, but keen to appropriate the symbolic association with initiation and sexual health, they adopt dance routines from the less secretive stages such as the well-known *domba* 'python dance'.[20] Even women who have not gone through initiation participate in these songs for the purposes of AIDS education.

For project designers and peer educators alike, the use of traditional songs is important for the legitimation of the projects in terms of ascribing 'Vendaness'. The fact that historically *malende*, *tshigombela*, and *tshifhase* have been employed extensively to construct and articulate social commentary on contemporary affairs (Kruger 1999) does not exclude them from being associated with an idealised, conservative, long-lost past. It is the power associated with this imagined history that peer educators try to capture when using traditional songs. Precisely because of their historical role in channelling social critique, most educators are enabled in transforming them into part of the AIDS education repertoire.

Original Songs

The last category into which peer educators group their songs is that of 'originals' (*zwa mathombo*). Some educators have become prolific song writers, creating original songs that are performed during weekly public performances in which the composers showcase their talents. As one peer educator wrote in her diary:

I have been busy writing a new song for the project. Today was a great day for me as we sung it [at the public performance] and everything went well. It's nice to use our own songs, we can really say, 'That is my song, I wrote that and now you are all singing it to learn that AIDS kills'. The only problem is when some others get jealous and say they wrote it. (Diary D, pp. 33–4, in Tshivenda)

Some years ago a group of educators at Ha-Rabali embarked on a project to record and sell their own songs commercially, but lacking

---

[20] Listen to a *domba* 'python dance' at http://www.cambridge.org/us/9781107009912.

financial support the project stagnated in the early stages. This was an attempt at making some extra income, rather than making a 'musical break' from the social and economic status offered by a job in the government. Nonetheless, many peer educators are talented writers, and although their melodies may be based on fragments of other popular compositions from the genres outlined above, the songs in this last category are widely accepted as original.[21] Ownership of the song symbolises ownership of the knowledge within it. As I suggested above, however, song writers are encouraged by coordinators and FAP staff to keep the lyrical complexity to a minimum. Some songs, such as 'Jealous down!', only have one line; focusing rather on harmony, melody, and dance, through which a simple message can be framed in complex symbolic terms.

Jealous Down![22]

Jealous down! Khondomu ya shuma!   Stop being jealous, use a condom!

This song, so I was told, emerged spontaneously from a drama performed by peer educators at Tshikombani in 2004. It relayed a version of the regional trope in which suspicion and jealousy encompass sexually promiscuous behaviour. A woman asks her husband to use a condom, as she suspects that he has been having an extra-marital affair. The husband responds to her request by beating her, claiming that she is jealous of his success and that the real reason for her desire to have safe sex is that she had been unfaithful to him and is afraid that she would pass on disease. The wife ended the drama rehearsal by exclaiming in English 'Jealous down, man!' (meaning 'Stop being jealous!') and someone in the group began to place it in a melody, which was then given several layers of harmony, until the woman in the drama began to sing the lead part – and so the song was born. It is often performed after this drama during public performances, having literally grown out of it.

The incorporation of original creations into public performances thus presents the educators with an opportunity to showcase their ownership of biomedical AIDS knowledge in a way that does not appear confusing to the audience. When writing their own songs, the educators thus focus on telling people what to do, as opposed to why they should do it. In this way the songs are intended to act as teaching devices. When a public performance includes songs such as '*Ri do I fhenya*' (We will conquer

[21] See Barber (1991) for an analysis of the contested nature of innovation versus tradition in African oral arts. Barber's analysis of Yoruba oral poetry demonstrates the ways in which *Oriki* simultaneously mark boundaries and transgress them, whilst blending innovatory aspects with well-established trends of tradition – much like the peer education music outlined in this chapter.

[22] There is some debate as to whether this song is actually 'original', in that the phrase it is built around seems to be heard in different contexts throughout South Africa. Nonetheless, the peer educators claim this version as their own.

it) or '*Muimana*' (Pregnant woman), the facilitator will ask the audience questions after the song about the lyrics: 'What are the three ways to prevent AIDS?' 'Why did the woman in the song take out blood?' 'What is Nevirapine?'

Ri do i fhenya – We will conquer it

Vho mme na vho khotsi na vhanna ri a fhela	Mother, father and children are perishing
AIDSE ngoho yo ri dzhenela (x2)	Really, AIDS has entered into us
lu a lila, lushaka,[23] '*AIDSE i bva ngafhi?*'	The nation cries 'where is AIDS from?'
A ri divhi, rothe yone I a vhulaya (x2)	We don't know, but it's killing us all
Ndi tharu ndila dzi ne na nga i thivhela	There are three ways to prevent it[24]
Dzone, ngadzo ni do vha no i fhenya (x2)	With them, we can conquer it
Ri do i fhenya! (x4)	We will conquer it!

<u>Muimana (Pregnant woman)</u>

Nne ndi muimana,	I am a pregnant woman
Ndo ya hangei sibadela	I went over there to the hospital
Sibadela tsha Silomu	the Siloam hospital
Nda dzhiwa malofha	I took out blood (got a blood test)
Nevirapine!	Nevirapine!

Context and Content

For peer educators in Venda, the way in which their message is delivered is very important. Specific songs are chosen to be adapted not just for the ease with which lyrical changes might be implemented in them, but for the pre-existing message in the song, dance, rhythm, or entire genre. Perhaps there is an element of pragmatism – in that music is a cheap and effective way to pass on information in rural South Africa – but this necessity has been turned into virtue. Symbolic association with music of the struggle, as we saw in songs such as '*Khondomu ndi bosso!*' and '*Aidse*', has immediate and obvious implications – placing peer educators at the centre of the contemporary struggle against AIDS whilst invoking the powerful spirit of a mass agitprop social movement to which many of their audience belonged.

The choice of specific struggle songs is not random, and the use of praise and funeral songs that seek to elicit emotional responses in those who hear them is deliberate. Moreover, although church music is also an obvious choice, by replacing 'Jesus' with 'condom' in 'Condom is Number One!' peer educators make a flagrant attempt to use shock tactics in a generally conservative religious environment. Condoms become

---

[23] The word *lushaka* refers to a patrilineal kinship group but can be extended to all one's blood relations. The peer educators use it to refer to 'the Venda nation'/all Tshivenda-speaking people.

[24] This refers to the now infamous ABC of AIDS prevention: Abstain, Be faithful, and Use a condom.

sacred, worthy of worship and sacrifice, with the eventual gift of life over death. The association with tradition (*mvelele*) reveals another important dynamic of the peer education experience. By appropriating specific genres such as *malende*, *tshifhase*, and initiation school music and dance, AIDS education is veiled symbolically in 'Vendaness'.

For the educators – and project designers – this serves to legitimate the performance and its raison d'être. The manner in which peer educators use music to deliver biomedical discourse can thus be seen as an attempt to transform AIDS education into a medley of messages and, by extension, themselves into a motley crew of warriors against social injustice with sacrosanct associations, legitimated by a play on culture. In doing so, they have cobbled together a *bricolage* of historically constituted meanings and present them in one coherent performance in which each musical tradition takes on a new significance in the context of AIDS prevention.

The content of the songs is as important as (if not more important than) the method of delivery. It demonstrates a sound understanding of basic biomedical knowledge and services offered by the government and AIDS-related organisations like the FAP. For a group of unemployed and under-educated women who live close to the poverty line, this knowledge (and the ways in which it is learned and presented) is often experienced as empowering in that it demonstrates significant differences between them and other unemployed women in the area. With regular government contracts for voluntary counselling and testing (VCT) and home-based care (HBC) being implemented by the FAP, this demonstration of knowledge brings them closer to a job 'in the government', with its associated rise in status and economic security (see Chapter 4). For at least a few, this promise of paid work has been realised.

The singing of these songs, then, invokes a dual notion of hope; hope that the 'nation will not perish' and hope that they may benefit from the situation by progression into employment. It is a public display to their friends and neighbours of their transition from 'sitting around doing nothing, waiting on God to help me' into a more respectable, proud, and ultimately employable quasi-social worker. To this extent the songs of peer educators and their weekly performances provide spaces in which they construct and project a distinctly positive identity through which they strive to negotiate positions of power and authority in adverse, unfavorable circumstances (cf. Erlmann 1996; Coplan 1994). Singing and dancing are central to their hopes for social and economic advancement, and highly skilled creative performances increase an educator's chance of promotion through the ranks.

Accordingly, performance presents the peer educators with a certain ambiguity, from which they attempt to exploit personal 'cover' from the experiences they sing about. As we see in Chapter 7, their public confessions to being experts on illness are important. By singing about them as a group – and not talking about them as individuals – they seek the protection offered by performances in other contexts, such as the safe transference of ritual knowledge in Chapter 3. As we will see however, they have only been partially successful is achieving this.

The songs presented above thus represent more than the salient mechanism by which peer educators in Venda seek to transfer AIDS-related knowledge. But to what extent do they actually fulfil this primary, pedagogic task? If project designers and advocates of peer education promote the use of songs as an effective and culturally appropriate process of transferring knowledge, does the evidence from Venda suggest the success of such a strategy? Are the songs heard and understood as the educators and project designers intended them to be?

In the following chapter, I address these questions by broadening the analysis to consider other musical interpretations of HIV/AIDS. This will allow me to develop an argument based on the construction of sexually transmitted illnesses in Venda aetiology. I shall show how blood, dirt/pollution, sexually transmitted infections, 'deviant' behaviour, and medical science have been strung together to provide historically constituted explanations for HIV/AIDS under the wider 'folk' cosmological concept of *malwadze dza vhafumakadzi* (the illnesses/sickness of women).

6 Guitar Songs and Sexy Women

A Folk Cosmology of AIDS

Peer educators are not the only people who sing songs about AIDS in Venda. It is also a popular theme in the male-dominated solo genre known as *zwilombe* (singular, *tshilombe*). Exploring this genre facilitates a critical appraisal of the peer educators' efforts through a wider ethnographic lens; it demonstrates the extent to which Venda men and older (initiated) women frame the educators' actions in terms of a dynamic 'folk model' (Good 1994) of sexual illness. This model of understanding, albeit expressed through a male genre of *zwilombe*, is rooted in and parallels the knowledge recounted in the female initiation schools recently bolstered by King Tshivhase's engagement with the African renaissance. This model captures peer educators – and the biomedical knowledge they tout – in a web of suspicion and blame, labelling them as vectors of the virus. As experts in biomedicine, their conspicuous knowledge of contraception (and to a lesser extent abortion) translates, in the folk model, as a reflection of their own intimate experience. They are thought to be acquainted with the regulation of their own reproductive capacities in unnatural and inherently dangerous ways. They are thus thought to be contaminated with blood-bound pollution, and are constructed as constituting a threat to fertility that places them at the very heart of the perceived crisis of social reproduction.

Folk models or indigenous knowledge systems (IKS; see Chapter 4) represent 'a culture's collective body of accumulated knowledge and wisdom' (Liddell et al. 2005: 624). Whilst this definition may suggest that 'a culture' has a fixed way of understanding the world, indigenous systems of knowledge are, of course, fluid and open to the incorporation of outside elements. This is especially the case in the representation of illness. Southern African folk models have readily incorporated elements of biomedical explanation since their earliest exposure to them. Notions such as pollution, infection, bacteria, or dirt have long been common proximate causes of ill health, answering the 'How?' beyond which witchcraft and ancestral vengeance generally provide ultimate explanations for the 'Why?'

In Venda, as in other regions of Southern Africa,[1] elements of the biomedical model of AIDS bear remarkable similarity to the representation of sexual illness in indigenous knowledge systems.[2] Both focus on blood, semen, and sexual transmission. This remarkably isomorphic set of representations has been brought to bear upon, or used to explain, social settings in a way which has yielded gendered and generational patterns of blame. Women – and specifically young women – have been held responsible for generating a build-up of pollution through slack moral practices (cf. Bujra 2000a; Baylies 2000), which are perceived as symptoms of a wider neglect of traditional authority. In Venda, we can trace this pattern of blame through songs performed by older men. In this way, intergenerational conflict dovetails with gendered patterns of blame, and the socio-political coordinates of a perceived moment of emergency are charted through musical expression. Again, the focus on songs here is not arbitrary; the *zwilombe* genre to which I now turn has a history of commentary on controversial topics, a theme that is raised again in the following chapter.

Zwilombe: 'The Prophet Musicians'

Zwilombe is the collective noun for a specific group of male musicians in the Venda region. Defined by Blacking (1965: 28) as 'wandering minstrel[s]', they perform with guitars, *dende* (a gourd bow), *tshidzholo* (an elongated zither), and lamellaphones or 'thumb pianos' (*mbila*). Linguistically, the term *zwilombe* is constructed from the same root as the term for *malombo* rites of affliction (*u lomba* – to fetch something from far away or to borrow from a spirit), and *tshilombe* musicians are thus associated to a significant extent with the invisible world of the ancestors that is strategically avoided in peer education songs. Extending this, it has been suggested that *zwilombe* are spiritually sanctioned and 'consequently present themselves as the voice of ancestral spirits or God' (Kruger 1999/2000: 22). From this position of relative power, *zwilombe* musicians construct models for and of social reality that constitute:

---

[1] See Heald (1995; 2006), Ingstad (1990), de Bruyn (1992), McDonald and Schatz (2006), Posel (2005), Liddell et al. (2005), and Niehaus (2007).
[2] Farmer (1988; 1990; 1994; 2006) has documented the ways in which AIDS became incorporated into the pre-existing folk model of illness in Haiti. His work is particularly interesting as he conducted research on the subject there before AIDS was known in the area, and documented the ways in which it was incorporated, and the role of narrative and rumour in the reaching of consensus. He looks mainly at AIDS as a 'sent illness' in terms of sorcery accusations. Although he does provide an analysis of blood-related illness and female morality (1988), he does not connect this directly with the aetiology of AIDS, as much of the material on Southern Africa has.

a comprehensive, long-tem strategy which attempts to influence the attitude and behaviour of people in the promotion of an ordered, supportive social environment... they are prophet-musicians who act on spiritual command... their instruments become 'spirit', symbolic extensions of religious authority. (Kruger 1993: 510)

Historically, every royal courtyard is said to have had a *tshilombe* whose job consisted of using his inherited talents to entertain the king and his royal councillors through song and dance (ibid.). However, *zwilombe* is not a conservative social institution engaged in the promotion of patriarchal or hereditary structures of political power. The association with ancestral authority expressed in song by travelling minstrels who mostly perform for beer or *folla* (tobacco or marijuana) has made *tshilombe* musicians very marginal figures. This marginality, coloured by their self-attributed 'madness' (Kruger 1993; 1999/2000), allows them to be openly critical where others would not dare. As we shall see in the next chapter, this allows them to speak openly about death without being implicated in the cause.

During the volatile political climate of the independent homeland era (see Chapter 2), *tshilombe* musicians exploited their peripheral status to make scathing attacks on the violent and corrupt ministers in the Venda government:

Ngevhala ndi Vho-Ravele	There is Mr Ravele, struggling to eat
Vho vhulaya na vhone Vho-Mphephu	He killed Mr Mphephu
Vha tshi nyaga tshidulo a shangoni la Venda	He was after the presidency of Venda
Ri la ri vhanzhi u zwimbela dzi a talula	Many ate, only one became constipated
Havha Vho-Ravela vhone vho dzhia hetshi	This Mr Ravele took the position
Tshidulo tsha president P. R. Mphephu	of President P. R. Mphephu
A si zwavho, vho tou renga	It is not yours, you just bought it
Ndi kwine vha ndzhie.	It is better to kill me by ritual murder.

(Kruger 1999/2000: 20)

In this way, as spiritually sanctioned social commentators with a desire for an 'ordered social environment' and a tendency towards articulating criticism, *tshilombe* musicians write and sing songs on pressing concerns of the day. They perform at beer halls, parties, and other public occasions. At the 2005 annual *tshikona* (national reed pipe dance) festival in Thohoyandou, several *zwilombe* with a variety of hand-made instruments patrolled the periphery of the dancing arena, in the area where traditional beer (*mahafhe*) was being sold. An inebriated *tshilombe* staggered towards me and began to perform a song in Afrikaans (presumably for my benefit) with a musical accompaniment on his bashed guitar. He wanted me to sponsor a song for a jam-jar (*scale*) of *mahafhe*. I agreed, asking him to sing about the activities of *zwilombe*. His improvised chorus, this time in Tshivenda, was so impressive that I gladly paid the price:

Nne ndi lilombe!	I am a big, powerful *Tshilombe*!
A no ngo zwi vhonna naa?	Didn't you see?
A tho ngo tou nanga hovhu vhutshilo	I did not choose this life
Ndi ndevhe dza midzimu	I am the ears of the ancestors
Ndi milomo ya vho makhulu wanu!	I am the mouth of your ancestors
Ndi bambiri na milenzhe	I am a newspaper with legs
Ndo shwika shango lothe!	I have been over the entire country!

This impromptu performance revealed not only the spiritual sanction invoked by *zwilombe*, but also the non-optative acceptance of what they see as their fate. It also demonstrated the ways in which their songs, and social commentaries, are often improvised for the benefit of their audience (see Barber 1991). Indeed, although based on recurring themes and phrases that constitute a core to each song, *tshilombe* lyrics are rarely standardised. Songs last at least ten minutes and precise lyrics may be difficult to recall, especially given that most song performances follow the consumption of much beer, sometimes adding to the flow of consciousness of lyrical composition and at other times seriously hindering it. Melodies, on the other hand, are more likely to remain consistent in repeat performances.

The song '*Zwidzumbe*' (Secrets) was performed for me on various occasions (the first in 2000) by the famous and prolific *tshilombe* musician Solomon Mathase. Mathase is well known in South African ethnomusicological circles, having been the subject of extensive writings by Jaco Kruger from the early 1990s (1993; 1999; 1999/2000; 2002; 2006; 2007). A *Mukoma* (petty headman) of Ngwenani ya Themeli village 10 kilometres north-east of Thohoyandou, he is a well-known character in the area. Although he works during the day as a maintenance man at the University of Venda, he is to be found in the evenings and weekends wandering the paths between beer halls in and around his village, guitar slung over one shoulder, three faithful dogs never far behind. In 2009, he had achieved a significant degree of local fame by recording the soundtrack for a popular amateur Venda movie (a comedy) called *Tshovhilingana 4*, for which he claimed he had yet to receive any payment. On the back of his *Tshovhilingana* fame, Solomon recorded a solo album, *Nne na Vhone* (Me and You). It was awarded the 'Best Venda Traditional Album (2009)' at the South African Music Awards in Durban, and the first single ('*Ntshavheni*') rapidly became a local favourite.[3]

---

[3] To say that Solomon Mathase's '*Ntshavheni*' became a local favourite is perhaps an understatement. The song tells the story of a man who was 'eaten' by prostitutes in Johannesburg, and returned home without a cent to his name. Following the extensive airplay the hit received, it is now common for Tshivenda-speakers to refer to someone who is totally broke as '*Ntshavheni*'.

As a petty headman, on the lowest rung of traditional authority, Solomon expresses his loyalty to King Tshivhase through music. In songs such as '*Ha-Tshivhasa*', Mathase declared his complete support for Tshivhase's bid to be officially recognised as a king, and implored others to do the same. King Tshivhase duly returned the compliment by awarding Mathase an award and a cash prize for his loyalty and success. In 2010 Solomon released another album, in which the king plays backing keyboards – cementing the relationship between the two in a mutually beneficial relationship that, according to Solomon, 'is the highlight of my career'.

'*Zwidzumbe*' was originally entitled '*Ri Tshimbilanayo*' (We walk with it) (see Appendix B: lines 36–7). Through it, Mathase complained that promiscuous women were 'carrying AIDS around with them', infecting men and 'the sons of the nation'. He called on them to adhere to the laws of 'God's country', in which they walk without giving due thanks or deference, causing the nation to perish (*lushaka lu khou fhela*; Appendix B: line 23) in the process. This general theme is remarkably similar to that of a song by *tshilombe* Mmbangiseni Madzivhandila, recorded by Kruger (1993: 348–56), which notes how promiscuous girls, with an insatiable sexual appetite, are blamed for harbouring and spreading the HIV virus.

When I met up with Solomon in 2004, I asked him to perform '*Ri Tshimbilanayo*' again so that I could make a digital recording for my PhD thesis. He informed me that he had been thinking about the song a lot, and it was now called '*Zwidzumbe*' (Secrets). We met many times over several months, and I became a regular visitor to his homestead, which was often a hive of musical activity during the weekends. Solomon, like his fellow musicians, claims to be an adherent of ancestral religion rather than Christianity. He makes regular sacrificial offerings to his ancestors, and engages in acts of traditional healing. We made several trips deep into the bush to Ha-Makuya (see Map 4) in my pick-up truck so that he could collect various parts of trees and shrubs for use in relation to my own, his family's, and his friends' general and spiritual well-being. Instructions for which plants to choose came in the form of encounters with ancestral spirits in dreams. Nonetheless, he often uses the life of Jesus in metaphor, and clearly has great respect for a Christian God: 'It is not my place to tell others who their God is', he once told me. 'How do I know that when I speak with my ancestors, God cannot also hear us?'[4]

---

[4] This is not to suggest that the concepts of God in ancestral and Christian theology are counterposed against each other, although there may be grounds for claiming this. Although their respective adherents have been distinguished clearly as social and class

He performed many songs during each musical session that I participated in, but always made a point of playing his *nyimbo ngaha Aidse* (song about AIDS), announcing each time to his audience that they must remain quiet in order that 'Mr Fraser' should hear his account (*tshitori zwavhukuma* – 'the *real* story') of the epidemic. He played it slightly differently each time, adding changes in the lyrical composition or the structure of the guitar accompaniment.

The central themes, however, remained consistent with the version I recorded in 2000. Solomon's performance of '*Zwidzumbe*' is not just a powerful articulation of the extent to which AIDS has been incorporated into the conservative and patriarchal folk model of sexual illness. The song also provides a lucid and eloquent account of the crisis perceived by older generations: that young people are not respecting the moral code of the elders/ancestors; and that young girls in particular are straying from patriarchal control, resulting in widespread sexually transmitted illnesses. In this way, '*Zwidzumbe*' is a musical expression of the extent to which Solomon and his peers feel a deep dysfunctionality in post-apartheid society, wrought through generational and gendered disarticulation. As he sings towards the end of the song, 'If you are a child, you must listen to the rules' (Appendix B: line 102).

In the song, Solomon shifts between imitating the voices and opinions of young, old, male, and female actors, simulating gossip and social situations in which AIDS, and the causes of sexual illness, are discussed. Through this process, he poses questions and provides answers to construct a complex representation of the ways in which HIV/AIDS is understood by the majority of rural Venda men and older (initiated) women.

The extract below is taken from a recording at Mathase's homestead at Ngwenani ya Themeli in June 2005 (see Figures 6.1 and 6.2) and the entire song can be heard at http://www.cambridge.org/us/9781107009912. A full translation is presented in Appendix B and the extract below begins at 8 minutes 50 seconds on the website track. Stylistic shifts in Mathase's voice are a feature of his performances. Here he moves from imitation of the bold statements made by young people, who appear to be mocking the concerns of their elders, to snatches of almost whispered gossip as elders discuss the cause of a specific death. This change in pitch and timbre is significant for the argument to be made in the next chapter: it is suggestive of the ways in which talking about AIDS – and other causes of death – is constrained by a series of conventions rooted in the distinction between private and public domains.

groupings and by their divergent practices and political affiliations, the concept of God in ancestral religion is not incompatible with that of Christianity.

186　AIDS, Politics, and Music in South Africa

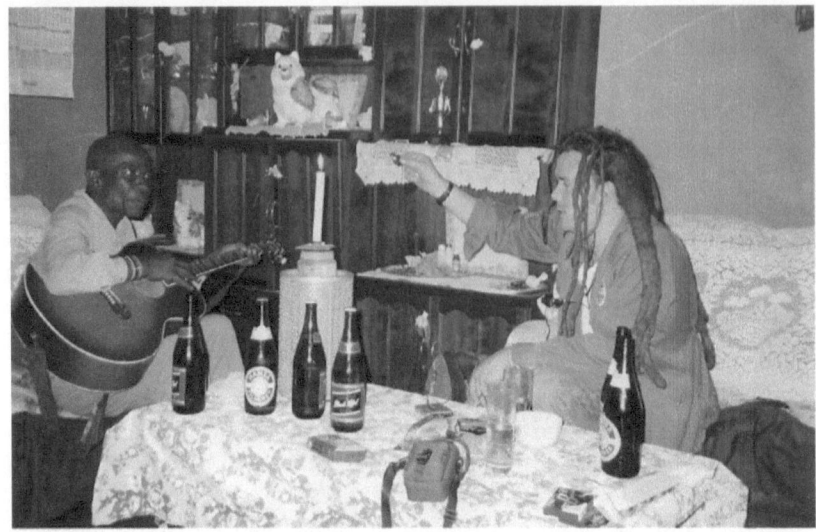

Figure 6.1. Recording *'Zwidzumbe'* at Solomon Mathase's home, June 2005.

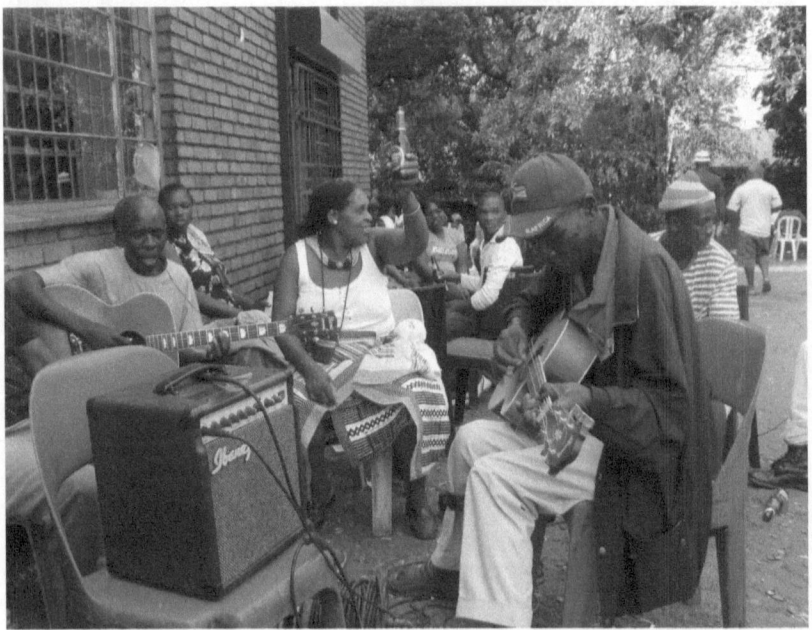

Figure 6.2. Solomon Mathase performing *'Zwidzumbe'* at Mapita's Tavern, July 2010.

Zwidzumbe (Secrets)

(65) *Houla mudulu, nda ndi sa mufuni zwone,*	That grandchild, I really loved him,
na u la nwanawanga,	and that other child of mine,
nda ndi sa mufuni zwone	I really loved him/her,
(66) *Mara u pfi o vhulwa nga yenei Aidse*	But they say he/she was killed by AIDS
(67) *Vhone, vhopfa uri zwone ndi zwifhio?*	You, what did you hear?
(68) *U la munwe ari hupfi hai!*	No! He slept with a woman
O tou wela	Who was unclean after an abortion
(69) *Munwe ari hai!*	Another said No!
Thiri o vha a khou pfana	Isn't it that he slept with
Na u la musadzi wa Vho-mukenenene?[5]	The wife of Mr so and so?
(70) *Nwana wa Vho-mukenenene, vhone vha*	The child of Mr so and so ...
(71) *Muthemba ula?*	Do you really trust her?
Ari thiri u tou nga o vha o bvisa thumbu?	Didn't she have an abortion?
(72) *Munwe ari hai!*	Another said no!
Thiri o vha a na zwilonda nga nnyoni?	Doesn't she have sores on her vagina?
(73) *Munwe ari hai!*	Another said no!
O vha otou vhifha muvhilini	She was pregnant ('ugly in the body') [Now speaking as a practising traditional healer]
(74) *Ngoho mara zwone*	Really, but honestly,
Zwa vhukuma ndi zwifhipo?	Which one of these is the truth here?
(75) *Tshihulwane, o vhuya a dida*	Really, she visited me,
Na kha nne ari ndi mufhe mushonga	So that I could give them medicine
(76) *A tshiyo pfana na nwana wa Vho Mukenenene*	When he fell in love with that daughter of Mr so and so
(77) *Thumbu a yongo fara*	But she could not conceive a child
(78) *Mulandu ndi zwilonda*	The problem was these vaginal sores
Zwe zwi la zwawe ndi li a 'gokhonya'	They led to her getting '*gokhonya*'
(79) *A vho ngo vhona na ula*	Didn't you see that one,
Nwana wawe wa u thoma, o mbo di lovha	Her first child died
(80) *O vha o funa o ya hanengei*	She should have consulted
ha Vho Nyatshavhungwa	Mrs Nyatshavhungwa.[6]
Thiri na vhala vha a zwikona?	Isn't she the one who can deal with these difficult things?

---

[5] Mr Mukenenene actually translates as 'Mr so-and-so'.

[6] This refers to a specific group of traditional healers called *maine*. *Maine* with the name Nyatshavhungwa specialise in adolescent illnesses. Tshivenda speakers distinguish between four different types of traditional healer. An *inyanga* is responsible for overall spiritual protection from witches, may practise witchcraft on his/her own account, and is commonly consulted to explain sources of misfortune. *Inyangas* divine by means of interpreting the patterns in which *thangu* (ritual bones/stones/shells) fall onto the floor, and they can also administer medicine (*mushonga*) for good luck with money, women, exams, et cetera. A *mungome*, who is usually Shangaan and attached to a specific royal court, is normally consulted when a relative dies, and can identify the killer by interpreting *thangu* in a divining bowl (*ndilo*). A *maine* (family doctor) does not use *thangu*, but learns through dreams which herbs can cure specific illnesses. Clans may hold allegiance to a line of *maine* for generations. The last category is *vhaporofhiti*, prophets in Zionist, Apostolic, and Pentecostal faith-healing churches who combine healing with church leadership and often replace herbs with holy water. Of course, these categories are frequently breached and an *inyanga* may claim to be able to cure various illnesses, whilst a *maine* may offer spiritual protection. This is explained by the fact that it is not the prerogative of individuals to be traditional healers; instead, their actions are controlled by ancestors who provide guidance through the medium of dreams.

Malwadze dza Vhafumakadzi: The Illnesses of Women

In this section of the song, Solomon raises closely related key issues from which we can sketch the parameters of a Venda AIDS aetiology. They are abortion/contraception (*o tou wela* or *u bvisa tumbu*), notions of socially unacceptable promiscuity, and the role of the *inyanga* in treating conditions such as vaginal sores (*zwilonda*, leading to *gokhonya*). These are connected, and I will deal with each in turn.

First, towards the end of the song, Mathase makes an explicit connection between AIDS and the woman who 'could not conceive a child'; a reference to the use of the contraceptive injection or pill. In his own words:

> When a woman is sleeping with a man, the bloods are not the same. This has not really been a problem unless you were sleeping with a prostitute who had too many mixtures in her blood and could always give you illness. The problem now is that women are using the pills and injections from the doctors... they get them at the clinics... I have seen them trying to hide it. When women use the pills to prevent a pregnancy, she will get pimples and wounds and smelly discharge from her vagina. You know women every month they have their period, now after taking the pill the periods disappear, so where does the dirty blood go?! It gets into their veins, they cannot conceive and they get this AIDS or whatever. Then the man gets inside her without knowing and catches it. (Interview in Tshivenda, Solomon Mathase, 1 August 2005. Tape 1, Side 2: 50–end)

This idea of 'mixed' or dirty blood which ought to have been taken out of the female body through the menstrual cycle is widespread. Throughout Southern Africa, it is linked to notions of pollution, sexual taboos, and social and physical illness. For Karanga-speakers in the Ndanga and Bikita districts of Zimbabwe, it is known as *svina* ('dirt') and avoidance of it is fundamental to the maintenance of fertility and sexual health. It is thought to be in particular abundance before the first period after a woman gives birth, and thus sex is highly taboo during this time (Aschwanden 1987: 21–3; Ingstad 1990: 33, among Tswana). In Malawi, some traditional practitioners have also conceptualised the symptoms of AIDS as a direct result of female transgression of blood-related sexual taboos (Lwanda 2003). Similar observations have also been made in Botswana (Ingstad 1990; de Bruyn 1992; Heald 2006). In other regions of South Africa women's bodies are also conceptualised as highly suitable places for harbouring 'dirt'. As Leclerc-Madlala (2002) has shown in KwaZulu-Natal, menstrual blood is intrinsically connected to notions of pollution and sexual health. She suggests that this wider complex of meaning has been mobilised to provide non-biomedical explanations for the AIDS epidemic and that 'women's promiscuity' (ibid.: 91) is widely regarded as being primarily responsible for the unhealthy contamination of blood (cf. Ashforth 2005: 160). In this context, widespread belief that sex with a virgin can cure or prevent HIV infection must be understood in terms of pre-menstrual purity as the flipside to the dangerous mixing of, or interference with, bodily cycles thought to be of the natural order.

Such connections between diseases of the blood, pollution, and the female body are of long standing in Venda. Writing about conception, Stayt comments that

> a child receives its flesh and blood from the mother, and sensory organs and bones from the father... probably because of the respective colours of the menstrual flow and the semen... all illnesses connected with the blood thus come from the mother's side of the family. (Stayt 1931: 260–1)

For Solomon Mathase, then, as for many others in Southern Africa, the natural cycles that remove pollution from the female body are central to healthy individual (and thus social) reproduction. The introduction of methods of contraception such as the pill and the injection put this system in danger by regulating the flow in ways perceived as unnatural that result in the trapping of 'dirt'. Women who use – or are suspected of using – contraception thus harbour dams of dangerous pollution that will eventually make them ill – and also infect men who come into intimate contact with them.

This sickness can take a variety of forms, such as *zwilonda* (line 72; open genital sores that resemble the third phase of syphilis), *gokhonya* (line 78; also known as *lukuse*, through which a woman's children die in infancy),[7] *tshidzwonyonyo* (a red, burning rash on the genitals similar to thrush), or *tshimbambamba* (through which a woman develops yellow pimples in the genital area that burst during sex and cause a white, smelly discharge similar to gonorrhoea). This complex of sexually transmitted infections is known in Tshivenda as *malwadze dza vhafumakadzi*: the illnesses of women. Explained by the 'experts' (peer educators) as a blood-borne infection transmitted through sexual intercourse, HIV/AIDS has been incorporated readily into this framework of knowledge. In the same way, at some point in history, syphilis was incorporated as *thusula* and gonorrhoea as *doropo*. The ways in which these sexually transmitted infections are explained through the biomedical lexicon render them more or less compatible with the folk cosmology of sexual sicknesses.

---

[7] *Gokhonya* is usually found in women after a difficult or problematic birth such as that induced by caesarean section. Symptoms include the child refusing the mother's milk and red marks on the child's head and neck. White pimples will be found inside the mother's vagina, and the conventional cure involves the *inyanga* scraping the vaginal sores with a razor and mixing the resultant fluid with the mother's urine and a mixture of three herbs. This potion is then given to the child in a milky drink and it will be healed. The mother, however, must undergo several more rites of purification.

Second, the evidence above demonstrates the ways in which menstrual blood and abortion can be constitutive of pollution that leads to the onset of HIV/AIDS. This has also been documented in other parts of the region. Auslander, for example, states that certain Ngoni women who have become economically independent in Zambia 'are said to become pregnant and self-abort continually, thus altering their "wombs" in such a manner as to infect with AIDS those who cohabit with them' (1993: 182). The connection here – between specific women with a desire for economic independence and the use of fertility-blocking biomedicine perceived as beyond male control – is important in the context of peer educators' apparent upward social mobility. But it would be misleading to suggest that we can understand the current situation solely through recourse to fluctuations in economic or social status.

In line 68, when Mathase sings about the woman who *o tou wela* ('fell deep inside of something'), he is referring to an abortion that has not been conducted in the 'correct' manner. For Mathase and his peers, the act of abortion in itself, whilst not encouraged, is not taboo. However, the process of *u bvisa tumbu* (abortion – 'to take out the stomach', line 72) must be conducted in strict accordance with principles of good practice in which the womb must be cleansed with specific herbal remedies to render it (and the woman) clean, and thus fertile again. In Solomon's own words:

A girl can get pregnant and she goes to the doctors for an abortion, you know, maybe the father of the child is an important person, or her father may be a pastor [in the church] or whatever, you know, these things do happen here in Venda. She goes to the doctor, they give her the pills and the baby dies. In our culture we have medicine that can also do that and then cleanse the womb out because when she does this it is contaminated with many diseases that should be treated. But they do not get the treatment from the *inyanga*. They are afraid maybe he will talk [about the abortion to others], so they just let the diseases build up until a man gets inside and catches that AIDS or whatever. These things are not even a secret. Venda boys are told all of this at *murundu* [the male circumcision lodge]. (Interview in Tshivenda, Solomon Mathase, 1 August 2005. Tape 1, Side 1: 75–90)

A traditional healer (*inyanga*) made this connection more explicit during an interview:

[I]t [AIDS] is the poison from the aborted child. You see, there are many types of medicine that can cure these things, they circulate around the body, and the waste is taken out in urine or faeces. None of these tablets affect the bones; they stay in the flesh and veins only. Now, in abortion, after one month or so, that tablet, the medicine that destroys the entire foetus, with bones and cartilage combined, it becomes a liquid. What remains is the bone solution, which remains inside the body of the woman as poison. The bones cannot be destroyed, they remain within. Only the blood comes out if she menstruates. Then we must put the medicine inside her and leave it for some few days until she is clean again. If she does not come to us for treatment, then the next male comes in with his penis, and catches it [AIDS].... Yes, it's osmosis, when the penis gets erect, it gets warm, the pores open up, all the poisonous gases in her womb will give him AIDS. The carrier, the first carrier [of AIDS] was the woman who aborted a child and did not get cleaned. (Interview, E. Maphanda, 7 August 2000)

The same *inyanga* (who also works as a part-time life insurance salesman) articulated his points in a poem. He sent copies by airmail to Tony Blair, the Queen, and Bill Gates in the hope that they would provide funding to develop his herbal infusion that acts as the post-abortion purifying agent mentioned above, and also thus as a cure for AIDS. The last three stanzas of the poem, written in fluent English, read:

> AIDS, AIDS, AIDS, revenge of the unborn,
> The white man is unaware you are the remains of the foetus,
> Yes, AIDS is the poison from the aborted child,
> Our ancestors have identified the *muti*, the signs and the symptoms.
>
> Black nurses and doctors have become sell-outs,
> The custom they buried for a foreign culture,
> When ours originated with the creator,
> Who is in all science and all life.
>
> He did hide the healing power in herbs,
> And Christianity failed to align faith and creation,
> The vagina is related to Rwanda and Kosovo.
> The pussy being known for pleasure, instead of progeny.

A copy of the entire poem is attached in Appendix C.

Maphanda's account of AIDS is interesting in the context of Stayt's 1931 observation, quoted above. When abortion disrupts the natural process, he tells us, it is the male essence (the white bones) of the foetus that is resistant to the medicine. The embryonic bones fester to become the gases which are said to cause AIDS. This suggests that sexual illness cannot be traced to blood alone; disruption of natural cycles also renders maleness as potentially polluted. Indeed, as I have already shown, although the folk model attributes pollution to women, a dichotomous distinction between the genders is inadequate here. It is young, often promiscuous women – rather than those who follow conservative, patriarchal norms – who are blamed by men and older women alike. The important divisions here are thus as much generational as they are gendered, and this becomes clear when we consider the dynamics of knowledge and experience that are in play at this juncture.

A 'Folk' Cosmology: Knowledge and Assumed Experience

Like scientific explanations, any folk model is a code of understanding that has been constituted in an historically and culturally specific setting. As we have seen, the incorporation of AIDS into Venda aetiology draws consistently from relatively recent, 'outside' influences on the model. It refers to reproductive technologies – the contraceptive pill and injection, the 'morning after' pill – procured in clinics and hospitals. Whilst the folk model refers to biomedical knowledge, however, it does so in a way that renders science guilty of causing the build-up of pollution. Peer educators are key players in this knowledge transfer. They have introduced a competing body of scientific knowledge that, like the folk model, claims to hold the key to healthy sexual and social reproduction at a time when unprecedented numbers of people are dying.

Is it coincidence, then, that AIDS is associated, through the folk model, with the people and places who have openly named it? I deal with this question directly in the following chapter, but for now it should be underscored that the doctors, nurses, and outside experts – with their methods and medicines that disrupt the pathways through which female bodily pollution is managed – are inseparable from folk understandings of AIDS. The contraceptive pill, the injection, and biomedical processes of abortion are inextricably implicated in the controversy. These agents of biomedicine cause the unhealthy accumulation of pollution in female bodies that aspire to transcend patriarchal constraints on their fertility – and possibly even their socio-economic positions. It is not, then, that these relatively recently arrived technologies have been rejected by those adhering to a folk model of sexual illness. Rather, they have become central to an explanatory paradigm that gives historical and cultural meaning to AIDS.

The evidence currently in question raises a third issue: the role of certain women in facilitating the spread of AIDS and other sexual diseases. In '*Zwidzumbe*', Solomon Mathase sings of the young girl who cannot be trusted (lines 70–2). The protagonists in his dialogue are unclear whether she has aborted a child, possesses *zwilonda* (genital sores), or was ever pregnant. Venda girls' initiation, as already demonstrated, is explicitly concerned with the maintenance of conservative female sexuality, based on systems of gendered and generational authority. This system of authority exists within a wider patriarchal environment, however, and thus legitimises – and is legitimised by – ideal values such as virginity until marriage, appropriate sexual relations, and fertility. These are defined in contrast to 'deviant' forms of behaviour such as extramarital affairs and promiscuity, which are thought to cause illness and thus disrupt harmonious social interaction.

Connections between ritual knowledge of the *vhusha* girls' initiation and the widespread, commonsensical articulation of the Venda aetiology of sexual health are important for my argument because they link folk cosmology with the contemporary political economy of traditional leadership discussed in Chapter 2. This association between sacred knowledge and everyday practice has resonance with anthropological approaches to ritual knowledge taken by Barth (1975; 1990; 2002) and Lambek (1993). Both of these authors are concerned with the uneven social distribution of ritual knowledge, its transfer between discrete and hierarchical social groups, and the extent to which 'traditions' or 'corpuses' of knowledge are bounded or fluid.

For Barth, knowledge is that which constitutes 'what a person employs to interpret and act on the world' (2002: 1). A person's stock of knowledge structures their understanding and purposive ways of coping with their lived environment. Barth's analysis is concerned primarily with the transfer of ritual knowledge in the seven complex stages of male initiations among the Baktaman of Papua New Guinea and in sacred temples presided over by priests of Bali Hinduism. Knowledge, he contends, is consistently characterised by 'three faces'. These appear together simultaneously in every performance and transaction of knowing, and allow him to build a model for the comparative analysis of different knowledge traditions and to account for 'marginal change' within them. The first of these 'faces' is a body of substantive assertions and ideas about aspects of the world: a 'corpus' of knowledge. The second is a characteristic set of media through which it is instantiated and communicated; and the last is the social organisation within which this takes place (2002: 3; cf. 1975). In different traditions of knowledge and over time in a single tradition, these three faces interconnect in various ways.

For example, Baktaman initiation is centred on secret rituals that deal with growth, fertility, and ancestral support. The validity of this knowledge is dependent upon its having been received from the ancestors under constraints of secrecy (1975: 217). The secret initiation of young men thus provides the validating organisational format for the reproduction and transmission of ritual knowledge. This process of initiation, through which men are restricted to certain responsibilities and prohibited from others, can take an entire lifetime. In this way the gradual release of ritual knowledge impinges on social organisation. Barth compares the different stages of initiation to the image of Chinese boxes: constructed with multiple levels, with each organised to obscure the content of the next. The communicative medium that embodies and transmits this knowledge depends upon a combination of secrecy and danger for its heightened experiential capacity and efficacy; and the corpus of assertions woven from analogies with the natural and social world is intended at once to mystify and reveal. Although, as the secret lore of the ancestors, theoretically this corpus should be unchanging (cf. La Fontaine 1985), Barth identifies regional and historical processes of 'marginal change' through the inconsistent pragmatics of performance and the variable memory of ritual leaders.

Interdependent traditions of knowledge and their uneven social distribution are also of central concern in Lambek's analysis of ritual knowledge in Mayotte, near Madagascar. In comparison to Barth, however, Lambek is explicit that

> things in Mayotte do not fully tie together... there is not a hidden order beneath the surface just waiting for the foreign anthropologist with his or her sophisticated intellectual technology to be mined... [rather] there are a plurality of unities, lying always just ahead. (1993: 379)

Following Schutz (1964), his analysis is based on the distinction between the 'expert', the 'well-informed citizen', and the 'man in the street' (1993: 69). The expert's knowledge is limited to a specific field, but therein it is clear and distinct. The man in the street has a working knowledge of many fields (or 'branches' in Barth's terms) through which he can react to typical situations to achieve typical results. Well-informed citizens fall in between these two categories in the amount of knowledge they seek, and they assist in its legitimation through periodic critical evaluation. The three most salient fields of knowledge ('traditions' in Barth's terms) in Mayotte are Islamic textual knowledge, the cosmology of sorcery, and spirit possession. At any given time, an individual's knowledge belongs in all three categories in relation to different fields. An expert in possession can be a man in the street in textual knowledge, and vice versa. Lambek is thus concerned not only with the relative quantity of people's knowledge, but 'the reasons they are acquiring it and their relationship to it' (1993: 69). Experts maintain levels of professionalism and attempt to secure legitimacy through the practice of secrecy. This is evidenced by a healer who, in the process of teaching a student, voices his concern that 'If it [the knowledge] becomes public, then people will not be able to become well' (1993: 296). The success of the cure is predicated on the restricted nature of the knowledge.[8]

The gradual release of secret knowledge (the corpus) by a powerful and spiritually sanctioned group (the experts) through processes of initiation (the communicative medium) to those who are in various states of

---

[8] Lambek makes a distinction between objectified and embodied knowledge, both of which exist in dialectical relation to each other in each of the disciplines. Islamic knowledge is primarily objectified in the text, but in the process and performance of learning is embodied through prayer and proverbs. Possession knowledge is primarily embodied through the practice of knowing how to become possessed, but ultimately objectified through the coding and observance of strict taboos that characterise the embodied experience.

liminality is, of course, familiar anthropological territory.[9] What, then, can we take from these accounts to help us make sense of knowledge transfer and its opposite, secrecy, in Venda? Three points need to be underlined. First, both authors stress that the acquisition and accumulation of ritual knowledge are based, fundamentally, on experience. For Barth this is the experience of long-term initiation and the revelation of ancestral knowledge. For Lambek, it is either the experience of reading and learning the Islamic texts or the embodied experience of becoming possessed. Second, for this knowledge to be transferred, conditions of secrecy must be ensured. Its value comes from the fact that it is not readily available in the public domain, and thus 'experts' are charged with the responsibility of maintaining the corpus and securing the appropriate conditions for its reproduction and, by extension, the regeneration of complete individuals. Third, both Lambek and Barth emphasise the inherent danger of knowledge, and the protective space offered by a ritual environment for its safe and complete transferral. In Mayotte 'it is bad to know too much... people with knowledge are both respected and suspected' (Lambek 1993: 7).

Returning to the Venda material against this comparative background, we can now address questions raised about connections within the folk model of sexual health between ritual knowledge and common sense. Those in possession of specialist knowledge – like Noriah and the ritual experts at the Dopeni project – are, in Lambek's terms, the 'experts'. Those with a working understanding of the basic principles, who assist in legitimating the knowledge though periodic critical evaluation – like Solomon Mathase, those of his ilk, and older (initiated) women – are '(wo)men in the street' or 'well-informed citizens', who remain ignorant of ritual specificities but for whom the basic principles of the ritual knowledge – how to avoid pollution – are commonsensical.

Folk cosmologies are not static, but are subject to periods of 'marginal change' (Barth 2002). In the case of Venda folk understandings of sexual health, it is not within the ritual context that legitimate knowledge is amended. As we saw in Chapter 3, ritual experts are loath to incorporate biomedical concepts into the ancestrally sanctioned initiation curriculum. The negotiation of a 'folk model' vis-à-vis biomedicine occurs, rather, through strategic appropriation of biomedical science by those – like Solomon Mathase – who maintain a working knowledge of the system but are not held responsible for its successful transfer to future generations.

It is within the realms of this working knowledge that men and older (initiated) women locate the coordinates of association through which

---

[9] See, for example, Turner (1969a); La Fontaine (1985); Comaroff (1985); Bloch (1992).

they blame certain young women in their midst for the crisis in sexual and social reproduction. They are the women who 'mix blood' to cause illness, those who interfere with the natural cycles of menstruation to regulate fertility, or, as Solomon calls them, the 'sexy women'. Eurocentric notions of promiscuity or prostitution are not necessarily appropriate here. Hunter (2002), Wojcicki (2002), and Thornton (2008) show how multiple concurrent long-term relationships that involve complex transactional negotiations and a certain degree of commitment between men and women (often younger girls) are commonplace and often viewed as socially acceptable.

In Venda, this is manifest in the social institution of *farakano*, through which a married man may have a secret lover (*mufarakano*; plural *mafarakano*).[10] This term is used to distinguish a secret wife or lover from both an official wife (*musadzi* or, respectfully, *mufumakadzi*) and a girlfriend (*cherrie*). So long as a man provides material goods to the woman's homestead, and the woman is not married, it is quite acceptable for a child to be born of the relationship. A wealthy man may have several *mafarakano* and may even propose marriage to one, if the circumstances are favourable. However, such relationships are generally kept secret and only discussed with groups of close friends.

A *mufarakano* is very different to the 'sexy women' of the song. These are beer hall prostitutes who offer quick-fix 'survival sex' (Wojcicki 2002) for on-the-spot cash. This kind of trade in sex is relatively common throughout Venda, especially in the vicinity of the larger towns of Thohoyandou, Makhado, and Musina. Its purveyors are regularly demonised in the media for lurking outside beer halls and hotels, soliciting business from passing men and encouraging them to visit motels for illicit sex. This stigmatisation has generally focused on the fact that many commercial sex workers are under-age illegal immigrants from Zimbabwe. Numerous articles in tabloids such as the *Daily Sun* warn men against the dangers of such girls who, they suggest, not only spread disease, but may even steal from you and then accuse you of rape. Nonetheless, in rural shebeens and beer halls (especially at month end when men are known to have disposable income) many Venda girls and women engage in such sexual transactions.

Unlike a *mufarakano* who may bear her lover's children, the girl in Solomon Mathase's song (cf. Appendix B: lines 13–18, 38–41) is suspected of using the contraceptive pill or injection to prevent pregnancy. She and others like her, it is implied, are likely to have had an abortion

---

[10] The meaning of this term seems to have changed in the recent past. Van Warmelo (1989: 207) states from data gathered in the 1930s that it derives from the verb *u gwanda* (to be entwined like wild, thorny weeds) and that it refers to the 'mutual aid set up of man and woman "just living together"' (ibid.).

and failed to have their womb cleaned (*o tou wela*). For Solomon Mathase and his peers, she represents the type of 'deviant' woman who is responsible for spreading the illnesses of women (*malwadze dza vhafumakadzi*). While not necessarily a full-time commercial sex worker, she may be occasionally involved in such transactions.

Alternatively, and importantly, she might have been rumoured to be using the pill or have had an abortion. As Mathase put it in the quotation above:

This [dirty blood] has not really been a problem unless you were sleeping with a prostitute who had too many mixtures in her blood and could always give you illness. The problem now is that women are using the pills and injections from the doctors... they get them at the clinics... I have seen them trying to hide it.

In addition to full- or part-time sex workers who have 'always' been bearers of illness, then, there is the more recent category of women using biomedical techniques to regulate their fertility. With their prolific knowledge of biomedical concepts, declared publicly on a weekly basis through songs, peer educators fall directly into this recently constructed category. They are guilty through association; caught in the web that connects publicly expressed knowledge with assumed experience.

If connections are drawn between extensive familiarity with the biomedical model and its practical use, we must see these in the wider context of the more general links between knowledge and experience. As I argued above, anthropological approaches to ritual knowledge have highlighted the fundamental nature of the experiential process through which claims to authoritative knowledge are facilitated. This was apparent in Chapter 3, where we saw that the powerful relationship between experience and ritual knowledge is integral to the hierarchy of authority in *vhusha* initiation. I also suggested that it is pervasive throughout social relations pertaining to ritual contexts more generally, and can be seen to operate in discourses of the occult, rituals of affliction, prophet-led Christianity, and traditional healing. In this way, it transgresses religious and political boundaries in the maintenance and transference of potentially dangerous, but essential, ritual knowledge.

Just as experience is intrinsically connected to the generation of legitimate and authoritative ritual knowledge, so the reverse applies: knowledge is assumed to be based on experience. Solomon Mathase assumes that the peer educators' biomedical repertoire is based on experience of such medicine. For Solomon and similar traditionalist males, and for initiated women, it is inconceivable that the peer educators' claims to biomedical knowledge, like the ritual experts' claims to ritual knowledge, would not be rooted in experiential processes of it.

Folk Cosmology and the Resurgence of Tradition

As the next chapter illustrates, it is very rare for anyone openly to discuss illness, death, or its causes in either scientific terms or folk cosmology. However, gossip and backstage rumour play an important part in the circulation of illness representations in general, as did the songs of peripheral artists like Solomon Mathase and other *zwilombe*. But these concepts, as part of a wider body of knowledge, are formalised, and to some extent regulated, through the institutions of initiation and healing. Whilst the role of traditional healers in the promotion of non-biomedical representations of AIDS in the region has received limited attention (see, for example, Ingstad 1990; Ashforth 2000; 2005), the role of initiation has yet to be explored in this vein.

The relationship between these two institutions is best conceptualised in terms of the relationship between those who have 'expert' knowledge and the functional capacities of the 'man in the street'. The *vhusha ya vhatendi* (the Christian *vhusha*) and the *vhusha ya musanda* (royal *vhusha*) are both based on the moral code (*milayo*) that is symbolised through the tricolour symbolism of red (unintentionally reflected in the uniforms of peer educators), white, and black. This ritual knowledge enshrines the centrality of blood-related taboos, sexual/social health, and fertility. It is also concerned with the centrality of traditional medicine in treating sexual illness. Thus, an important and currently overlooked means by which alternative conceptualisations of AIDS are transmitted to young people in South Africa, and reinforced in older generations, is through initiation schools.

The recent surge in official attempts to increase female initiation has, as I have argued, reinforced the hierarchical authority within the *tshivhambo* ritual hut. This has, by extension and possibly inadvertently, bolstered the authority of the ritual knowledge upon which that hierarchy is based, and thus the authority of the 'working knowledge' of the ritual corpus that is accessible for general consumption. When men like Solomon sing about dirty blood, *zwilonda* and 'breaking the rules' (see Appendix B, lines 102–5), they are articulating the values and moral codes not only of traditional healing and initiation, but of the patriarchal and conservative order of which they are a part. This is based, fundamentally, on respect for ancestors and thus on generational and patriarchal authority.

The extent to which AIDS in Venda is understood by men and older women through the folk model should thus be seen in this wider, contemporary political context. Ignoring the decisions of traditional leaders to increase the frequency of female initiation schools would be equivalent to building an understanding of AIDS in rural South Africa without a cornerstone. Folk understandings of AIDS are inseparable from notions of an African renaissance that have become central to strategies for the consolidation of power in response to the nationally instigated competition for paramount kingship. In this way the African renaissance has indeed promoted 'African solutions to African problems', and *Thovhela* Tshivhase's implementation of ANC policy has served to legitimate a corpus of ritual knowledge over which, paradoxically, he has little influence.

Non-scientific understandings of AIDS must not be thought of as mystical, lingering hangovers from a pre-scientific yesteryear but – at least in part – as the dynamic manifestations of the contemporary political economy in post-apartheid South Africa. Like belief in the occult, folk representations of AIDS are:

not archaic or exotic phenomena, somehow isolated or disjointed [from] historical processes of global political and economic transformation. Rather, these are moral discourses alive to the basic coordinates of experience, highly sensitive to contradictions in economy and society. (Auslander 1993: 168)

Conclusion: Towards a Medical Ethnomusicology?

The comparison between peer education songs in the previous chapter and *tshilombe* interpretations of HIV/AIDS has enveloped a wide-ranging discussion of the social relations mediated by access to various gradations of ritual knowledge and different forms of experience associated with them. To conclude this chapter, however, I want to return to the theme of music – and specifically to some implications of the discussion so far for the emerging sub-discipline of 'medical ethnomusicology'.

In a recent analysis of Ugandan performance genres, Barz argues that women's AIDS songs – similar to those performed by peer educators in Venda – have played a significant role in the country's allegedly impressive reduction in HIV transmission rates: both as therapeutic interventions in their own right and as media for AIDS education in remote regions.[11] It is likely that the songs described by Barz have played a role in this by instigating action among some who are exposed to them. They may have encouraged a pregnant woman to be tested for her child's sake if for no other reason, or convinced a commercial sex worker to manage her workplace hazards by using condoms or reducing the number of sexual partners. To be sure, at least in the Venda context, peer educators' songs

---

[11] HIV prevalence in Uganda decreased from 9.5 per cent of the population in 1997 to 5 per cent in 2001 (UNAIDS 2004 in Barz 2006: 11). Other data from antenatal clinics in Uganda suggest that the figures have fallen from 29.4 per cent in 1992 to 11.25 per cent in 2000 (O'Manique 2004). However, Allen (2006) has questioned the reliability of statistics recording Uganda's battle against AIDS. It is sobering to compare this to comparative statistics for South Africa; from 12.9 per cent in 1997 to 20.1 per cent in 2001 (ibid.). See Thornton (2008) for a historical ethnographic analysis of the differences between 'sexual networks' in the two countries.

have sparked conversations about antiretroviral medication or voluntary counselling and testing.

But the extent to which people, on hearing the songs, have followed the instructions given is questionable: one song can be heard in many different ways. There is little evidence in the AIDS literature that 'accurate' knowledge (whether presented in song, text, or radio) leads to behaviour change in African populations. As this chapter has illustrated, biomedical understandings can be reinterpreted and incorporated into conservative, patriarchal folk models of illness in a way which serves to further stigmatise the women who promote scientific understandings of AIDS.

As a contribution to the emergent discipline of medical ethnomusicology, then, this chapter highlights the inherent dangers of privileging songs that are rooted in bio-scientific worldviews over those which emerge from folk cosmologies of health and/or sickness (see McNeill and James 2009). It is only by recognising the interaction between the intended and unintended social effects of these two paradigms that we may begin to tease out the complex contexts and processes that give rise to musical performances upon which any medical ethnomusicology might be based. A similar recognition of the reciprocal interrelation between structural forces and local protagonists is necessary in order to understand how ethnomusicology in general might be repositioned in the setting of twenty-first century South Africa.

This brings us back, full circle, to Blacking's theoretical dilemma between music's dual role as a conservative force for equilibrium and a radical force for change. The evidence presented above provides us with ample opportunity to verify both of these possibilities. The songs of the peer educators, for example, have followed government policy in a reactionary manner that has not incorporated advocacy but deferred to the status quo. This is closely connected to the comfortable relationship between office staff and Provincial Department of Health, and peer educators have to a large extent acted as peripatetic advertisements for government services. On the other hand, however, it could equally be argued that in the cobbling together of their musical *bricolage* peer educators are engaging in a form of resistance against the patriarchal model that frames them as carriers of pollution. The use of songs from the struggle in this endeavour can be seen as an explicit statement of defiance and an attempt to embody the spirit of resistance. The very act of demonstrating knowledge of government services and the biomedical model is, for the peer educators, a demonstration of their ability and willingness to transcend their current peer group, to get a job in the government, and to realise their vision of an alternative reality.

Music's dual capacity was again apparent in Solomon Mathase's rendition of '*Zwidzumbe*'. His song clearly articulates concern over modern medical practices causing the build-up of pollution in young women.

He makes the powerful, albeit implicit, connection between knowledge and experience, to suggest that those who 'hide' birth control at clinics are negating traditional structures of authority and thus placing their fertility – and the nation's ability to reproduce – in jeopardy. Mathase's song is an articulation of attempted resistance against this, and as such it presents the case for folk cosmology in the battle to re-establish healthy social and sexual reproduction. *'Zwidzumbe'* thus also symbolises one of the most conservative forces in Venda, that of the ancestors and traditional authority. By reinforcing the role of pollution, cleansing, and the observance of taboos, Mathase echoes the ritual knowledge of the *vhusha* and *domba*, and, in the process, bolsters the conservative, patriarchal order upon which traditional and generational authority is based, and of which initiation is a part.

The picture that has emerged here is necessarily a complex one, pointing to similarities and differences that exist between alternative, but not necessarily 'rival', interpretations of AIDS in Venda. But overall the biomedical framework within which AIDS has been introduced to the region dovetails neatly with the folk model, and the fact that young women are the local bearers of this scientific model confirms the belief of many men and older (initiated) women that AIDS is indeed located within the explanatory paradigm of *malwadze dza vhafumakadzi*, 'the illnesses of women'.

This throws light on the new-found positive identity sought after by the peer educators, outlined in the previous chapter. Whilst constructing their new selves they make it possible for others to simultaneously reconstruct them on several levels – not only with close connections to the biomedical circles from which the pill, injection, and condom originate, but – as I show in the next chapter – by taking public responsibility for AIDS. Any attempt at an AIDS-inspired 'medical ethnomusicology' should thus, at the very least, examine AIDS songs in their multi-faceted complex relationship with other songs about sexual illness. Failure to do so may lead to the damaging propagation of half-truths and misconceptions upon which so many mis-targeted AIDS interventions, such as peer education in Venda, have been modelled.

However – and finally – if we accept that the folk model influences sexual decisions made by men, then the condom may remain a feasible option to prevent contact with 'dirty' blood or gases that are believed to lead to AIDS. The ways in which men perceive their own risk of becoming infected with HIV must then be understood in terms of who the sexual partner is, and not how intercourse takes place. This illuminates a reported pattern of behaviour in which some men have unprotected sex with their wife or long-term partner, with whom they have established a relationship of trust, but use condoms if they are having a brief affair with a stranger or short-term girlfriend, or a casual encounter with a sex worker (cf. Stadler 2003). In terms of the patterns of blame enunciated above, it is the polluted character of the sex worker which explains why a condom is used in her case. Here we see again the overlap between folk models and bioscience that has yet to be exploited by policy makers (see also McNeill and Niehaus 2010). Would it be unthinkable to promote condom use in terms of avoiding 'pollution'? In what other ways could interventions be tweaked to incorporate folk conceptions?

As the next chapter shows, however, it may already be too late to save the condom's reputation from its association with poorly implemented intervention programmes. Condoms, throughout Southern Africa, have been blamed for causing AIDS.

7 'Condoms Cause AIDS'

Poison, Prevention, and Degrees of Separation

> These things, you must understand, there are some things we just do not talk about here in Venda. That is why there is so much gossip. (Chief Rathogwa of Fondwe village, 28 December 2004)

In this final ethnographic chapter, I tackle an issue that has been raised implicitly and explicitly throughout this book: the ways in which people speak – and do not speak – about AIDS.[1] This leads to a critique of the prevalent notion that South Africans are engaged in a mass act of 'AIDS denialism'. To develop this, I again widen the lens of analysis to consider AIDS not just as a sexually transmitted infection, but as a source of perceived unnatural death. I argue that the complex social processes that create and maintain the avoidance of open conversation around HIV and AIDS must be understood in the wider context of conventions through which causes of death are, and are not, spoken about. By invoking silence, coded language, and obfuscation, 'degrees of separation' are constructed that create a social distance between an individual and the unnatural cause of another's death.

The construction of AIDS as a 'public secret' (cf. Mookherjee 2006) must thus be seen in the context of strategies that are intended to negotiate limited responsibility as opposed to a blanket denial of reality. What has been understood as 'denial' is, rather, a direct protest of innocence. Indeed, the public silence around AIDS demonstrates the very real acceptance of the problem and the seriousness with which it has been met. Nonetheless, the conviction that Southern Africa is gripped by macro-level AIDS denial has influenced policy makers profoundly and has been equated with the need for more peer education and empowerment programmes in order to 'break the silence' – the official title of the Thirteenth International AIDS Conference held in Durban in July 2000. In this chapter, I suggest that unless our understandings of the avoidance of open conversation are grounded in a more sensitive appreciation of the relationship between language and folk aetiologies, then the breaching

---

[1] A version of this chapter has been published in the journal *African Affairs* (see McNeill 2009). It is reproduced here with permission from Oxford University Press.

of this public silence in the form of female peer-group education will continue to produce potentially counter-productive consequences.

This argument has far-reaching consequences for the social position of peer educators, particularly for the effectiveness of their strategy in promoting condom use. Building on the argument made in the previous chapter, I show that proponents of the folk model, in conjunction with powerful, parallel social forces, attribute blame to the peer educators not only on the basis of their connections to 'the illnesses of women', but also through the manner in which they breach the public silence around causes of death. When understood through the relationship between publicly expressed knowledge and assumed experience, this acts to confirm what many people suspect: that peer educators are indeed vectors of the virus. The combined effect of these processes has profound implications for the way in which people ascribe meaning not only to the peer educators, but to their central symbol of prevention in the pervasive belief that 'condoms cause AIDS'. The particulars of this accusation vary, but a common explanation is that if condoms are filled with warm water and left overnight, or in direct sunlight, small, white 'worms' hatch inside. Contact with these worms allegedly results in the transmission of the virus. As Epstein (2007: 148) has recently pointed out, the notion that condoms cause AIDS is widespread: 'Many people [in Southern Africa] attribute the epidemic to condoms themselves.'[2] This is not an irrational myth but is underpinned by a certain cultural logic rooted in a folk model of illness. This logic has tended to render peer education impotent.

The ethnographic gaze is here refocused to present an analysis of a parallel phenomenon that similarly has unnatural death at its core: a spate of alleged poisonings. The socio-cultural pressures that impinged upon public discussion around the poisonings are fundamentally related to the reasons why people do not speak openly about AIDS. The comparison between the two 'silences' highlights the extent to which the avoidance of publicly expressed knowledge about causes of death in general is central to understanding the reasons for peer education's limited success.

Secrecy and Denial

In the vast literature on HIV/AIDS in Southern Africa, the avoidance of open conversation that surrounds the pandemic is written about in terms of secrecy, stigma, and denial. 'It is difficult to see what is happening, harder to measure, easiest to deny', argue Barnett and Whiteside (2002: 5). This echoes the sentiments of many other commentators on the topic who have resorted to the explanatory paradigms of denial and stigma to make sense of the powerful influence that HIV/AIDS seems to have

---

[2] See also Pisani (2008: 148), Thornton (2008: 199), Rodlach (2006: chapter 7).

on the ways in which people talk – or more commonly do not talk – about it.³

One of the main objectives of peer education in Southern Africa is to combat what has been termed 'communal denial' (Lwanda 2003: 122). A distinction ought to be made here between this communal denial, a term coined by Lwanda to describe the situation in Malawi, and what can be thought of as 'individual denial'. The former refers to concerted efforts, allegedly made by communities, to suppress the reality of increasing deaths brought on by AIDS. The latter refers to individual, cognitive processes through which HIV-positive persons may delay acceptance of their status. These have been discussed comprehensively in the medical literature (see, for example, Soler-Viñolo et al. 1998), and they undoubtedly play into wider communal processes of shame and stigmatisation. Nonetheless, for the purposes of this chapter, 'AIDS denial' refers to the widespread refusal to name AIDS as a cause of death and the associated unwillingness to talk openly about it in public settings.

To understand why so many people choose not to talk openly about HIV/AIDS in rural South Africa, it is crucial to look beyond notions of shame and stigma. This is not to reject the importance of these concepts, but rather to suggest that they must be contextualised within the wider framework of ways in which death in general, not exclusively AIDS-related, is avoided as a topic of public discussion.

Clearly, notions of secrecy are central to this analysis. And yet the classic sociological account of secrecy by Simmel (1950) has had remarkably little impact on the AIDS literature. A reason for this may be that Simmel essentially analyses secrets in an overtly functionalist manner as tools for the maintenance of group cohesion – restricting the distribution of knowledge to specific groups over time as, for example, we saw with ritual knowledge through the *vhusha*. Recent anthropological work on secrecy and silence, however, has taken more notice of Simmel's work,⁴ raising themes remarkably similar to those that emerge in connection with AIDS. Mookherjee (2006), for example, provides an analysis of the extent to which the rape of certain Bangladeshi women, socially recognised as 'war heroes', remains a 'public secret' that is intrinsically connected to structural power arrangements. It is widely known and yet rarely spoken of. The notion of a public secret is particularly apt in relation to AIDS in South Africa, and I adopt Mookherjee's term intermittently while also borrowing Stadler's notion of public silence (see below). West (2003) raises similar issues when writing of the silence endured by

---

³ See, for example, Herdt (1987), Campbell and Mzaidume (2001), Reid and Walker (2003), Schneider (2002), Stadler (2003), Campbell (2003), and Delius and Glaser (2005).
⁴ See Robbins (2001) for a recent account of secrecy in relation to a millenarian movement's notion of time and narrative in Papua New Guinea.

survivors of torture in colonial Mozambique, and the subsequent failure of FRELIMO to provide official spaces for them to speak about, and thus heal, their experiences of brutality – though they have continued to speak about it 'at home'. This parallels the situation in Venda, where private and public domains entertain very divergent ways of talking and not talking about ways of dying.

In the South African context, the disinclination to discuss AIDS openly has been thought of in terms of public silence – a concept used recently by Stadler (2003), who conducted research in the Bushbuckridge region of Limpopo Province, approximately 250 kilometres south of Venda. He used the term to compare ways in which AIDS can be acknowledged privately by families as a cause of illness or death, but publicly shrouded in secrecy. Although this term, like the notion of a public secret, remains problematic for several reasons to which we shall return, it is nonetheless useful as a starting point from which we may reach a more composite understanding of the social processes involved.

The term 'indirect communication' is favoured by Lambert and Wood (2005; cf. Hendry and Watson 2001) in analysing processes of coding through which, they argue, the word AIDS is avoided by Xhosa-speakers in the Eastern Cape to circumvent disrespect. Since AIDS is associated with socially unacceptable sexual promiscuity and bodily forms of pollution, it shows 'respect' to avoid mentioning it. Along similar lines, a central tenet of Mbeki's denialist stance was his perceived underlying assumption that bio-scientific AIDS discourse constructed Africans as promiscuous and lustful (Posel 2005). Niehaus (2007) has challenged this emphasis, however, by suggesting that AIDS stigma in the Bushbuckridge area is not attributable to its association with sexual promiscuity, but arises because people living with AIDS are seen as 'dead before dying', in the anomalous domain between life and death.[5] The evidence from Venda demonstrates that AIDS stigma cannot be understood as primarily rooted in either sex or death – for they are two sides of the same coin.

The twin notions of sex and death are intimately connected through the widespread belief in the existence and efficacy of witchcraft. Greed, suspicion, jealousy, and insatiable sexual and material desire have combined to produce what Ashforth (2004; 2005) calls an AIDS-induced epidemic of witchcraft in the post-apartheid era. Paul Farmer (1990; 1994; 2006) has provided a lucid account of similar processes in Haiti, in which he discusses the way in which sorcery and voodoo have been invoked in

---

[5] More general studies of AIDS stigma have been offered by Stein (2003), Reid and Walker (2003), Deacon et al. (2005), Deacon (2006), and Parker and Aggleton (2003). They draw to varying extents on cross-cultural and trans-historical comparisons with other illnesses (plague, leprosy, cancer, tuberculosis) that produce symptoms similar to AIDS (cf. Sontag 1990).

patterns of accusation around cases of AIDS. The similarities between the Haitian cases and the Soweto ethnography provided by Ashforth are striking. Both have made important contributions to our understanding of AIDS through the paradigms of witchcraft and sorcery, in which the illness can be 'sent' by a jealous enemy. Farmer's wide-ranging analysis was pioneering in this field, and made connections through a 'geography of blame' that encompassed the political and unequal economic relationship between Haiti and America, and the individual accusations made in the village of Do Kay. Despite a tendency to reduce the spread of AIDS and sorcery accusations to patterns of economic inequality, Farmer's work leaves the reader with a solid historical and political account of AIDS in Haiti, and reflects the humanity of his informants in an 'anthropology of suffering'.

All this has added a welcome nuance to literature on the topic. Yet, whilst social and cultural patterns of stigmatisation are key to understanding the ways in which meaning is attributed to HIV/AIDS, they do not adequately explain the processes through which people avoid open, public conversation about it. What does this so-called public silence mean for those who choose not to discuss AIDS openly in their everyday conversations? If AIDS stigma can be blamed on its intimate associations with immoral sex, witchcraft, or the living dead, then the relationship between this stigma and any denial of the existence of AIDS becomes unclear. Denial does not seem an appropriate term: these ethnographic accounts demonstrate that South Africans actively avoid the conspicuous display of AIDS-related knowledge for complex, historically grounded reasons. But why did this silence develop in the first place, why does it continue in the face of widespread HIV/AIDS education campaigns, and what is the relationship between the two?

Answering these questions requires two preliminary contextual observations. First, there is a literal and figurative invisibility of causes of death in Venda. For example, on receiving news of someone's death, it would be unthinkable to enquire publicly about the cause: the bearer of the news would never admit, in public, to knowing the answer. Should the conversation veer towards this topic, vague euphemisms and obfuscation are used consistently between friends and acquaintances in all manner of public social situations. This is exemplified every weekday evening, between 8.30 and 9 p.m., when listeners to the hugely popular Phalaphala FM (South Africa's only Tshivenda radio station) are subjected to the *dzivhadzo dza mpfu* ('funeral announcements') – a roll-call of people who have died the previous week and will be buried the coming weekend. This information is supplied directly to the radio station by grieving families, and the daily announcements follow a strict formula: name of the deceased, place and date of birth, employment history, names of surviving close kin, date of death, time and place of prayer meetings and funeral. On no occasion is a cause of death alluded to in this procession of information. Further examples of this reluctance to reveal the cause of death include two academic theses, written by Venda anthropology students in the late 1990s, that took as their topics 'A changing view of death in a Venda village' (Mavhungu 1998) and 'The role of women in burial societies' (Rambau 1999). In neither document was there any reference to cause of death in the numerous, but selectively detailed, case studies.[6]

After death, the secrecy is likely to intensify; most notably with the 'cause of death' entry on the death certificate. South Africa does not yet have a national register of AIDS deaths, nor is it a notifiable disease (Stadler 2003: 129; Schneider 2002). For this reason, AIDS-related deaths are often officially recorded in much more nebulous terms. I give four examples of people I personally knew to have died of AIDS-related illness:

Male, born 1965: cause of death: hypertensive stroke.
Female, born 1978: cause of death: natural causes.
Female, born 1975: cause of death: gastroenteritis.
Male, born 1970: cause of death: chronic illness.

This pattern of secrecy and euphemism continues at funerals, during which religious and community leaders inevitably improvise variations on the same theme; 'a long sickness', 'an illness', 'an ailing/failing physique', or a 'recent lack of health'. This phenomenon has been incorporated into Solomon Mathase's song, '*Zwidzumbe*', which I discussed in Chapter 6 (Appendix B: lines 119–20):

A huna ane a nga takadza	No one can ever please
Shango lothe	The whole world
Kani ha ndi zwone zwo itaho	Maybe this is what causes
Uri vhafunzi vha zwifhe	Ministers to tell lies
Mavhidani	At the graveside

A rather different situation has been reported in other parts of South Africa. Lambert and Wood (2005) point out that at Xhosa funerals in the Eastern Cape religious leaders make a customary 'cause of death' speech at the graveside, and that other causes of death may be mentioned so long as AIDS is avoided. In Bushbuckridge, Stadler (2003: 129) notes that mourners at a funeral referred in comparatively more explicit terms to 'OMO' (a popular brand of washing powder with three letters), or

---

[6] Recall here the lyrical composition of the *ludodo* through which initiates in the *vhusha* (Chapter 3) attempted to incorporate AIDS into the ritual curriculum. Following instruction to talk about things that are prohibited in conventional conversation, they immediately invoked detailed knowledge of deaths and poisonings.

'a House In Vereeniging' – spelling out HIV without explicitly saying it. Whilst this was not the case in Venda, and whilst these two examples allude to quite different social processes, they nonetheless raise important and difficult questions that relate to degrees of separation between codes of insinuation and the explicit naming of a cause of death, to which I return in due course.

The congregations at funerals I attended in Venda, like those discussed by Stadler, were generally aware of the fact that their friend or relative had been HIV-positive and had died from an AIDS-related illness. References made to 'sickness' and 'many *cherries*' to some extent constitute a code within which AIDS-related mortality can be spoken about respectfully in public without ascribing a specific cause of death and thus without invoking social stigma against the deceased or their family. Although this is important to recognise, I suggest here that such arguments avoid a crucial wider question: why does the naming of a specific cause of death invoke social stigma?

The second – and closely related – contextual point to be recognised is the widely held belief throughout Southern Africa that no death (with the occasional exception of the very old or very young) is natural (cf. Liddell et al. 2005: 693; Ashforth 2005: 80). All but the most devout Christian families will harbour suspicions that someone was responsible for their relative's early passing. Talking about Shona conceptions of death in Zimbabwe, Aschwanden states that 'serious diseases or death are, *as a rule*, ascribed to people or spirits' (1987: 17, my italics). Likewise, in Soweto, 'any death' according to Ashforth (2005: 70) 'is an occasion for the speculation of witchcraft'. However it does not follow that every AIDS-related death is blamed on the malicious actions of a specific person. In Venda, and throughout Southern Africa, the cause of death has come to be accredited to physical contact with particular things: condoms.[7]

The Case of 'Seven Days' Poisoning: Big News and No News

Poison: An Introduction

Tshivenda speakers use several words to describe poison, depending on the source of the substance and the social context of the conversation. *Vhutungu* refers exclusively to poison from the natural world, such as

---

[7] Since the 1930s, witchcraft accusations have been illegal in South Africa. This has led to a widely felt but largely unarticulated anxiety that although there are growing instances of unnatural deaths, the historically conventional recourse to justice remains prohibited (cf. Geschiere 1997 in Cameroon). As authors such as Niehaus (2001a; 2001b) and Ashforth (2002) have shown, it is not uncommon for people in post-apartheid South Africa to believe that the state is actively involved in protecting witches by continuing the prohibition against accusations.

snake or spider venom. Although an unfortunate person may be poisoned by *vhutungu*, for example by standing on a spider or being stung by a wasp, this class of poison is rarely used with intent by humans to poison another person. One exception to this is when the animal is believed to have been sent by a witch – underlining the distinction made in Chapter 6 between proximate and ultimate causes of illness.

The descriptive terms for poison which is not of the natural order include *mulimo* ('evil drug'; as in the phrase *u na mulimo* – he kills people in secret/he is not to be trusted) and *tshefu*, although these are widely seen as 'deep' Tshivenda words which are used mostly by elders or in the royal dialect in company of a king. The most commonly used words for poison that does not occur naturally as venom, but which can be obtained for the purpose of harming someone or something, are *mushonga* and its colloquial variant *muti*. *Mushonga* literally means medicine, drug, or anything imbued with magic, but it is a highly ambiguous and versatile category with a diverse array of applications in everyday life.[8] Biomedical treatments such as penicillin, antiretroviral drugs, prophylactics, and even spectacles or hearing aids are referred to colloquially as *mushonga*. In its most common form in Venda, *mushonga* is usually a collection of herbs, roots, twigs, or dried animal parts which can be kept close to the body as an amulet, or hidden in the homestead (mostly in the thatched roof above the entrance to the main hut) for the purposes of ritual/spiritual protection. It can be passed down from specific ancestors or bought from an *inyanga*, and can be used towards positive or negative ends.

In its least common but most notorious form, *mushonga* can be the organs of a human body, taken during a '*muti* murder' in which the victim has body parts removed whilst he or she remains alive, usually being left to die from loss of blood. Human *muti* is widely believed to be very powerful in the pursuit of financial wealth or political influence, and has reportedly been used in Venda since pre-colonial times (Kirkaldy 2005: 177, 219–22). At various times in recent history, before and during the transition from apartheid to democratic governance, alleged periodic escalations of *muti* murders in Venda have received limited attention from academics, and have prompted government enquiries (Le Roux 1988; Ralushai et al. 1996). However, in a comparative historical analysis of Lesotho and Venda, Murray and Saunders (2005: 306) suggest that the evidence does not support the great increase in *muti* murders that Venda is widely believed to have endured from the 1980s. Rather, they suggest that it was the political circumstances at the time that gave *muti* murders a new significance, and caused them to garner so much attention. Nonetheless, their wider occurrence throughout South Africa has been theorised by Comaroff and Comaroff (1999) as part of an 'occult

---

[8] See, for example, Engelke (2005), Ashforth (2000; 2005), Niehaus (2001a), and McGregor (2005).

economy' through which magical means are manipulated towards material ends (see below).⁹

Mushonga, then, is a term which can mean various things in different social and historical contexts. Nonetheless, the diverse manifestations of *mushonga* outlined above, except where the term is used to describe biomedical treatment, have one important property in common: secrecy. To ensure their efficacy, herbs from an *inyanga* must be hidden. They are often carried surreptitiously in a pocket, stored with sacred objects, or stashed in the roof of a house. If *mushonga* fails to attract the desired wealth, female companion, or good luck, then an *inyanga* may explain to the unsatisfied client that the medicine was not adequately hidden. The power of *mushonga*, as we shall see, ultimately lies in the web of secrecy that surrounds it, as is evident in the abundance of gossip and rumour through which attempts are made to explain its origin and efficacy.

In the spate of alleged poisonings to which I now turn, the poison at the centre of the controversy became known as Seven Days, after the length of time a victim could expect to live after ingesting it. Although the precise nature or source of Seven Days never became public knowledge, competing explanations circulated through rumour and gossip. The local *Limpopo Mirror* newspaper and radio presenters on Phalaphala FM commented on and contributed to this, but the silence on the ground that reflected a pattern of not talking openly about Seven Days persisted until the panic had passed. It was big news and no news simultaneously. Then, as I was told one day in late 2005 after raising it with a friend in conversation, it had become 'old news'.

Seven Days: Early Gossip

I first became aware of Seven Days in August 2004. Nyamuka,[10] a friend who has a steady job as a domestic worker for a white family, was finishing

---

[9] The commercial availability of human body parts from corrupt hospital workers and undertakers is a lucrative activity in South Africa. In 2004 an SABC exposé in the series *Carte Blanche* not only ascertained the extent of this trade but pointed to Venda, and Tshivenda speakers, as central in it. Such 'cold' body parts, however, do not have the power of 'hot' *muti*, taken whilst the victim is still alive. There is a massive element of risk involved in committing ritual murder. If the user of human *muti* is caught, his/her life will be immediately at risk from lynch mobs that descend on the homesteads of suspects and apportion a variety of punishments. If police are seen to be inefficient in their capture, or involved in a conspiracy of silence to protect the murderers, then large-scale protest may escalate into rioting in which roads are blocked and shops looted. Recently, the Venda region has experienced a sudden and abrupt moral panic around the perceived increase in the incidence of ritual murder, reminiscent of the late 1980s. This has led to numerous calls for independent investigations into the matter. Whilst there is no space here for an adequate discussion of this phenomenon, or its recent increase, it would appear to be connected to a simultaneous flurry of xenophobic activity against illegal Zimbabwean migrants, and possibly also fluctuations in the local politics of several Apostolic Faith Mission churches. There has been extensive local media coverage of this. See articles, letters, and archives at <www.zoutnet.co.za>.

[10] A pseudonym.

up early on a Friday afternoon. Knowing that she dreads the 30-minute walk uphill, through the forest to the main road where she meets her taxi, I suggested that she need not rush as I would give her a lift home. I was heading in that direction anyway and I genuinely enjoyed my conversations with her. She accepted the lift and headed off to the garage where she washes after the day's work in a deep clay sink before donning smart clothes for the public eye. Nyamuka is almost 50 years old, and her husband lives in Johannesburg with a second wife. He occasionally comes home to be with his children, but does so with the younger, prettier wife, who then sleeps in the marital bedroom. This cuts Nyamuka to the bone, but she is powerless to change it – and, even if she could, the upheaval would simply draw more attention to her embarrassing, but not uncommon, situation. She has four children, and each of her two teenage daughters has a child fathered by the same youth, who is a promising star in a local football team. The daughters have left school to care for their children and both collect government child support grants. With Nyamuka's wage, her husband's remittances, and the state welfare payments the family is not poor, and is comfortable enough to be building a three-room extension to their house.

I could tell that Nyamuka was going to a funeral that weekend by the smarter than usual frock that she carefully tucked under her as she climbed up into my *bakkie*. 'Who is it this time?' I asked. She snorted at my cheeky opening gambit. 'A relative, down past Tshakhuma.' As I have mentioned, my habit of offering lifts to friends and strangers was more than altruistic. In the absence of an audience, notepad, and tape recorder, such conversations felt more natural, but even with friends like Nyamuka, whom I have known for ten years, talking about the dead was always a risky business.

Slowly the details of her story emerged. Nyamuka's sister's daughter (*muduhulu*)[11] had died the previous weekend after her own wedding celebration two weeks earlier. She had married a relatively well-off local man who owned shares in a prominent local bus company. A known womaniser, he had many secret wives (*mafarakano*), some of whom were present at the ceremony. One, Nyamuka explained, was helping with the preparation of the wedding meal. Exactly a week after the wedding, the bride died whilst vomiting white froth and blood. She had been sick since the ceremony, but perfectly healthy before it. The *mufarakano* who had been helping to cook was now nowhere to be found, and it was assumed that she, motivated by jealousy, had poisoned the bride.

This story in itself was by no means extraordinary in that alleged poisonings, often involving jealous lovers, are a common trope in the region. The first words of advice proffered to me by Harold Lemke,

---

[11] The actual relation was Nyamuka's father's third wife's second daughter's first-born daughter. Nyamuka is from her father's second wife, and within the terms of Venda extended family, a sister's daughter is called *muduhulu*.

founder of the Forum for AIDS Prevention (FAP), explained that 'If a Venda wants to kill you, he will not shoot you, he will poison you'. The threat of being poisoned is pervasive and longstanding in Venda (Stayt 1931). Writing with specific reference to the elaborate tasting etiquette of royal courtyards in the late 1920s, Stayt comments that 'as in the old days this [poisoning] was a favourite method of disposing of an enemy, every chief lives in constant dread of meeting his death by poison' (ibid.: 204). The communal manner in which food is eaten by men in public is justified in symbolic terms of emic group politics centred on suspicion and the need to engender trust. Indeed, towards the end of July 2005, I myself was the target of an attempted poisoning. Fortunately, amid the chaos of a feast, a vigilant friend who became suspicious warned me not to swallow the next mouthful of my beer, but to taste it for anything different. The sharp, metallic, sulphurous taste was clearly toxic and left me salivating profusely for hours.[12]

Radio dramas and the Tshivenda soap opera *Muvhango* regularly write poisonings into their scripts. On my occasional visits to Matatche, the local prison, to visit an old friend, I was struck by the manner in which guards would accept food parcels for inmates only if the visitor ate a portion first. A friend who works there explained that this became protocol during the 1980s when the incidence of politically inspired poisoning in the area was particularly high. Legendary accounts tell of elaborate plots through which numerous high-profile politicians, activists, and traitors met their deaths by being dealt a fatal dose of toxin. As we saw in Chapter 2, the period from 1979 to 1994, when Venda was an 'independent' homeland, provided a political climate fraught with longstanding grudges, promising fragile yet unrealisable new alliances, and featuring underground revolutionary movements. In this climate, many politicians are said to have been poisoned. Within this context as well as during the period since Venda's reaggregation into the new South Africa, the suspicious deaths of many traditional leaders, successful businessmen, and (un)successful lovers have been told in detailed narratives that conclude with some form of poisoning.

Nyamuka's story, however, got more animated as she told me of two other deaths in the area that same week of healthy people who had died exactly one week after attending a funeral together. She was in the process of explaining how dangerous it now was to eat at public functions when we stopped to collect an elderly neighbour who was heavily laden with firewood. The tiny old woman squeezed up next to us in the front cab of my truck and the conversation changed swiftly to pleasantries. Nyamuka did not have to explain that she could not be heard talking with me about

---

[12] The friend in question here was the late Humbulani Nekhavhambe, to whom I dedicated this book.

death and poison. She later explained it through the proverb '*U vhonwa zwi a vhonwa, zwi a ila u amba*': there are certain things you are permitted to see or have an opinion on, but it is prohibited to be heard talking about them.

Seven Days in the Beer Hall

On the Friday night after Nyamuka related her tale, I met as usual with my drinking buddies at Mapita's, the local tavern. Mapita's is advertised as a 'complex', and qualifies for this title as it boasts a well-stocked (if overpriced) shop, a payphone, butchery, tavern, and *braai* (barbecue) area at the back nestled under huge, old trees. Mapita's is situated at the bottom of the main road which cuts up into the Thathe Vondo tea plantation, a large enterprise employing thousands of seasonal tea pickers and which, in mid-2005, was rumoured to be closing down.

Just behind Mapita's, the modest Mutshindudi River provides young girls and women with the water for evening cooking and washing, which is laboriously carried up the hill in plastic containers to homesteads in the surrounding villages. As evening sets, the men who drink take up their places in the tavern with their friends. Some play cards, others partake in animated games of chess or the Venda version of solitaire, *mufhufha*. My group of friends at Mapita's, an eclectic mix of farmers, teachers, musicians, traffic police, artists, full time *mahafhe* drinkers, and civil servants, prefer just to talk the night away.[13] Conversation skips from women to football, chiefs to riddles, Johannesburg to Scotland, and, inevitably, back to women. The only females around are girlfriends (*cherries*) – actual or potential; although sex workers drop in occasionally, it is not a regular spot for them. A polite, respectful man does not drink beer with his wife in public, and Mapita's tavern, as my father was told during a visit, is a 'gentlemen's bar', frequented by men and generally avoided by youngsters who prefer the more lively nightspots towards Thohoyandou.

It was still light outside when I saw the *Mirror* article on the counter of the butchery. The headline read:

TAPS OF POISON

Mysterious tablets in water taps spark poison scare

Itsani – Mystery and secrecy surround an alleged attempt to poison the communities of Itsani, Maniini, Tswinga, Tshakhuma and Muledane during past

[13] Such a diverse group of men, differing in age, class, and status, would not normally be in the same drinking group. Since my initial visits to Venda in 1995, however, these men have joined me at Mapita's, initially to impart their knowledge of Venda to me. In my absence, they drink within their own peer groups, but in my presence we form a loose cohort.

weeks, after it was allegedly found that unknown tablets were inserted in some of the public taps in the area. According to several members of the communities, they discovered unidentified white and red poison pills in their public taps. Although they are taking as many precautions as possible, the community members are living in fear for their lives.... The tablets are called 'seven-days tablets' in the community which means you will live for only seven days after consuming one... community members are living in fear and were pleading with anyone with information regarding the poisoning of their water to report it. (*Thulamela Mirror*, Friday, 27 August 2004 – see Map 4 for the geographical distribution of these villages)

I read it intently, twice, and stuffed the already ripped copy into my bag. As I was stashing the bag behind the seat of my truck, the five o'clock news on Phalaphala FM was reporting the same feature. Seven Days was big news, and I made a mental note to finish my conversation with Nyamuka.

The drinking circle was busy that night as it was month-end and government workers were paying off their small beer and cigarette debts to the teachers, who received their wages in the middle of every month. Mashamba, a close friend who had received his pay, bought me my first beer, and as usual delivered it unopened. If a beer is delivered already open, then the bearer should take a taste of it before handing it over. This convention serves to prove that the bottle has not been poisoned. It is common for beggars to be sent to buy beer: they can manipulate this by returning with an open bottle and consuming as much as possible in one gulp, to the anger of the sender and the general amusement of everyone else.

As Mashamba sat down next to me, he leant over and whispered that if I had to go to the toilet tonight I must not leave my bottle on the table. This was unusual in that the large bottles – known as 'quarts' or *ngolongolo*, after the noise made when drinking from them – were usually shared between two or three of us. When I whispered back asking why, he answered that, tonight, we would just leave the room at the same time. As the night progressed I waited for discussion to turn to the front-page story. I rarely raised topics of conversation at Mapita's, choosing instead to participate in whatever was on the agenda. But the heightened state of alert in the group that night was starting to make me uncomfortable. I noticed that some of the guys were even sitting with their thumbs firmly capping the tops of their bottles, and, eventually, I asked why. Although I assumed that everybody knew the answer to this question, I wanted to know more about it. There was no response, and my discomfort grew.

Mashamba signalled that we should visit the toilet (which consists of a pungent brick wall behind the butchery), where he scorned me for asking such a question in public. As one of my closest friends, he took pride in ensuring that I was fluent in Tshivenda and flawless with male protocol, and I protested that I was unaware of having breached the code. 'Some things', he said, 'we just *do not talk about*. It is very dangerous to know too much about these things'. Then, as if to contradict himself, he leaned forward and whispered to me that he had overheard people talking on the taxi, saying that Seven Days had originated in a mortuary outside Sibasa. Body parts (spinal cords) were being ground into a paste and then left to dry in the sun. It was this deadly mixture, in powder or tablet form, that people were calling Seven Days. One of the men we were drinking with worked as a driver for that very company and, although Mashamba doubted that we were in imminent danger, he said we must be very careful. 'These guys can even hide that *mushonga* under their fingernails.' By the time we got back to the circle, the driver in question had left for a nightspot towards Sibasa. Mashamba looked at me with a 'told you so' expression, and the subject was dropped.

Seven Days in the Village

September 2004 was a particularly hectic time in my host village of Fondwe. Chief Rathogwa had decided to hold a celebration that would coincide with the national public holiday on the first day of October. The public holiday was in recognition of Heritage Day, and Fondwe was to observe this by organising its own Fondwe Day. The plans included a variety of traditional dancing, praise poetry, a small beauty pageant, many speeches from prominent community members, and, inevitably, a feast. In the month leading up to Fondwe Day our homestead was the centre of attention as people came and went at all hours of the day making arrangements and delivering notes for my host, Zwiakonda, who is the official messenger to his elder brother, Chief Rathogwa. Then disaster struck.

Someone reported to Zwiakonda that he had discovered his dogs and chickens dead, with white foam coming from the mouth. His neighbour, an elderly man, had found white powder under the rim of his water tank and when he fed it to a stray dog with bread, it died within the hour. The news that Fondwe had been targeted by Seven Days spread rapidly.

Clearly concerned that his planned feast could backfire with horrific consequences, Chief Rathogwa held an emergency meeting of the royal council. It was agreed that on the following Sunday the weekly public meeting (*khoro*) should be upgraded to an emergency *tshivhidzo*, and that all the old ladies from the village would be summoned and interrogated by the chief or a member of the council as to what they knew. Old women, it was generally agreed, knew everything that was going on, and would appreciate the urgency of the situation with a mature wisdom. It is also possible that the chief suspected certain elderly women of involvement.

That Sunday, as planned, the *khoro* convened at 6.30 a.m. As we arrived, the customary distribution of *mabundu* (a non-alcoholic traditional maize drink) was conspicuous by its absence, and men of all ages and ranks slowly went inside the large council hut. The seating arrangement consists of concentric wooden benches around the inside wall, and a stage on the right-hand side where the chief sits on a throne with two chairs on either side of him – one for each of the four headmen. It was a full house, and some men were forced to sit on the cement floor. As we took our seats inside and began the preliminary business, the old women began to gather outside. The chief addressed us and reiterated the seriousness of the situation, waving a copy of the newspaper article to reinforce his point. He spoke of the recent attempted poisonings and openly criticised the secretive manner in which they were being treated as 'dangerous and child-like'.

He was clearly concerned that Seven Days would claim a victim at the forthcoming celebrations, and was determined to thwart what he saw as a threat to his power. Before calling the old ladies, he asked if any of the men present knew anything. Roughly five minutes of total silence passed – the only noise coming from men readjusting their posture for comfort on the thin wooden benches, or to take the occasional nip of snuff. He then asked what kind of *mushonga* Seven Days was, and again was met with silence. Shaking his head into his right hand, he summoned the old ladies with his outstretched left arm.

Unless they are called for a specific purpose, women do not attend the council. In the presence of the chief it is expected that they enter on their knees. They shuffled in, keeping their heads bowed towards the floor, and filled the space that had been prepared for them in the middle of the circle. For almost two hours, the old women were subjected to a mix of elaborate praise and sharp questioning, but this thinly veiled flattery failed to induce a single one of them to break silence by offering the desired information. Seemingly angry and frustrated, the chief stormed out of the council hut, pledging to everyone present that he would discover those responsible for bringing the poison to Fondwe, and deal with them severely. We were then informed that the meeting was over.

Far from being an error of Chief Rathogwa's judgement, the holding of an emergency council was his method of returning the warning to whoever was threatening his power. When I interviewed him some weeks later, he explained:

I knew that my people would not talk on that day, in front of me and everyone else, but I also knew that they would listen, and they did [listen] because no one was poisoned at our celebration. These things, you must understand, there are some things we just do not talk of here in Venda. That is why there is so much of this gossip.... It has been like that for a long time. (Interview, Chief Rathogwa, Fondwe Musanda, 28 December 2004)

Researching and Explaining Seven Days

Over the course of the next few months, many clandestine stories circulated about people who had attended funerals, weddings, parties, or beer halls and died within seven days of consuming food or drink there. My research assistants and I endeavoured to establish the source of and any patterns in the rumours. The original plan was to start at the hospital where the victims mentioned in the *Mirror* article had been taken, and to track down the media liaison officer who had said that samples of the poison were being tested to confirm what substance had been used. My primary research assistant, Mushai, absolutely refused to get involved in this, arguing that it would appear as if he was venturing to procure a sample for his own use. As we will see, this was much more than a feeble excuse.

The proposed solution to this difficulty was to go together to the royal courts of the villages mentioned in the article and ask permission to talk with people in their own homes. He agreed on the condition that I organised someone to invite and introduce us to the different areas, as it would appear dubious were we to appear unannounced. I contacted a longstanding colleague from a youth NGO who was an active member of the civic association at the village of Tswinga. After I had waited a week for his response, he contacted me to explain that he had made inquiries, and that it would be pointless for us to go there: no one knew anything about Seven Days in his village. I tried several other contacts in Tshakhuma (where I knew many HIV/AIDS peer educators) and Muledane (where a friend had a secret lover), and we drove without invitation to Itsani where I had played in a soccer team in 1995. People denied all knowledge of the events. Even the media liaison officer at the hospital and the local police refused to furnish us with any information, claiming to be 'bound by agreements of confidentiality'.

Seven Days was no news, and yet it was big news at the same time. This avoidance of open conversation had evolved in parallel with the willingness demonstrated by certain people and institutions to talk openly about the suspected poisonings. Newspapers and radios reported it widely. A late night phone-in show on Phalaphala FM devoted an entire evening to it, but the few people who ventured to phone and comment refused to reveal their identities. Village leaders raised the topic at council meetings, and local politicians discussed it in various addresses to the public and in ward meetings. Those with spiritual authority such as traditional healers and prophets of African Independent Churches professed to sacrosanct knowledge of a panacea either through herbal antidotes, all-night prayer sessions, or holy water. *Zwilombe* musicians, living in the human world but with privileged access to the ancestral one, wrote it into song texts that were performed in beer halls throughout Venda:

Ngoho Mudzimu mara vhathu vhanzhe	Really, but it seems many people
Vha vha divha uri	Know all about
Mavhege maduvha ano	Weeks [Seven Days] these days
Kha thogomele vhatuni,	Take care in public,
Vhana wa mavu,	Children of the soil,
Ri khou fa rothe.	We are dying together.

(Solomon Mathase, untitled song)

And yet among the general public Seven Days was referred to strictly in whispers. Some of my contacts in the villages got back to us with anonymous snippets of gossip, explaining that they wanted to help my research but they did not really know anything. Recognition of this widespread reluctance to speak removed my initial worry that it was to me, specifically, that people were reluctant to divulge their knowledge. Meanwhile, we were picking up on the wealth of gossip and rumour that was circulating quietly between friends and families at home, in taxis, at beer halls, in churches, and at washing places in the shallow rivers. There were very distinct patterns in this backstage whispering. It consisted mostly of clustered speculation and allegation through which specific groups and things were named as responsible for inventing, selling, and using Seven Days.

There is a long history of debate in anthropological literature regarding the role of gossip and rumour. Recent attempts have been made to create a distinction between gossip as '[taking] place mutually among people in networks or groups' (Stewart and Strathern 2004: 38) and rumour as 'unsubstantiated information, true or untrue, that passes by word of mouth' (ibid.), but the difference here does not appear to be clear. As I have argued elsewhere, there are specific social contexts where gossip becomes rumour, but the precise dynamics through which this occurs are almost impossible to identify (McNeill and Niehaus 2010). Max Gluckman's (1963) classic anthropological account of gossip and scandal among Haitian villagers and others suggested that gossip is 'functional' and conducive to group solidarity through the reinforcing of norms and enshrining of group membership. To gossip is to be a member of the group, and an anthropologist comes to understand the significance of gossip in the process of becoming acculturated. Gluckman's ideas about gossip were criticised. Paine (1967) argued from his Makah Indian ethnography that gossip is more about individuals seeking to forward their own interests through the denigration and exclusion of others than it is about the fortification of group solidarity. Brenneis (1984) shows both processes at play in an account of gossip in an acephalous society, in which he argues that gossiping is 'also an event in itself' (1984: 496) and not just 'about' something else. From the ethnographic cameos presented above, we can see that gossip both fosters group membership and simultaneously excludes some from the group. As Mashamba and I whispered his explanation for Seven Days, our common interests were affirmed in the same process which excluded the funeral car driver and his Shangaan bosses.

Connecting the notions of silence, secrecy, and gossip in a manner more useful for the current argument, White argues that silence can often be pregnant with 'eloquent assumptions' about local knowledge (2000: 77). In response to this, gossip and rumour reveal the 'intellectual world' (ibid.: 86) of fears, fantasies, and ideas that constitute themselves around silence in the telling and retelling of things which cannot be spoken about openly. In this way, the gossip and rumour about the taboo topic of poisoning offer an intriguing insight into the anxieties and apprehensions of contemporary life in post-apartheid Venda.

Patterns of rumour mongering about Seven Days revealed an 'occult economy' (Comaroff and Comaroff 1999) in which global processes took on localised incarnations, but through which the seductive allure of international ('millennial') capitalism was eclipsed by the enduring realities of mass poverty. Magical means, claim these authors, are invoked to manipulate the market and bring wealth to those who would otherwise be structurally excluded from it. In criticisms, it has been pointed out that relatively few of those disappointed by their failure to accrue untold wealth have actually resorted to the use of magical means to improve their material circumstances, and that occult economies are not characteristic only of the post-colonial era (cf. Falk Moore 1999). This critique notwithstanding, the Seven Days data from Venda demonstrate that 'occult economy' is a useful analytical tool to further our understanding of the rumoured allegations. Although the majority of people may not engage directly with such economies in order to accrue an income, this does not prohibit them from entertaining the notion that magical means are manipulated on a daily basis to procure material ends.

There were two frequently occurring explanations for Seven Days. The first, as mentioned above, alleged that the poison was derived from human body parts, processed in a Shangaan-run mortuary. In this version of events, Seven Days, associated with stories of hearses speeding through the night on surreptitious missions, involved the extraction of money from people through the costs of organising a funeral, while depriving them in a more psychic sense through a kind of grave robbery. The concoction of spinal cord and secret (Shangaan) *mushonga* in pill or powder form could, it was rumoured, be purchased from the night drivers, although no one I spoke to knew how much it cost.

The second, more common explanation suggested that the poison was derived from the local tea estate, either in the form of an industrial fertiliser or the condensed residue of old, rotten, tea leaves.[14] It could be purchased for extravagant prices, according to this explanation, from tea-estate workers. The Department of Trade and Industry had recently announced the imminent closure of the two large tea estates that had been established under the National Party in the early 1960s to create the illusion of development in the Venda homeland (see Chapter 2). After years of generous subsidies from the apartheid government, the tea estates had eventually been exposed to global market forces under the ANC-led democratic dispensation. This radical and unexpected swing in ANC fiscal policy from left to right under the leadership of Finance Minister Trevor Manuel caught many by surprise in its seeming contradiction of the Freedom Charter signed 50 years previously. However, as we saw in Chapter 2, it was a result of the need to implement a neoliberal framework that would encourage 'confidence' in the South African economy and thus strengthen its currency.

To a large extent, this has been a successful approach, but the bitter and predictable side effect was a rising tide of unemployment (Daniel et al. 2005; Southall 2007). With the complete removal of state subsidies, the overall growth of the South African economy and subsequent increase in value of the rand on the global currency exchange, the Venda tea estates began recording huge losses. They simply could not compete on the global market, and in 2000 they were partly taken over by Liptons, a multinational private enterprise with tea estates throughout Southern Africa. However, before long cheaper tea became available from Malawi, Uganda, and Kenya, and by 2004 the Venda tea estates were no longer financially viable. Liptons backed out and the government refused to provide further financial assistance. Since the venture had employed a core staff of almost 1,000 and up to 3,000 seasonal pickers, its closure and the subsequent loss of employment had severe and abrupt effects, socially, economically, and politically, throughout the region.[15]

---

[14] There is an interesting comparison here with Mark Auslander's work (1993). He reports that chemical fertiliser was rumoured to be used as poison by Ngoni people in Zambia.
[15] This played directly into the hands of *Thovhela* Tshivhase, ever the optimist, who announced at the time that the Tshivhase Development Trust (TDT – see Chapter 2) was lobbying for subsidies to provide funding and infrastructure to plant a macadamia farm on the land. This became another string to his bow in the competition for *Khosikhulu*. By 2009, the TDT had secured private investors and government subsidy, and the tea estate was officially reopened as a branch of Tshivhase's development apparatus, securing thousands of jobs in the region. However, early optimism that the tea estates could be run as a successful business venture has been marred by allegations of corruption, and high productivity has proved difficult to maintain: the Rooibos tea packed and sold from the Tshivhase Tea Estate in Venda was being sourced and transported by road from Cape Town. Still, in 2010 the tea estates were – at least officially – running at a profit.

That the deadly potion believed to cause death in seven days was thought to be readily available – at a price – from redundant tea-estate workers points to a series of inverse connections between the elusive bounty of the market and the harsh reality of poverty. Democracy has enriched only the few (often previously privileged), whilst the majority languish in poverty. The division is exacerbated by a deepening inequality between rich and poor. The hunger, anger, and despair brought on by the redundancies, just when black South Africans were being told to enjoy their freedom, culminated in a physical phenomenon that killed quickly and secretively. But it nonetheless enriched those who sold it. Tea, the commodity whose cultivation had promised to provide a sustainable quality of life for so many, had become embroiled in an economy of the macabre, morphing from a source of life, health, and wealth into a source of potentially sudden death.

And yet, rumours about the origin of Seven Days fail to explain why people felt the need to adhere to a strict, but unspoken code in which open, public dialogue was avoided. To make sense of this, it is helpful to return in more detail to the so-called 'public silence' about AIDS in Venda, and the ways in which it has been breached by peer educators. There are multiple connections between AIDS and Seven Days, all building on the fundamental link that both concern and are suspected to be the cause of new modalities of unnatural death, and both are avoided in open conversation by the general public. To breach 'public silence' is problematic for participatory AIDS education, its protagonists the peer educators, and the technologies they advocate.

'Condoms Cause AIDS': The Breaching of Public Silence

The sections above demonstrate that whilst Seven Days was 'no news' in that it was constructed as a public secret, it was simultaneously 'big news' in that the media reported it, musicians sang about it, leaders raised it in public meetings, and it gave rise to gossip and rumour that speculated about and sought to explain its origin and efficacy. We also saw at the start of the chapter the extent to which open conversation around AIDS is avoided, and Chapters 4, 5, and 6 laid bare the extent to which peer educators systematically break this public silence through the weekly performance of public shows during which they sing songs and act out dramas to promote behavioural change.

At the start of 2005, I issued a random selection of peer educators with diaries and encouraged them to record a regular commentary of their experiences not only of volunteering, but of their daily lives and the micro-politics of their homesteads and villages. One of the most salient topics to emerge from this experimental methodology was their acknowledgement of, and discomfort with, the labels assigned to them by many people in the communities where they work.

Quote 1

[A]s a peer educator most people look and see that I am teaching the community about AIDS and sexual illness. If we tell them, they will look and say 'This one, she must be infected; she is the one who is positive.' Others ask 'How can you teach us about [blood] testing and counselling when you cannot tell us if you have gone for the test yourself?'

Quote 2

Our job really, it is not easy. Last week we went to [the village of] Dopeni for house meetings; we have not been there for some few months now. On the way walking there we were joking that the entire village will be infected now because of our absence! When we got there no one would let us past their gate, they would just hide and pretend to be not at home... they do this because they think *we* will infect *them*!

Quote 3

I have just come from a public meeting. At least this one was better than others, because there was a small group watching us and some youths even joined in. I really enjoyed that. We were all happy. It is so boring when no one comes to the meetings. Another group of men in the *shebeen* [beer hall] refused condoms from us. They say that 'These condoms cause AIDS, if we fill them with water and leave them in the sun, you will find worms inside there, and these worms will get inside if you put on that condom, and the worms give you AIDS.' They think like that, these Venda men of ours.

Quote 4

I heard women at the mill at Mandala saying we were working for the Americans, and they said that they had sent AIDS because it means the 'American Institute to Destroy Sex'.

The above quotes demonstrate clearly that peer educators have been socially constructed by many in their target communities as vectors of the virus that they have been charged with preventing: and that they are fully aware of this. As I argued in the previous chapter, one important explanation for this is the extent to which the folk model of sexual illness in Venda has incorporated biomedical discourse, and aligned the young, female, educators with *malwadze dza vhafumakadzi*: the illnesses of women.

But another, fundamental flaw in the peer education model is that it is exclusively oriented towards encouraging these already stigmatised women to breach the public silence around AIDS. Their public performances and home visits are acted out against the backdrop of deeply entrenched patterns of not speaking about causes of death. As self-styled experts on the topic, peer educators have a detailed and very conspicuous knowledge of a suspicious and mysterious source of mortality that – like other causes of death – is rarely spoken of in public. Through their regular, open confessionals of this knowledge, they actively create an intimate connection between themselves and the virus. Combined with the existing connection from the folk model of sexual illness, this has established a pervasive belief that peer educators are implicated in the spread of HIV. The reference to 'Americans' (Quote 4) speaks to the frequent visits of white (European and American) evaluation and fact-finding teams representing international donor agencies. They possibly refer to my presence as well. 'Americans', however, referring to the 'West' in general, are also thought to be experts in the science of AIDS, and through this association are implicated in its invention, rapid distribution, and devastating consequences (cf. Rodlach 2006).

By publicly naming AIDS, the peer educators have put an easily recognisable name onto an otherwise elusive face. This is not to suggest that this malign presence is thought to remain powerless if not named openly; indeed avoiding mention of AIDS – and other causes of death – is a recognition of their efficacy and great power (cf. Ashforth 2005; Stewart and Strathern 2003). However, the practice of consistent public naming radically alters the dynamics of power that maintain the patterns and processes of indirect communication, and shifts the focus of attention directly to the female peer educators. They are then held responsible for mediating a malign power and are placed in the vulnerable situation of being potentially implicated in harbouring and distributing a source of perceived unnatural death. The very public nature of the Project Support Group programme of participatory AIDS education – and many others like it in Southern Africa – leaves peer educators with no choice but overtly to breach the so-called public silence and to demonstrate their intimate knowledge on a weekly basis.

Indeed, this is their raison d'être. Of course, some people (such as groups of close family, close friends, and those associated in some way with the public health or voluntary sectors in Venda) do recognise their role as volunteers and their attempts to reduce infection rates by raising awareness. However, the majority of 'men in the street' with a working knowledge of the folk model of sexual health would perhaps agree with a comment my research assistant overheard on a minibus taxi as he alighted to join me at a public performance: 'These women', said one old man to the other, 'they just know *too* much... and the way they throw it around... how do they know these all things?... Yes, they must be the ones spreading it'.

The widespread assumption that they are implicated in this way impinges directly on their ability to perform the tasks assigned to them by project funders and designers. Families often refuse them entrance to the homestead for informal house meetings (Chapter 4; and Quote 2 above) and public performances are just as likely to scare people away as to attract their participation (Quote 3).

It is notable here that whilst peer educators are blamed for spreading the virus, their counterparts working in home-based care (HBC) are not. Of fundamental importance to HBC volunteers is the ability to act surreptitiously and keep impeccable standards of confidentiality. The socio-cultural environment in Venda is not yet conducive to disclosure (McNeill and Niehaus 2010).[16] In this context positive people live a public life of secrets. It is unheard of for clients to be open about their HIV status, and the frequent visits of FAP workers to a specific homestead can raise the suspicion of neighbours and lead to disastrous consequences for the family.

A well-known example of persecution is often cited as evidence for why it is advisable to remain silent about being positive. Not far from Siloam Hospital, in 2002, a local man and his family, all of whom were HIV-positive and some of whom were sick, were visited by a stranger. The stranger introduced himself as a new FAP health worker, and stated that he was there to document the family's current situation, as a new funder from overseas had donated money that had to be distributed to those families most in need. The clearly sick man posed for pictures outside his crumbling hut with his four daughters, and told the stranger of their concerns that the community would discover the truth behind their ailing health. The following Friday, the headline in the local newspaper screamed 'AIDS hits Venda', under which pictures of the man and his daughters were surrounded by text in which his confession was printed. He had been duped. The visitor was not a representative of the NGO, but a ruthless journalist. As a result of the family's exposure, the children were stoned by teachers, parents, and other school children alike as they tried to enter the village school. They were denied access to washing places at the river, and could not collect water from the communal tap unless they went under the cover of darkness. Their father was beaten almost fatally, and their crumbling hut was burnt to the ground along with their meagre possessions. By the following Thursday, when I went with some FAP workers to bring the family to a safe house in another village, they had disappeared; leaving behind only a letter to their support worker explaining why they had no option but to flee. No one has seen or heard of them since, and no one wants to be the next victim of a witch hunt in which their lives could, quite literally, be destroyed.

Thus, although HBC volunteers have recognisable uniforms and large bags in which to carry food parcels, Bibles, and medication, they often

---

[16] This is largely due to the fact that the Treatment Action Campaign (TAC) is yet to make its presence felt in the region. Unlike other regions in South Africa, an openly HIV-positive identity in Venda is not yet an option for people living with AIDS.

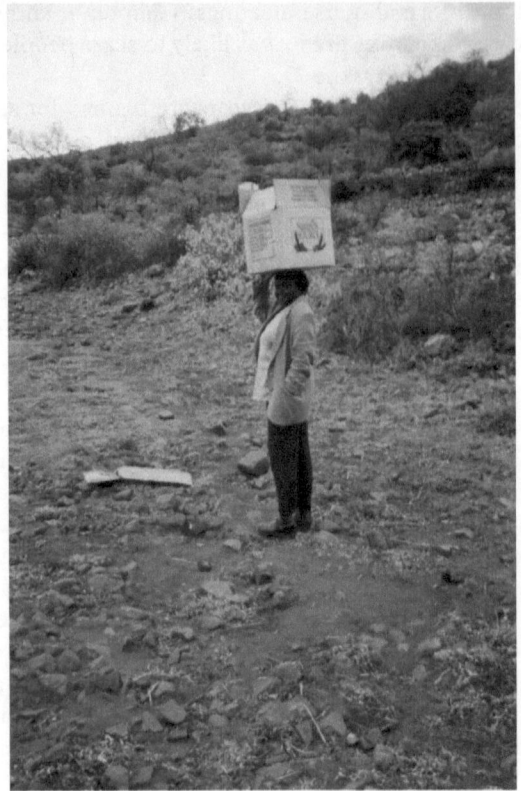

Figure 7.1. A home-based care worker, on a home visit at Ha-Rabali. Note the lack of uniform and inconspicuous cardboard box.

work in casual clothes and take any provisions in an inconspicuous suitcase or cardboard box so that suspicious neighbours can assume that they are visiting relatives rather than 'AIDS people' (see Figure 7.1). As a volunteer approaches the client's homestead, they often greet them loudly using kinship terms such as '*Malume!*' (uncle) or '*Mazwale!*' (sister-in-law), pretending to be relatives who have recently returned from a visit outside of Venda. By working within the principles of established family networks in this way, HBC volunteers have developed webs of secrecy and trust through which they conduct their daily business. To some extent the sensitive nature of their work leaves them little option but to be surreptitious if they have the best interests of the client in mind. Nonetheless, their conventional methods of working keep rumour and (hopefully) disease stigma to a minimum for both the client and the carer. Clearly, in village settings where gossip is rife and living conditions are often claustrophobic, this level of deceit is an unsustainable method of gaining access to patients. It functions, however, as an initial diversion and makes the clients feel more relaxed with the visiting volunteers who, in time, may choose to become more open about their true purpose if the situation becomes conducive.

Peer educators, on the other hand, leave people in no doubt as to the nature of their activities. The hundreds of thousands of free condoms that educators distribute on a daily basis cannot escape this process of association; indeed they have become its symbol. If 'Americans' (Western biomedical scientists) are the world experts on AIDS, if they teach the peer educators (local 'experts') the importance of condoms, and if both of these groups are thought to be involved in the spread of HIV, then why should the essence of what causes AIDS not also be found in the very thing that they both insist everyone must use? It would, in fact, following this logic, be very strange if it was not. A central tenet of prevention – the condom – has thus been implicated in the spread, as opposed to the containment, of HIV. For many people, the condom they take home from a public performance remains imbued with the same powerful association that links the educators with infection – and by extension is thus often said to 'cause AIDS'.

Degrees of Separation

The ethnographic examples given above, then, outline the dynamics of two quite different phenomena: Seven Days poison, rumoured to emerge from a defunct tea estate; and AIDS, rumoured to be an 'American Institute to Destroy Sex'. The two kill in different ways. One is a white or red tablet that infects water supplies, food, or drinks, and will run its deadly course within a week. The other is a mysterious virus that kills slowly and can be passed on during sex or even through the worms that many people believe lie dormant in sealed condoms. Both, however, are believed to have equally fatal effects. A form of 'public silence' developed around both of them that reflected the general avoidance of discussing openly any cause of death.

The failure to speak clearly about AIDS in South Africa is thus related fundamentally to the same social processes and pressures that prevented public confessions of knowledge about Seven Days. The refusal to mention AIDS as cause of death, or the proclivity elsewhere in South Africa to refer to it euphemistically out of respect for grieving families, are not anomalous. Such reluctance is a safety precaution, collectively undertaken by individuals to protect themselves from the constant threat of guilt by association. If someone were to have come forward with information about Seven Days in the royal council hut or in the beer hall, or had in other ways made him/herself a public 'expert' on the topic, then it is highly likely that s/he would have been suspected of implication in the poisoning. My research assistant's refusal to enquire about Seven

Days at the hospital was not a mere excuse: it was based upon the fear of being seen as attempting to procure a sample for his own use. 'Why else would I want to know about such things', he asked me, 'unless I wanted to use it against you?' Likewise, to ask someone bringing news of death about its cause would be to exhibit an unhealthy preoccupation with, and knowledge of, fatal illness.

I suggest here that by invoking silence, coded language, and obfuscation, 'degrees of separation' are constructed that forge and maintain a social but simultaneously metaphorical distance between an individual and the unnatural cause of another's death. The indirect communication, the refusal to name a cause of death, is the direct protest of innocence. Lambert and Wood's (2005) suggestion that avoidance of the term 'AIDS' circumvents a social stigma being attached to the family of the deceased is instructive here. But this is a partial and inadequate explanation of events. The elementary reason for avoiding the term 'AIDS' is that such avoidance creates the crucial social distance between those who remain silent and the death itself, thus refuting any potential involvement in it. The act of refusing to name AIDS, then, is just as important for the individual making that choice as it is grounded in any motivation to protect or respect the mourning family.

It is in this context that the 'fictitious kinship' invoked by HBC volunteers takes on a more discernible significance. They greet their housebound, dying patients as though they are visiting relatives – not treating someone for an AIDS-related illness. On the approach to a homestead, and when departing, they make no open acknowledgement of the true purpose of their visit, and no one asks them to elaborate. Of course, people 'know' what is going on, but such knowledge is also widely recognised as dangerous (cf. Lambek 1993) and conversation relating to it is restricted, remaining within the realms of 'gossip'. In adapting the practice of AIDS-related palliative care in this way, the home-based carers actively separate themselves from the illness that will inevitably claim their patient's life.

Perhaps this facilitates a more nuanced understanding of the mourners reported by Stadler in Bushbuckridge who used the three letters of 'OMO' washing powder to code the cause of death (HIV) in that instance. This is hardly a code, in that it is quite clear what is being suggested – people know what is being referenced. To refer to HIV as OMO, in this sense, is to state the obvious. Nonetheless, more ethnographic detail would be required to identify who said this, and in what context (whispered to a friend or said loudly to a stranger), and thus to map the necessary distance required in a particular case if potential implication in the death is to be negated. It is the common desire and tendency secretly to allocate blame that is responsible for saturating this so-called public silence with meaning.

However, given the data above, it may be misleading to think of the situation in terms of 'public silence' at all. As we saw with the case of Seven Days, some institutions and individuals could and did speak openly about the controversial poisonings without incurring blame or appropriating suspicion. The media reported the case in newspapers and on the radio, but neither journalists nor their corporate bosses were implicated in the controversy. Those with political power such as chiefs and headmen, in the run-up to village feasts, scolded their subjects for refusing to disclose information, and local politicians raised it in addresses at public gatherings, but they nonetheless evaded involvement. *Tshilombe* musicians incorporated it into their songs, but their spiritual sanction and strategic claims of 'madness' (Chapter 6) placed them in an ambiguous but authoritative social position beyond blame. Traditional healers and self-made AIC prophets claimed to have antidotes and protection prayers for the poison, but their powerful spiritual connections also permitted this. Whilst it is true that the most powerful people can also be the biggest witches (cf. Geschiere 1997), they can also manipulate their positions of power to bolster their own assertions of innocence. None of these authoritative and powerful actors were associated – through rumour or gossip – with Seven Days. The social and political positions they occupy permitted their public comment on suspicious forms of supposedly unnatural death at a time when the general public could only whisper about it for fear of implication.

Peer educators, on the other hand, do not occupy powerful or authoritative social positions from which they may speak openly about such issues without incurring some extent of blame. Indeed as young, mostly unmarried women, positions of power, influence, and authority generally elude them. Against the background of an overtly gendered aetiology that blames young women for harbouring and spreading sexual illness, their public forays into participatory education act as a magnet for accusation.

This brings us back to the recurring theoretical theme raised in Chapters 3, 5, and 6: the symbiotic relationship between knowledge and experience. Having demonstrated the importance of the links made between experience and knowledge in female initiation (Chapter 3) and the reversal of this with the assumption of experience based on extensive knowledge of biomedical approaches to blocking female fertility (Chapter 6), we can now add another layer of analysis. Cutting through the links between knowledge and experience is another variable: that of potential recourse to power and authority.

It would appear that knowing about a cause of death (as revealed by open acknowledgement of it) leads to potential implication in (that is, experience of) the fatality. Likewise, the opposite of this is also valid; a lack of knowledge about Seven Days, like a lack of knowledge of AIDS, is equated with a lack of experience and is expressed by avoiding open conversation. The 'degrees of separation' between guilt and innocence in the cause of a death, as outlined above, are rooted in claims to authority and influence. Depending on these, people may either employ gossip or openly converse.

It is this parallel dynamic that forced Mashamba to whisper his accusation that Seven Days originated in a Shangaan mortuary, and that permitted Chief Rathogwa to openly demand more knowledge of it. It allowed Solomon Mathase to sing about Seven Days in beer halls throughout Venda, whilst no one in the Fondwe council hut would admit to knowing anything about it. It prevented my research assistant from making enquiries, whilst the radio and newspapers reported it widely. The connection between knowledge and experience, in the open discussion of death, can be transcended or ignored by those with sufficient recourse to authority or power, whilst others, in the knowledge that they would be suspected if they were seen to know 'too much', have little option but to change their behaviour accordingly.

Peer educators' breach of the norm is to engage in open conversation without the necessary power or influence to do so safely and thus render themselves – and the condoms they swear by – open to guilt by association where others may negate this conjunction.

The majority of people in Venda, however, are not forced by interventional policy to breach this conventional means by which those who need to can avoid the use of 'deadly words' (Favret-Saada 1980). Those, like Nyamuka, Mashamba, and my research assistant, who do not occupy positions of relative power or influence, must maintain their separation from AIDS as a cause of death through backstage gossip and rumour. This perhaps helps to make sense of Chief Rathogwa's advice to me: 'There are some things we just do not talk about here in Venda. That is why there is so much gossip.'

Conclusion

In this final ethnographic chapter, I have suggested that the explanatory trope of 'denialism' is inadequate for understanding public silence around AIDS in rural South Africa. Through an analysis of reactions to a spate of alleged poisonings, it has become clear that the refusal openly to discuss cause of death is strongly connected to a wider strategy of seeking distance from the phenomenon of unnatural death. Attributing this to a collective AIDS denial is thus unhelpful, concealing more about the social processes involved than it reveals. To do so potentially obscures explanations for the failure of AIDS prevention programmes, such as the meaning attached to conventional processes for the expression of innocence. I have suggested that the silence in question is closely related to causes of death in general, and is not AIDS-specific. What has been termed a consensus of denial is, then, perhaps closer to a mass act of self-censorship.

By understanding the silence around AIDS in these terms, this chapter has outlined the inherent logic behind a seemingly irrational belief across Southern Africa that condoms cause AIDS. Current AIDS education policies, dominated by the peer education model, have helped to construct female educators as HIV carriers: they have been trapped in the web that connects knowledge of a death with potential implication in the fatality. The free condoms that peer educators distribute are inseparable from the process of association through which peer educators have been framed. It is in this context that prophylactics and peer educators are perceived not as protective agents, but as deadly participants in the ongoing battle for successful reproduction.

8   Conclusion

The Perception of a Crisis Revisited

On the evening before I left Venda to return to London, my host, Zwiakonda, joined me in my hut for one last late-night chat. He had come to present me with a gift: a painstakingly prepared map of the village with family names on each plot of land written in colour-coordinated code that represented the number of people who had recently died in each homestead. He had worked on this in secret, at night, for months. Such a project – even if it was for an outsider's research – would surely raise suspicion that he was up to no good. The map demonstrated that, by his count, one in four of the homesteads in Fondwe had lost at least one life in the past three years: most of them were people under the age of thirty. 'I don't know what is worse', he said after presenting me with my farewell gift, 'that people are becoming rich funeral directors, or that directing funerals seems to be the only secure job to have these days'. Driving down the N1 highway from Venda towards Johannesburg airport the following morning, Zwiakonda's parting words were in my head. The reverse side of the billboards that had welcomed me to 'Africa's Eden' were now urging my swift return, but I could not help wondering – with his graphic representation of the death toll as memento and harbinger – how many of the people I had befriended would be there to welcome me back again.

Zwiakonda's concerns articulate two of the most pertinent apprehensions in post-apartheid Venda. Unprecedented numbers of young people are dying, whilst those who evade 'sickness' struggle to find secure employment. To enunciate this lament by evoking the spectre of funeral directors – parasitic and unwelcome, but nonetheless indispensable – seemed to embody the profound contradictions that map out the lived experience of contemporary post-apartheid rural South Africa. His comments represent the widespread perception that contemporary African affairs, in Venda and beyond, are caught up in a crisis of social and sexual reproduction that has been so prominent in the ethnographic encounters presented in this book: a crisis that has exacerbated social cleavages along gendered and generational divides, and that threatens to deliver a stillborn future (Comaroff and Comaroff 2004: 336).

In its widest sense, this book has been an attempt to encapsulate and analyse the internal dynamics of this perceived crisis of reproduction through ethnographic accounts of creativity and practice. The creative processes of writing and performing songs, improvising nuanced and euphemistic expressions in public conversation, and devising pragmatic transformations of the ritual process are all ways in which people attempt to mitigate a sense of emergency in their daily lives. This has revealed the micro-politics of individuals and groups engaged in attempts to create and recreate connections with seemingly contradictory forms of power. In this vein, King Kennedy Tshivhase's decision to promote 'tradition' in the battle for paramountcy against his historical rival – through a dominant discourse in which state sovereignty trumps traditional authority – has seen chiefly legitimacy tested through the concurrent scrutiny of the state, the kingship, and the citizenry. As a direct result of this 'traditionalism', further contestations in value – to be found at a level more local than that of national political influence – have erupted between ancestral and bio-scientific forms of knowing about, and dealing with, sexually transmitted infections that lurk within polluted bodies, given life by 'dirty blood'.

The ethnography in this book illustrates processes which transfer different types of ritual or healing knowledge in an attempt to regain control over reproductive capacities. These attempts have been met with varying degrees of success, and in charting them I have found explanations as to why some were less successful than others.

Sex and death have become inseparable, and the link between them constitutes a profound challenge to securing a stable future. Massive reductions in the extent of migrant labour have stripped men of what for many had been a socially recognised symbol of masculinity, whilst removing the remittances they sent from often distant workplaces to household economies once managed by 'stay at home' wives. In this way, the perceived crisis of social reproduction is a dual process hingeing, on the one hand, on a desire for continuity in social, political, and economic processes, and, on the other, on the urgently felt need to secure healthy physical, sexual, intimate relations. The pursuit of the latter, however, often leads to illness, undermining the former.

But crisis yields hope. The ethnography here shows that any sense of emergency is not necessarily or only experienced as a contradiction between opposed poles. The crisis can also appear in the guise of – and be converted into – opportunity, through engagement in a series of material and symbolic entrepreneurial activities. Indeed, in the absence of significant or realistic structural frameworks through which to earn a living in the post-apartheid era, the rural poor have been left with little option but to engage opportunistically in diverse and multiple forms of activity. Doing so, however, may inadvertently reinforce the perception of crisis.

Thus, King Tshivhase's 'traditionalism' – whilst of itself representative of his royal polity's strategy for the consolidation of power – gave rise to community-led projects in which female initiation was revived in commoditised form by groups of women affirming their ability to act meaningfully on the world. More to the point, they seek the means to earn a living by selling their knowledge of tradition. Through moral panics, poison scares are blamed on inventive – if immoral – individuals who convert tea-estate fertiliser and body parts into deadly toxin in exchange for unknown material or spiritual favours. At the same time, embedded in this landscape, the key players in the account offered by this book – the peer group educators – are involved in the entrepreneurial brokering of symbolic capital, rooted in a presumed experience of sexual illness, in a market through which the parastatal positioning of so-called non-governmental organisations makes it very likely that, out of all the actors in this account, they (or some of them at least) will eventually achieve their stated aim of employment. In doing so, the peer educators sing songs about AIDS, advertising their fluency in biomedicine and drawing on diverse genres of music. This has contributed to the social and cosmological construction of AIDS – and those who tout their knowledge of it – as multi-vocal signifiers taking on and reflecting different interpretations within power struggles that cut across and exacerbate divisions of gender and generation for the possibility of, and control over, a productive, healthy, future.

The peer educators, although seemingly strung into historically constituted patriarchal structures, thus engage in symbolic transactions, trading their assumed experience and history of sex work and disease for new, more employable, identities from the local NGO and their international funders. AIDS, in this sense, symbolically reflects the ambivalence of free market forces: it 'works' to provide some with a source of new opportunity and aspiration to social mobility, leading ultimately to a 'real job' and a better life – but it is more likely to instigate social and physical decay through the obstruction of processes that ought to ensure productive and reproductive capacities.

Tradition Revisited

The particular version of traditionalism that has taken hold in post-apartheid Venda is indivisible from King Tshivhase's preoccupation with the succession struggle for paramount kingship. I have stressed the importance of historical processes that shape the current political economy of traditional leadership in the region. In the contemporary political alignment, we find the influence of pre-colonial internecine feuds and the subsequent weight of colonial and apartheid governments that incorporated already divided chiefly structures into their systems of racially segregated governance. In the post-apartheid era, the role of chiefs in the democratic dispensation has been influenced by a global discourse whereby the *right* to tradition is guaranteed in courts and constitutions throughout the world. Moreover, a pressing concern for economic stability, which is dependent more on the confidence of international speculative capital than on a centralised national fiscal policy (Koelble and Lipuma 2005), has forced the ANC-led government into carving a niche for traditional leaders in the implementation of policy orientated towards social justice, whilst the government simultaneously sets about implementing its neoliberal agenda.

This agenda is pervasive, but it is not all-encompassing. It has given rise to aspirations towards success and wealth, encouraged by the state through policies connected to GEAR and black economic empowerment. The perceived need to partake in the new future of prosperity – to get a good job and drive a flash car – coexists with the drive for a revival in traditional practices, legitimated precisely because they are perceived to be 'of the past'. As we saw in Chapter 3, this seemingly contradictory set of principles is not necessarily experienced as ambiguous. This was personified in the image of Noriah, translating the roll-call of initiation graduates into a computerised database with the intention of writing more convincing funding proposals to donor agencies and government bodies. The traditional intersects with the modern in such ways – but at the intersection it is not necessarily experienced as anything new. Revived tradition rather enables one to make the most of an opportunity.

If the ways in which global, local, and historical elements have been incorporated into processes of traditionalism have been well documented in the literature, the intersection of these processes with the micro-politics of knowledge has perhaps been neglected. Kennedy Tshivhase's well-publicised claim that AIDS education has been incorporated into the *vhusha* girls' initiation provides a case in point here. His statement must be read on different levels of intent. First, in the most obvious terms of the recent succession challenge, Tshivhase sought to combine his impeccable struggle credentials with the promotion of African renaissance values and development projects in his region. He has to some extent been led into this strategy by the historical relationship between the royal houses of Tshivhase and Mphephu, and the increasingly autocratic party line of the ANC – which recently deployed him to be one of South Africa's representatives to the Commonwealth Secretariat. His assertion that AIDS education is a part of female initiation presented Tshivhase with an ideal opportunity to court the media and engage in an act of constructing himself as a dynamic leader with the ability to nurture tradition and development: simultaneously spinning the past and the present; seeking, but not necessarily achieving, legitimacy in the eyes of the citizenry, the state, and the kingship.

The chiefly promotion of initiation, however, has had implications beyond the battle for paramountcy. It has bolstered the corpus of ritual knowledge upon which initiation is based and thus fortified the stratification of female hierarchies within the *tshivhambo*. Through an ethnographic account of *vhusha*, we saw that this resulted in the forceful ejection of the biomedical model from the initiation ceremony: not only because it appeared as an esoteric code to the ritual leaders, but more importantly because the folk model of sexual health being transferred to initiates can also be seen to offer instruction in how AIDS and other sexually transmitted diseases can be avoided. In this way, biomedical knowledge not only posed a threat to older women's status, but contradicted directly the inherent wisdom of ritual, ancestral knowledge.

Thus, proponents of the folk model would agree with King Tshivhase that AIDS education is indeed part of female initiation – in that it teaches young girls the centrality of monthly ablutions and respect for blood-related taboos through which pollution can be managed and fertility maintained. At the same time, those who have the biomedical model in mind (most importantly, perhaps, members of the Nhlapo Commission) would concur that such teaching is, at least in principle, a good idea. In this reading, both the ritual experts at Dopeni and the initiates who caused controversy during *ludodo* were following what they understood to be chiefly instruction. But without the experience and authority to back up their knowledge, the initiates found themselves in a powerless state of liminality.

It is difficult to know whether Tshivhase had this in mind when making his claims – such direct questions are not permissible in his presence – but given his history of shrewd political manoeuvres it would seem quite likely that he did. Whatever the case, he would have to adjust to the reality that the secretive and gendered nature of *vhusha* knowledge and practice would prevent it from becoming open and accessible public property. It would not easily be turned into a repository for cases of action funded by policy makers and NGOs. Nor would it lead the Nhlapo Commission to uphold his claim to a 'dual kingship' in the former homeland.

Biomedicine as Ritual Knowledge

In shedding further light on a crisis – and in particular on how it is perceived – the arguments made in this book have brought together three analytical threads that have not intersected previously: the politics of tradition; an anthropological approach to knowledge; and health-related interventionism. The convergence of the three in a focus on AIDS in Venda has raised some pertinent issues for each thread of analysis, and for a broader understanding of AIDS in similar settings. The response of people in Venda to AIDS as a threat to the social reproduction of their lives has revealed some inescapable patterns. Salient amongst these has been the dialectical relationship between ritual knowledge and experience. In these concluding remarks, I draw together the discussion offered in earlier chapters to situate AIDS education within changing dynamics of the contemporary politics of knowledge, through which biomedicine has been reconceived as ritual wisdom.

As we have seen, the biomedical and folk models are not incommensurable. They represent different means to what is essentially a similar end: the restoration of a healthy society. If we consider the relationship between ritual knowledge of the female *vhusha* initiation and the folk model of *malwadze dza vhafumakadzi* (the illnesses of women) as equivalent to that between 'experts' and 'the man in the street', then processes of 'marginal change' (Barth 2002) in the body of ritual knowledge can be discerned. Scientific concepts are incorporated into a 'working knowledge' of the system, such as that held by *tshilombe* musician Solomon Mathase. This adds a new dimension: 'marginal change' of ritual knowledge is managed by those on the periphery of ritual control – actors whose agency is relatively unimpeded by the structural hierarchies that bind the dynamics of the *vhusha* initiation together.

This casts some doubt on La Fontaine's claim that 'ritual knowledge is antithetical to change' (1985: 189): change to the ritual corpus can occur, and does not necessarily entail its dilution or loss of authenticity. On the contrary, selective and strategic incorporation of external factors can act to strengthen a body of knowledge. Thus the incorporation of biomedical concepts into the folk model has not been random or arbitrary. Abortion and contraception have become central tenets in patterns of blame whereby they cause the dangerous accumulation of pollution in the female body that, by extension, has been associated with harbouring HIV/AIDS. In this way, the opposition between traditional and modern conceptions – which appear historically and materially quite different but yet make almost identical claims to restoring the balance of social reproduction – is, at least partially, resolved.

I have argued throughout that the relationship between ritual knowledge and experience is central to an understanding of the ways in which people in Venda perceive and respond to HIV/AIDS. But this argument presents us with one final problem. If, as has been established, ritual knowledge is rooted in experience, are we then to assume that the ritual leaders at Dopeni, who slowly released the secrets of initiation, revealing the folk model of sexual illness to the initiates, have experienced sexual illness or the loss of fertility about which they purport to be experts? Put another way, are the ritual leaders polluted by their knowledge of pollution? After all, I have been insistent that peer educators, through their conspicuous knowledge of all things biomedical, are assumed to be very experienced in them.

The answer to the question is no; the ritual experts are not assumed to be tainted by historical experience of the ritual corpus in this way, and the reason for this is to be found in the social context in which the transmission of knowledge is managed. As Barth (1975; 2002) and Lambek (1993) have shown – and as my own data have evidenced – the ritual context in which a body of knowledge is transferred must be strictly controlled, and central to this control is the inculcation of secrecy. This is not primarily through a desire to construct and maintain privilege, hierarchy, or the 'mystification' of unequal power relations in society, although such socio-political dynamics may well arise from it.[1] It is, rather, through a desire to protect a body of sacred knowledge that is fundamental to the maintenance of healthy social reproduction. Moreover, as Lambek and Barth argue forcefully, ritual knowledge is dangerous: in the wrong hands it is thought to result in undesirable consequences for an individual and the wider community of which she is a part.

It is the secret and controlled transfer of ritual knowledge, in the ritual context, that protects the experts and initiates from unmediated exposure to a dangerous, but nonetheless essential, body of knowledge. Following this line of thought, the corpus of ritual knowledge in the *vhusha* that refers to sexual health and fertility is explained to the initiates not as 'sexual health' or 'family planning', but as 'ancestral wisdom' (*vhutali wa midzimu*) (cf. La Fontaine 1985; Barth 1975). This is a fundamental and crucial euphemising of ritual knowledge that separates it from the experience of the initiate or agent, yet facilitates the transfer of skills that are necessary for the reproduction of healthy sociality.

But the analysis of peer education has pointed to a different set of dynamics. At the intersection of planned HIV/AIDS interventions, where the line between biomedical and folk traditions of knowledge remains a blurred one, the relationship between knowledge and experience takes a significantly different twist. If planned interventions are aimed at 'changing behaviour' and providing education, then this is to be achieved primarily through the transfer of knowledge. As should be clear by now, this is hardly a straightforward endeavour, and takes place on what have been aptly termed 'battlefields of knowledge' (Long 1992; cf. Cernea 1995).

---

[1] Broadly Marxist arguments such as that proposed by Bloch (1992) are inadequate for a full comprehension of the dynamics that a ritual such as *vhusha* gives rise to in the post-apartheid context. A crude Marxism that sees ritual as deceptive superstructural ideology dismisses culturally constructed worlds without understanding them. The challenge is to understand cultural meanings, but to step outside them as well – not simply to dismiss them as ideological mystifications, but to situate them in relation to historical processes, politics, and economic relationships (cf. Keesing and Strathern 1998: 320; Blacking 1985).

On this 'battlefield', the incorporation of medical science into the folk model has not been entirely a one-way process. Through it, the biomedical model has come to be perceived by men and initiated women as a corpus of ritual knowledge in its own right. Given the educators' repeated claims that 'their' knowledge, when applied to everyday behaviour, can prevent illness, treat infection, and regulate fertility, the perception of science as a ritual corpus, at least for those with a 'working knowledge' of the folk model, is self-evident. The peer educators' biomedicine falls into Barth's 'three faces' of ritual knowledge, outlined in Chapter 6: a body of assertions and ideas (science); a medium through which it is communicated (public performances); and an underlying social organisation (the role of young women in allegedly non-governmental organisations). The 'biomedical corpus' – as it could be termed – and the folk model are to some extent *experienced* as mirror images of each other.

Whilst the '(wo)man in the street' is expected to be knowledgeable about the folk model and interpret illness through it, s/he would not necessarily class herself as an expert with the ability or sanction to facilitate its complete transference. Thus, whilst Solomon Mathase sings so eloquently about the folk model, he does not see his position as granting the right to teach it to others (cf. Lambek 1993: 69). Such a process occurs in the safe ritual environment of initiation; to recall Mathase in Chapter 6: 'These things are not even a secret. Venda boys are told all of this *at murundu* [male circumcision lodge].' Through government-funded workshops, peer educators have become the undisputed ritual experts of their own 'biomedical corpus' of ritual knowledge, and through weekly public performances they seek to reveal and transfer it to the wider public, to create 'men in the street' who may legitimate their corpus as the ritual experts at *vhusha* do in transference of the folk model.

But the contrasting social contexts of these attempts to transfer knowledge have profound consequences. Whilst biomedicine is perceived as a ritual corpus of knowledge – and the educators try to convey it through the ritual medium of music – public performances are not regularly defined ritual spaces. Rather, they are thought of as profane, marginal settings of occasionally successful entertainment. For this reason, peer educators cannot be thought of as 'critics of crisis' as described by Victor Turner, involved in the implementation of ritual practice as redressive machinery for the resolution of a social drama (Turner 1957). By operating outside of a circumscribed, controlled, ritual environment, peer educators are deprived of the protection offered by secrecy or obfuscation: their corpus is not framed in the distancing terminology of 'ancestral wisdom' but in the immediate one of 'sexual health'. In a non-ritual context, peer educators thus operate without the bulwark of a ritual hierarchy headed, ultimately, by the ancestors. Whilst this may have served to regulate their experiential connections with dangerous knowledge, their performances – attempts at the complete transferral of a ritual corpus – at beer halls, clinics, and market places leave them exceptionally vulnerable to guilt by association in the web of knowledge and experience.

In addition, then, to their counter-productive associations with biomedicine explained in Chapters 5 and 6, and their public courting of untold causes of death that were the topic of Chapter 7, the policy of peer education in Venda also forces young women to attempt the transferral of the 'biomedical corpus' in exposed, non-ritual settings. If knowledge is rooted in experience, then this paradigm is mediated by two key variables: recourse to power/authority and the social context of knowledge transfer.

In the final analysis, then, it is the combination of these factors – knowledge, experience, power/authority, and context – that undermines the good intentions of policy makers in their design of participatory interventions for public health, and has essentially turned peer education programmes into powerful magnets for the attraction of social stigma. The peer educators, in fact, *cannot* 'sing about what they cannot talk about' without reinforcing the reasons why they could not talk in the first place. Music does not work, for them, as a means of transcending the connections between knowledge and experience; but it does advertise their services as quasi-social workers, fluent in biomedicine and thus ultimately more employable than they would otherwise be.

This book has demonstrated that young women are perhaps not the ideal candidates for AIDS education in Venda, and it points to a pertinent critique of the way the epidemic has been represented. From the policy maker's perspective, statistics show that young women are far more likely to become infected with HIV than any other demographic group in Southern Africa. Thus the logic of implementing peer education projects within this category has largely been taken for granted. The unintended consequences that result from these projects – some of which I have alluded to – are not immediately visible and may remain obscure to the evaluation teams that sporadically assess project success in terms of categories such as 'condoms distributed' and 'public meetings held'. Policy makers have thus reinforced the folk model of sexual illness in which men are less concerned with *how* they sleep with women, and more concerned with *who* the women they sleep with are. If peer educators endure their frequent association with the disease and the way they are blamed for it, their fortitude and resilience are mainly due to the potential for social mobility that their position gives them.

Like any study, this one should be honest about its limitations. This is an ethnography of AIDS with one glaring omission: the voice of those who are HIV-positive. This is as much an issue for my analysis as it is a symptom of the social forces that I have been at pains to explain. In the absence of pressure groups such as the Treatment Action Campaign (TAC), the Venda region has failed to develop a secure framework within which people can be open about their status. Even among the peer educators, who promote the virtues of early testing for the benefits of treatment, not one has publicly affirmed her status. Of course, this is related to the widespread assumption that they are already carriers of the virus, and to their general intentions of 'moving on' from the projects, but their unwillingness to test and disclose their HIV status clearly cannot make it easier for others to do so.

Meanwhile, peer education continues to be one of the most prevalent forms of AIDS education in the world. I hope that, in some way, the data and analysis presented here can contribute to a more nuanced policy, or at least increase understanding of why some current approaches fail.

There is no 'collective denial' of AIDS in South Africa. Biomedical and folk models are not incommensurable. The political economy of traditional leadership is fundamental to understanding the meanings people weave around the virus. Policy makers ought to initiate the process of taking African worldviews seriously by thinking about prevention interventions in local terms.

Only then will condom be the boss.

Appendix A: Songs on Accompanying Web Site

Songs referred to in the text that can be heard by logging onto http://www.cambridge.org/us/9781107009912:

1. '*Tshikona*' – Recorded at *Vhuhosi*, Nengwenani ya Themeli, July 2005.
2. 'The Great *Domba* Song' – Tsianda, May 2005.
3. '*Nya Vhasedza*' from the *vhusha* initiation – Tsianda, March 2005.
4. '*Vho i vhonna naa?*' – Peer educators, Ha-Matsa, June 2005.
5. '*Daraga*' – Peer educators, Tshikombani, May 2005.
6. '*Khodomu Ndi Bosso*' – Peer educators, Ha-Matsa, June 2005.
7. '*AIDSE*' – Peer educators, Tshakhuma, August 2005.
8. '*Zwonaka*' (commonly heard version) – Tsianda, March 2005.
9. '*Zwonaka*' (peer education version) – Ha-Matsa, July 2005.
10. '*Khondomiza!*' – Peer educators, Ha-Matsa, June 2005.
11. '*Jojo Tshilangano*' – Peer educators, Tshakhuma, August 2005.
12. '*Ri do i fhenya*' – Peer educators, Ha-Matsa, June 2005.
13. '*Muimana*' – Peer educators, Tshikombani, May 2005.
14. '*Jealous Down*' – Peer educators, Tshikombani, May 2005.
15. '*Zwidzumbe*' – Solomon Mathase, Ngulumbi, June 2005.

All songs recorded by and copyright the author.

Appendix B: *'Zwidzumbe'* (Secrets)

Written and performed by Solomon Mathase

[Opens with Mathase taking the persona of a nurse at a clinic]

(1) *Huna mashango fhano Venda o vhaliwa* (x4)	There are many villages here in Venda, and they are all counted
(2) *Khavhaye sibadela vha dodi vhavhudza vhone* (x2)	Go to the hospital, they will tell you so
(3) *Huna mashango o vhaliwa hafha kiliniki*	There are villages, counted here at the clinic
(4) *Vhari tshone ndi tshidzumbe na tshone ndi tsha vhone vhane wee!*	They say it is a secret, just for them [those who are sick]
(5) *Hetshi ndi tshidzumbe ndi tsha vhone vhane wee!*	[They claim that] this is their secret
(6) *Thinga ambi munganga nga uri na nne ndo do shuma wee!*	I will not talk/gossip, my friend, I am just here to work

[Now talking as himself – as *Tshilombe*]

(7) *Khavha do pfa muthu a tshi khou toda u vhulahisa munwe muthu*	Listen now, someone is leading another into troubles
(8) *Ndi Khou pfana na munganga, ha nyagi u zwi amba*	I have a female friend, but she also does not want to talk [about it]
(9) *Vho nnese nazwino a vhanyagi u zwi amba*	The nurses, even now, they don't want to talk
(10) *Vho dokotela, nazwino, a vhanyagi u zwi amba*	The doctors [biomedical], even now, they don't want to talk
(11) *Ndi Khou nyaga u amba nga AIDS*	Now I want to talk about AIDS
(12) *A vhanyagi u zwi amba*	[Even though] they do not want to tell

[Now talking as a woman]

(13) *Vhasadzi rifela masheleni lupfumo wee!*	Women, we die because of the love of wealth
(14) *Kha rife, ri fhelele nga uri tshelede ri khou itoda*	Let's all die, because we want money

[Woman speaking to woman]

(15) *Tshelede ndi khou itoda munganga, sa kanudi yela hafho*	I want money, my friend, just go there yourself [to get it – to sell sex]
(16) *Nne tshelede ndi khou toda soku ndi...*	I want money, let me just...
(17) *Hei, AIDS, ndi kwine ndi do fa nayo wee!* [2 mins 22 secs]	This AIDS, it is better that I just die with it
(18) *Ngauri ndi khou toda tshelede heee!*	Because I want money!

[Woman speaking to long-term boyfriend with whom she lives]

(19) *Ndi do u itani fhedzi, nga uri fhano mudini a hu liwi na tshithu, a hu liwi na tshithu munganga. Ndi musi ndi mafhungo ashu ro no kwatisana, ngauri ndi vhudziwa zwa uri nne athishumi munganga*	I will just take it [have sex outside the relationship], because in this house we have nothing to eat, nothing to eat my friend. It is because of that business of ours, after we quarrelled – making each other angry – and I am always being told by you that I do not work.

244

Appendix B

[Speaking as himself again]

(20) *Vhashavha na u isa zwilonda*	They run away and leave open sores [ulcers or a shallow festering spot associated with sexually transmitted diseases – lesions associated with HIV]
(21) *Vhashavha na ala malwadze*	They run away with those illnesses [sexually transmitted]
(22) *Vhashavha na zwila zwithu zwe vhari, vha sokou a zwina ndavha*	They run away with those things they say are just useless
(23) *Na nne, ndi fa luthihi, lushaka lukhou fhela*	And me, I will die [only] once, the nation is vanishing ['getting finished']
(24) *A ri zwifuni mungana a ri divhani matshelo ro kuvhangana!*	We do not like it my friend, and we will not like it tomorrow when we are gathered [i.e., at your house for your funeral]
(25) *Zwipfisa mbilu vhutungu mungana naguri na inwi no tuwa, a hee*	It is very painful in my heart, my friend, because you are now also gone

[Singing as the dead woman]

(26) *Ndo dzhia tshelede, ngau nga vhusiwana* (x2)	I took the money, because of poverty

[Now referring to a rich man with many 'girlfriends']

(27) *Mulovha ni tshi di khoda niri a ni fhedziwi*	Yesterday, you boasted that you can never get finished [money-wise]
(28) *Na dzhena lonzhi, ndi inwi, ndi inwi*	And entering the lounge, it is you, it is you [who buys all the beer]
(29) *Na dzhena hodelani, ndi inwi ndi inwi* [**4 mins 4 secs**]	And entering the hotel, it is you, it is you
(30) *Na dzhena dzithekhisini, ndi inwi, ndi inwi*	And getting into taxis, it is you, it is you
(31) *Navhuya na fhata na nndu, ndi inwi, ndi inwi*	You came back [from migrant labour] to build a house, it is you, it is you
(32) *He ila nndu yanu ina opositizi!*	And this house of yours, it even has upstairs!
(33) *No vhuya no renga goloi na yone ndi Pajura*	You even bought a car, it was a Pajero
(34) *Vhafhasi navhone a ni tsha vha funa*	The ancestors, you no longer love them
(35) *Vhanntha, ni nyaga 'vho ne . . . '*	You pray to the Christian God, high up in the sky
(36) *Aidzi ritshimbilanayo, ritshimbilanayo, ri tshimbilanayo* (x3)	AIDS, we walk, we walk with it, we walk with it
(37) *Ahee, ritshimbilanayo, Nne, Aidzi, Vhari Vha tou I rengisa, vhari vhatou rengisa vhone vhane*	We walk with it, me, AIDS, they say they sell it because you buy it
(38) *A thi fi, nne ndi ndothe* (x2)	I will not die alone. [This is the name of a Radio Thohoyandou production – '*Ndi do fa na vhanzhe*', I will die with many – from 1986/8, when AIDS was first dramatised for radio. The story line featured a young temptress called Munaka (Beauty) who discovered she was HIV-positive after selling sex in beer halls, and endeavoured to sleep with as many men as possible to pass on the virus before she died.]
(39) *Aidzi, vhatau rengisa*	AIDS, many people are selling it
(40) *I tou rengiwa wee! Sa makipukipu*	And they buy it! Just like popcorn
(41) *I tou rengiwa wee! Sa masimba, kha la Venda Kha la Venda wee!* [**5 mins 45 secs**]	And they buy it, like crisps here in Venda, here in Venda

(42) *Madokotela, itani! Vhe lushaka lu khou fhela*	[Biomedical] doctors, just do it [make medicine] – the nation is getting finished
(43) *Ndi tou livhuwa Mudzimu, munwe ari*	I thank God, someone said,
(44) *Kha la Venda ndi tou tshimbila na mashango*	Here in Venda, I will walk around the villages
(45) *Vhatshimbila na mivhundu vha dzhena Mahosini*	They walked around the villages, even entered the King's court
(46) *Vha do zwiwana ngauri thuso a I ho*	They will just find out that there is no help [for them] there
(47) *Vhono di lenga* – [in English] –	'You are late, you are late my friend. Come here! It is much better, can I help you maybe... get ready, 15 days or 20 days, or 100 days. Can I help you? *Ndo vha thusa?*
(48) *Nga Lwa hashu zwiya konda wee* (x2)	In our language, it is difficult.

[Now he is speaking as a traditional healer – Solomon is a practising *inyanga*]

(49) *Ndi do dzhia zwidongo na lugwane ndi tshiyo tala miri thavhani*	I will take broken pieces of pot [*zwidongo* – clay pot for storing mixtures of medicinal herbs – also used as a ritual object in *vhusha*, *domba*, and *murundu*] and a shovel when I go looking for herbs in the mountain
(50) *Hezwi ndo dzula ndo rali thina na goloi ndi yodzhia ila mushonga mashangoni*	As I sit here, I don't even have a car to drive there and get that medicine from far away parts of the country
(51) *Ha-Makuya ndi kule* (x3) [**7 mins 21 secs**]	Ha-Makuya is far [a region of Venda in the remote north-eastern corner, associated with powerful traditional medicines. It borders with the Kruger National Park and Zimbabwe]
(52) *Khavha mmbeuele*	Just look for me/help me to look for it
(53) *Vhone, U khou lovha*	Hey you! He is dying
(54) *Muzwala, u khou fa, khonani khonani na lushaka shangoni*	Cousin, he is dying, my friend, and the nation (listen to me)
(55) *Ri tshimbilanayo* (x4)	We walk with it
(56) *Hetshi tshigero*	These scissors [i.e., it is cutting people down]
(57) *Vhakegulu vhari ndi yone 'Ace', a vha tsha ri Aidzi, vhari 'Ace'*	Old women, they say it is 'Ace' [the mealie meal flour] they don't say 'AIDS', it is 'Ace'
(58) *Ende u tshivhudzisa vhari houla o liwa ngani?*	And when you ask them what killed him? ['what ate him?']
(59) *Vhari 'Ace'*	They say 'Ace'
(60) *Vhatuka vhana vhutuku vha khou fhela*	[Shortened version of the proverb *vho tou konyolela matanda ndevheni*, they break sticks into small pieces and put them in their ears – i.e., the youth no longer hear the words of wisdom from their elders; the young kids are 'getting finished', perishing]
(61) *Vhana vhutuku nga mirole*	These kids are young in years
(62) *Vhana vhutuku, vhakegulu vha khou gungula na vhakalaha*	The young kids are making the old women and old men grumble/worry/complain
(63) *Vhotou u gungula vhari ri vhulungwa nga nnyi muduhulu – ni khou lovha!*	They complain and ask their grandchildren 'who will you be buried by?' as you are dying.

[Now speaking as young people in response to the elders]

(64) *Vhari ri khou lovha ri do vhulungwa nga nnyi?* (x3)	They say we are dying, and ask who will bury us

[Speaking again as parents/grandparents, engaged in gossip about the cause of a recent death] [**8 mins 50 secs**]

Appendix B   247

(65) *Houla mudulu nda ndi sa mufuni zwone, na u la nwanawanga, nda ndi sa mufuni zwone*
That grandson – I really loved him. And that child of mine, I really loved him/her

(66) *Mara u pfi o vhulwa nga yenei Aids*
But they say he/she was killed by this AIDS

(67) *Vhone, vho pfa uri zwone ndi zwifhio?*
You, what did you hear?

(68) *U la munwe ari hupfi hai! O tou wela*
That other one, he said no! He slept with a woman who aborted a child [*o tou wela* – the phrase for an abortion that was not properly cleaned/purified out by specific herbs]

(69) *Munwe ari hai! Thiri o vha a khou pfana na u la musadzi wa vho-mukenenene?*
The other one said no! Isn't it that he was in love with that woman of Mr so and so?

(70) *Nwana wa vho mukenenene vhone vha.*
The child of Mr so and so ...

(71) *Muthemba, ula – ari thiri u tou nga o vha o bvisa thumbu?*
Do you really trust her? That one says isn't it that she had an abortion? [Folk model – if a man sleeps with a woman who has had an abortion but was not properly 'sterilised' with the correct herbs afterwards, then the man will contract a potentially fatal illness. It is believed that an *inyanga* can kill the foetus easily, but it takes a lot more effort to clean the womb after this has occurred, returning the woman to the proper 'cleansing' menstrual cycle.]

(72) *Munwe ari hai! Thiri o vha a na zwilonda nga nnyoni?*
Another one said no! Isn't it that she had sores in/on her vagina?

(73) *Munwe ari hai! O vha otou vhifha muvhilini*
Another said no! She was pregnant [was ugly in the body]

[Turning to speak as himself – as an *inyanga* – now, and moving away from the gossip above]

(74) *Ngoho mara zwone zwa vhukuma ndi zwifhipo?*
Really, but honestly, which one of these is really the truth here?

(75) *Tshihulwane, o vhuya a dida na kha nne ari ndi mufhe mushonga*
They even visited me in a very respectful manner so that I could give them *mushonga*

(76) *A tshiyo pfana na nwana wa Vho Mukenenene*
When she went to fall in love with the child of Mr so and so

(77) *Thumbu a yongo fara*
But she could not conceive a child

(78) *Mulandu ndi zwilonda zwe zwi la zwawe ndi li a 'gokhonya'*
The problem was the sores [*zwilonda*] which led to '*gokhonya*'

(79) *A vhongo vhona na ula nwana wawe wa u thoma, o mbo di lovha*
Didn't you see her first child? It died

(80) *O vha o funa o ya hangeni ha 'Vho-Nyatshavhungwa'. Thiri na vhala vha a zwikona?*
She should have consulted Mrs Nyatshavhungwa. Isn't she the one who can deal with those difficult things?

(81) *Na vhala Vho-Jimu, fhedzi nne nda mulaya*
And [she should even have visited] Mr Jim [another local *Maine*], but at this time it was me who advised her

(82) *U fhedza, hanefho nne nda vhosokou pfa ndi 'dabadaba'*
After all that, I just ended up like a lunatic [*dabadaba*] [i.e., my advice was for nothing; she was just wasting my time]

(83) *Mathikho! hou la nwana ndi dabadaba*
Ooh! That young girl became a lunatic

(84) *A mbodi enda a vha a tshi khou dzedza hangeni, onoya lonzhi*
She started to spend nights at the beer halls

(85) *Nne nda tou mugaida, nda tou mufha na munwe mushonga*
I advised her, and gave her the correct mushonga

(86) *Nda mbodi da na tshila tshinopfi Tshirole*
I even gave her *Tshirole* [a specific medicine to assist in her social and physical development]

(87) *Nda mbodi mugwela nda muthusa*
I even dug up muti [from tree roots] that helped her

(88) *Mathiko! hezwi a khou tavha mukosi o onovha hange 'bodelotshitolo na lonzhi' hone ndo tou zuza fhedzi nda ndi songo muitela zwothe*

Hee! When she makes noise like that [i.e., started to regain health], she was happy in the beer hall, but this medication was just my first step for her to follow – I did not give her the entire sequence/dosage.

(89) *Na zwino mushonga wahone khuyu zwino nne ndi khou mangala hu tshipfi hai na zwino vhula vhulwadze hokunda nga usapfa!*

Now, I still have that medicine I was going to give her, and it was amazing to hear when they say that illness is beyond healing [i.e., she is dead], and all because she *did not listen* to me!

(90) *Arali o vha o ita hezwi ro vha ri tshi do divha ro muthusa fhedzi ha rido ita hani?*

If she had followed this [advice], we could have saved her, but what can we do? [N.B. Similarities with failure to follow a course of ARV medication.]

(91) *Zwino hupfi mbulungo ndi ya vhege idaho*
(92) *Ee, Yaa! Zwa zwisongo fanela*
(93) *Hee! ndi zwe zwi la zwilonda*
(94) *Ngoho havha vhana vhaano maduvha vhado fhela*

Now they say that the funeral is next week
It was not expected
It is because of these sores (*zwilonda*)
Really, today's children, they will perish.

[Solomon's friend now talking to him]

(95) *Vha do fhela ngani mungana?*

What will they perish by, my friend?

[Solomon's response]

(96) *Ndari huna vhulwadze ha zwilonda hafha nnyoni dza vhasidzana ende vhathannga a vhavhuyi vha zwithogomela*

Like I said, there is illness of sores [*zwilonda*] in girls' vaginas, and young men do not take care

(97) *Ndikhouri vha songo vhuya vha zwi ambi!*

Even you, my friend, please don't ever speak about it!

[Friend responding]

(98) *Mara vhone vhala ndi khonani yanga vho*

But that man is your friend [i.e., How can you keep quiet?]

[Solomon responding]

(99) *Arali wa tou vha sevhela vho hu si uri na munwe a dovhe vho*

Maybe if you just tip him off when no one else is around, that will be fine

(100) *Ai ndi a vhuya nda tou ralo ndido vhudza makhadzi wanu uri zwithu zwitshile?*

Ah! Will I have to report this to your auntie [that you are not listening] so that you will not die?

(101) *Hafha shangoni a vhanga koni u tshila*

Here, in this world, you cannot live

(102) *U nwana, thetshelesa milayo, thetshelesa milayo* (x3)

If you are a child, you must listen to the rule/laws

(103) *Midi yofhambana na malofha o fhambana, na mashango o fhambana*

Houses are different, and blood (i.e., family) is different, and villages are different

(104) *Ndi ngani hutshikhou pfi 'vhala mukalaha vhoshulwa mutodo?'*

Why is it that they say the old man was smeared with fresh cow dung? [Metaphorical comparison of old age with the smearing of dung on floors and walls to make them strong and fit for human habitation]

(105) *Ndingani hukhou pfi 'fhala mudini a huna lufu?'*

Why is it they are saying that 'in that household, there is no death'?

(106) *Vhavenda vha tshi amba vhari o dzhia shambo la hone*

Vendas, when they speak, they say yes, he has inherited the correct [pure] blood [skeleton] of the family [i.e., the child must bear resemblance to the father, making reference to socially acceptable ways of reproduction – not from casual sexual encounters with dangerous women, but within controlled, planned liaisons between different homesteads].

Appendix B

(107) *A vha vhoni nga ngei, hu tshi pfi huna Ha-Tshivhasa*
(108) *Hadovha nga ngeno hapfi hu na ngei Ha-Mathase*
(109) *Ha dovha hapfi hu na vhala vhanwe nga ngei vho*
(110) *U amba nga madzina ndi sokou lopola*

(111) *Fhedzi ngoho yone vha a idivha!*
(112) *Nne ndi khou amba ndi khouri English, Afrikaans, Tshizulu, Tshisuthu, Tshikhosa, Tshibeli, hotho hothe nne ndi ya vha dzhenela*
(113) *Hee, Hedzi nyambo dzothe dzi tshi tuwa dzituwa dzi tshikhou tou ya 'sitireiti', 'tswii'!*

(114) *Ngauri arali ndi khouri 'How are you', yo tou da sitirethi kha vhone*
(115) *Ari ndi khouri 'minjani' yo tou da kha vhone sitirethi, tswii!*
(116) *Arali nne ndi khouri 'hu itahani' ndi khouri na vhone zwotou da khavhone tswi!*
(117) *Nga uri Tshivenda na Tshikalanga, Tshizulu a tshidologiwi, u nga tou zwitalukanya!*
(118) *Vha do lovha mungana, nga u sapfa, mungana, khonani nga u safpa*
(119) *A huna ane a nga takadza shango lothe*
(120) *Kani ha ndi zwone zwo itaho uri vhafunzi vha zwifhe mavhidani*
(121) *Hafha shangoni lothe a huna mufunzi ane anga vha kwae*
(122) *Vha sokou tou pomokana, arali ha vha vhafunzi vhovha vhakhou da na zwavhukuma na rine ra ri do amba zwa vhukuma*
(123) *Ndi ngazwo mbilu yanga iya vhavha*
(124) *Ndo muvhulaya!*

Don't you see, there, he is a Tshivhasa (Subject of King Tshivhase)
And here, over here, this one is of Ha-Mathase (showing the differences between the two families)
And again, they say, there are also many other families [that are different]
But, to talk about all these names is just a waste of time ['talking shit']

And after all, you know the truth!
I am saying that it can either be English, Afrikaans, Zulu, Xhosa, Sipedi, everywhere – I will verbally attack the youngsters who do not want to listen.
All these languages, when they go [are spoken], they should go straight, direct to the point! [making the point that it is not just Venda youth who are dying – youth throughout South Africa no longer respect their elders' values]

Because if I am saying 'How are you' – then it is straightforward
And if I say 'Hello', then it is to the point!

And if I am saying 'How are you' it is coming at you straight to the point!
Because in Venda, Shona, Zulu, there is no need for translation, they can be easily understood!

They will die, my friend, because they are not listening
No one can ever please the whole world
Maybe this is what causes the pastors to tell lies at the graveside [i.e., covering up the cause of death]
In the entire world no pastor can be perfect

They just blame each other, pointing fingers; if the pastors were bringing the truth we would also be able to talk the truth
This is why my heart is so painful
I killed him! [Quote from contemporary reggae song by Colbert Mukwevho – in which I play rhythm guitar – commenting on the recent increase in witchcraft-related killings in Limpopo. It is used here as a metaphor for death, actual and potential, being all around – and also as a quote from the woman, Munaki, in the radio drama (line 38 above).

Appendix C: AIDS, AIDS, AIDS

By Edward Maphanda

AIDS, AIDS, AIDS, mysterious woe, bury the old and new alike,
The world trembles as no cure is found,
The stubborn child of the white man who ignores other cultures,
Though sex will be forever and forever sweet.

AIDS, AIDS, AIDS, one white man's threat, not known for long in other cultures,
Only reigns in white man's laboratories,
And being defeated, they give it a gigantic name,
To confront the black healer, now and again.

Muti, muti, muti, no not AIDS,
Muti, muti from healers of years upstream,
And still to go millions downstream,
Where AIDS was not called AIDS, the healer has his own words for the disease.

Ten days the healer needs to cure your AIDS,
Three bowel movements needed to cut off virus,
Virus seen in second and third movements,
One litre of tonic herbs and sex is forever and ever sweet.

AIDS, AIDS, AIDS, revenge of the unborn,
The white man is unaware you are the remains of the Foetus,
Yes, AIDS is the poison from the aborted child,
Our ancestors have identified the *muti*, the signs and the symptoms.
Black nurses and doctors have become sellouts,
The custom they buried for a foreign culture,
When ours originated with the creator,
Who is in all science and all life.

He did hide the healing power in herbs,
And Christianity failed to align faith and creation,
The vagina is related to Rwanda and Kosovo.
The pussy being known for pleasure, instead of progeny.

References

Achmat, Z. 2004. 'The Treatment Action Campaign, HIV/AIDS and the government', *Transformation* 54: 76–84.
Africa, S. 1992. 'The role, prospects and expectations of the TVBC intelligence services during an interim government period', *Strategic Review for Southern Africa* 14 (2): 78–94.
Allen, T. 2006. 'AIDS and evidence: interrogating some Ugandan myths', *Journal of Biosocial Science* 38 (1): 7–28.
Amnesty International. 1983. *South Africa: detention without trial and torture of detainees in Venda*. London: Amnesty International.
Anderson, A. 1999. 'The Lekganyanes and prophecy in the Zion Christian Church', *Journal of Religion in Africa* 29 (3): 285–31.
Appiah, K. H. 1992. *In My Father's House: Africa in the philosophy of culture*. London: Methuen.
Aschwanden, H. 1987. *Symbols of Death: an analysis of the consciousness of the Karanga*. Gweru: Mambo Press.
Ashforth, A. 1990. *The Politics of Official Discourse in South Africa*. Oxford: Clarendon Press.
—— 1997. 'Lineaments of the political geography of state transformation in twentieth-century South Africa', *Journal of Historical Sociology* 10 (2): 101–26.
—— 2000. *Madumo: a man bewitched*. Chicago IL and London: University of Chicago Press.
—— 2004. 'An epidemic of witchcraft? The implications of AIDS for the post-apartheid state', *African Studies* 61 (1): 121–45.
—— 2005. *Witchcraft, Violence and Democracy in South Africa*. Chicago IL and London: University of Chicago Press.
Auslander, M. 1993. '"Open the wombs!": the symbolic politics of modern Ngoni witchfinding' in J. Comaroff and J. L. Comaroff (eds), *Modernity and Its Malcontents: ritual and power in postcolonial Africa*. Chicago IL and London: University of Chicago Press.
Bähre, E. 2002. 'Witchcraft and the exchange of sex, blood, and money among Africans in Cape Town, South Africa', *Journal of Religion in Africa* 32 (3): 300–34.
Barber, K. 1987. 'Popular arts in Africa', *African Studies Review* 3 (30): 1–78.
—— 1991. *I Could Speak Until Tomorrow: oriki, women and the past in a Yoruba town*. Edinburgh: Edinburgh University Press for the International African Institute.

———— (ed.). 1997. *Readings in African Popular Culture*. Oxford: James Currey and the International African Institute.
Barnett, T. 2004. 'HIV: A challenge for Africa', *Anthropology Today* 20 (4): 1–2.
Barnett, T. and P. Blaikie. 1992. *AIDS in Africa: its present and future impact*. London: Belhaven Press.
Barnett, T. and A. Whiteside. 2002. *AIDS in the Twenty-First Century*. Basingstoke: Palgrave Macmillan.
Barth, F. 1975. *Ritual and Knowledge among the Baktaman of New Guinea*. New Haven CT: Yale University Press.
———— 1990. 'The guru and the conjurer: transactions in knowledge and the shaping of culture in Southeast Asia and Melanesia', *Man*, n. s. 25: 640–53.
———— 2002. 'An anthropology of knowledge', *Current Anthropology* 43 (1): 1–11.
Barz, G. 2006. *Singing for Life: HIV/AIDS and music in Uganda*. New York NY: Routledge.
Basset, M. 1998. 'Impact of peer education on HIV infection in Zimbabwe', *Sexual Health Exchange* 4: 14–15.
Bayart, J.-F. 1993. *The State in Africa: the politics of the belly*. Harlow: Longman.
Baylies, C. 2000. 'Perspectives on gender and AIDS in Africa' in C. Baylies and J. Bujra (eds), *AIDS, Sexuality and Gender in Africa: collective strategies and struggles in Tanzania and Zambia*. New York NY and London: Routledge.
Beall, J. 2005. 'Decentralising government and decentralising gender: lessons from local government reform in South Africa', *Politics and Society* 33 (2): 253–76.
Beall, J., S. Mkhize, and V. Shahid. 2005. 'Emergent democracy and "resurgent" tradition: institutions, chieftaincy and tradition in KwaZulu-Natal', *Journal of Southern African Studies* 31 (4): 755–71.
Beidelman, T. O. 1997. *The Cool Knife: imagery of gender, sexuality and moral education in Kaguru initiation ritual*. Washington DC and London: Smithsonian Institution Press.
Beinart, W. 2001. *Twentieth Century South Africa*. Oxford: Oxford University Press.
Bern, J. and S. Dodds. 2002. 'On the plurality of interests: aboriginal self government and land rights in South Africa' in D. Ivison, P. Patton, and W. Sanders (eds), *Political Theory and the Rights of Indigenous Peoples*. Cambridge: Cambridge University Press.
Blacking, J. 1959. 'Fictitious kinship amongst girls of the Venda of the northern Transvaal', *Man* 59: 55–8.
———— 1962. 'Musical expeditions of the Venda', *African Music* 3: 54–72.
———— 1964a. 'The cultural foundations of the music of the Venda', PhD thesis, University of the Witwatersrand.
———— 1964b. *Black Background: the childhood of a South African girl*. London: Abelard Schuman.
———— 1965. 'The role of music in the culture of the Venda of the northern Transvaal' in M. Kolinski (ed.), *Studies in Ethnomusicology*, Vol. 2. New York NY: Oak Publications.
———— 1967. *Venda Children's Songs: a study in ethnomusicological analysis*. Chicago IL and London: University of Chicago Press.
———— 1969a. 'The songs, mimes, dances and symbolism of Venda girls' initiation schools, Part 1: Vhusha', *African Studies* 28 (1): 3–35.

_____ 1969b. 'The songs, mimes, dances and symbolism of Venda girls' initiation schools, Part 2: Milayo', *African Studies* 28 (2): 69–107.
_____ 1969c. 'The songs, mimes, dances and symbolism of Venda girls' initiation schools, Part 3: Domba', *African Studies* 28 (3): 149–79.
_____ 1969d. 'The songs, mimes, dances and symbolism of Venda girls' initiation schools, Part 4: The great domba song', *African Studies* 28 (4): 120–44.
_____ 1969e. 'Initiation and the balance of power: the *tshikanda* girls' initiation school of the Venda of the northern Transvaal', *Ethnological and Linguistic Studies in Honour of N. J. van Warmelo*. Pretoria: Department of Bantu Administration, Ethnological Publications.
_____ 1973. *How Musical Is Man?* Seattle WA and London: University of Washington Press.
_____ 1985. 'Movement, dance, music and the Venda girls' initiation cycle' in J. Spencer (ed.), *Society and the Dance: the social anthropology of processes and performance*. Cambridge: Cambridge University Press.
_____ 1995a. 'Reflections of the effectiveness of symbols' in R. Byron (ed.), *Music, Culture and Experience: selected papers of John Blacking*. Chicago IL and London: University of Chicago Press.
_____ 1995b. 'The music of politics' in R. Byron (ed.), *Music, Culture and Experience: selected papers of John Blacking*. Chicago IL and London: University of Chicago Press.
_____ 1995c. 'Music and the historical process in Vendaland' in R. Byron (ed.), *Music, Culture and Experience: selected papers of John Blacking*. Chicago IL and London: University of Chicago Press.
Bloch, M. 1974. 'Symbols, song, dance and features of articulation', *European Archives of Sociology* 15: 55–81.
_____ 1992. *Prey into Hunter: the politics of religious experience*. Cambridge: Cambridge University Press.
_____ 1998. *How We Think They Think*. Boulder CO: Westwood Press.
Boyer, D. 2005. 'Visiting knowledge in anthropology: an introduction', *Ethnos* 70 (2): 141–8.
Bozzoli, B. 2000. 'Why were the 1980s "millenarian"? Style, repertoire, space and authority in South Africa's black cities', *Journal of Historical Sociology* 31 (1): 78–110.
_____ 2004. *Theatres of Struggle and the End of Apartheid*. Edinburgh: Edinburgh University Press for the International African Institute.
Brenneis, D. 1984. 'Grog and gossip in Bhatgaon: style and substance in Fiji Indian conversation', *American Ethnologist* 11 (3): 487–506.
Bruner, E. M. and B. Kirshenblatt-Gimblett. 1994. 'Maasai on the lawn: tourist realism in East Africa', *Cultural Anthropology* 4 (4): 435–70.
Buhlungu, S. 2002. 'From Madiba magic to Mbeki logic: Mbeki and the ANC's trade union allies' in S. Jacobs and R. Calland (eds), *Thabo Mbeki's World: the politics and ideology of the South African President*. Scottsville: University of KwaZulu-Natal Press.
Buijs, G. 2003. 'Presenting and re-presenting the past: African childhood recalled', Occasional Paper, *Tydskrif vir Nederlands en Afrikaans*, Stellenbosch University.
Bujra, J. 2000a. 'Target practice: gender and generational struggles in AIDS prevention work in Lushoto' in C. Baylies and J. Bujra (eds), *AIDS, Sexuality*

and Gender in Africa: collective strategies and struggles in Tanzania and Zambia. New York NY and London: Routledge.

―― 2000b. 'Targeting men for a change: AIDS discourse and activism in Africa', *Agenda* 44: 6–25.

―― 2004. 'AIDS as a crisis in social reproduction', *Review of African Political Economy* 102: 631–8.

Bujra, J. and C. Baylies. 2000. 'Responses to the AIDS epidemic in Tanzania and Zambia' in C. Baylies and J. Bujra (eds), *AIDS, Sexuality and Gender in Africa: collective strategies and struggles in Tanzania and Zambia.* New York NY and London: Routledge.

Bureau for Economic Research. 1979. *The Independent Venda.* Johannesburg: Hortotos.

Byron, R. (ed.) 1995. *Music, Culture and Experience: selected papers of John Blacking.* Chicago IL and London: University of Chicago Press.

Calland, R. 2006.*Anatomy of South Africa: who holds the power?* Cape Town: Zebra Press.

Campbell, C. 1998. 'Peer education and safer sexual behaviour amongst adolescents' in H. Moore (ed.), *Promoting the Health of Children and Young People: setting a research agenda.* London: Health Education Authority.

―― 2000. 'Selling sex in the time of AIDS: the psycho-social context of condom use by Southern African sex workers', *Social Science and Medicine* 50: 479–94.

―― 2002. 'The role of social capital in promoting or hindering HIV prevention: a case study of a South African mining community', *Proceedings of the Fourteenth International AIDS Conference,* Barcelona.

―― 2003. *Letting Them Die: how HIV/AIDS prevention programmes often fail.* Oxford: James Currey.

Campbell, C. and C. MacPhail. 2002. 'Peer education, gender and the development of critical consciousness: participatory HIV prevention by South African youth', *Social Science and Medicine* 55 (2): 331–45.

Campbell, C. and Y. Mzaidume. 2001. 'Grassroots participation in HIV prevention programmes', *American Journal of Public Health* 91 (12):1978–86.

Campbell, C. and B. Williams. 1998. 'Evaluating HIV prevention programmes: conceptual challenges', *Psychology in Society* 24: 57–68.

―― 1999. 'Beyond the biomedical and the behavioural: towards an integrated approach to HIV prevention in the South African mining industry', *Social Science and Medicine* 48 (11):1625–39.

Campbell, C., B. Williams, and D. Gilgen. 2002. 'Is social capital a useful tool for exploring community level influence on HIV infection? An exploratory case study from South Africa', *AIDS-Care* 14 (1): 41–55.

Cernea, M. M. (ed.). 1991. *Putting People First: sociological variables in rural development.* New York NY: Oxford University Press.

―― 1995. 'Social organisation and development anthropology', *Human Organization* 3: 340–51.

Chabal, P. and J.-P. Daloz. 1999. *Africa Works: disorder as political instrument.* Oxford: James Currey and the International African Institute.

Chabal, P. ―― 1983. *Rural Development: putting the last first.* London: Longman.

―― 1994. 'Participatory rural appraisal (PRA): challenges, potentials and paradigm', *World Development* 22 (10): 1437–54.

Clifford, J. 1988. *The Predicament of Culture: twentieth-century ethnography, literature, and art*. Cambridge MA: Harvard University Press.
———— 1997. *Routes: travel and translation in the late twentieth century*. Cambridge MA: Harvard University Press.
———— 2003. *On the Edges of Anthropology (Interviews)*. Chicago IL: Prickly Paradigm Press.
Cochrane, J. R. 1986. *Servants of Power: the role of English-speaking churches 1903–1930*. Johannesburg: Ravan Press.
Coetzee, E., H. Hawksley, and H. Louw. 2004. *Life Orientation Today*. Cape Town: CTP.
Cohen, D. W. 1991. 'La Fontaine and Wamimbi: the anthropology of "time-present" as the substructure of historical oration' in J. Bender and D. Wellbery (eds), *Chronotypes: the construction of time*. Stanford CA: Stanford University Press.
Comaroff, J. 1985. *Body of Power, Spirit of Resistance: the culture and history of a South African people*. Chicago IL: University of Chicago Press.
Comaroff, J. and J. L. Comaroff. 1987. 'The madman and the migrant: work and labour in the historical consciousness of a South African people', *American Ethnologist* 14 (2): 191–209.
———— 1991. *Of Revelation and Revolution: Christianity, colonialism, and consciousness in South Africa, Volume 1*. Chicago IL: University of Chicago Press.
———— 1993. 'Introduction' in J. Comaroff and J. L. Comaroff (eds), *Modernity and Its Malcontents: ritual and power in postcolonial Africa*. Chicago IL: University of Chicago Press.
———— 1999. 'Occult economies and the violence of abstraction: notes from the South African postcolony', *American Ethnologist* 26 (2): 279–303.
———— 2004. 'Notes on Afromodernity and the Neo World Order: an afterword' in B. Weiss (ed.), *Producing African Futures: ritual and reproduction in a neoliberal age*. Leiden: Brill.
———— 2009. *Ethnicity, Inc.* Chicago IL: Chicago University Press.
Comaroff, J. L. 1974. 'Chiefship in a South African homeland: a case study of the Tshidi chiefdom of Bophuthatswana', *Journal of Southern African Studies* 1 (1): 36–51.
Comaroff, J. L. and J. Comaroff. 1997. 'Postcolonial politics and discourses of democracy in Southern Africa: an anthropological reflection on African political modernities', *Journal of Anthropological Research* 53 (2):123–46.
Comaroff, J. L. and S. A. Roberts. 1981. *Rules and Processes: the cultural logic of dispute in an African context*. Chicago IL: University of Chicago Press.
Cooke, B. and U. Kothari. 2001. 'The case for participation as tyranny' in B. Cooke and U. Kothari (eds), *Participation: the new tyranny?* New York NY: Palgrave Macmillan.
Cooper, F. 2005. *Colonialism in Question: theory, knowledge, history*. Berkeley CA and London: University of California Press.
Coovadia, A. 2009. 'Courting morality: the fight to prevent mother-to-child HIV transmission' in K. Cullinan and A. Thom (eds), *The Virus, Vitamins and Vegetables: the South African HIV/AIDS mystery*. Johannesburg: Jacana.
Coplan, D. 1985. *In Township Tonight! South Africa's black city music and theatre*. New York NY: Longman.

―――― 1994. *In the Time of Cannibals: the word music of South Africa's Basotho migrants*. Chicago IL: University of Chicago Press.

Craddock, S. 2000. 'Scales of justice: women, inequity, and AIDS in East Africa' in I. Dyck, S. MacLafferty, and N. D. Lewis (eds), *Geographies of Women's Health*. London: Routledge.

―――― 2007. 'Market incentives, human rights, and AIDS vaccines', *Social Science and Medicine* 64 (5): 1042–56.

Crick, M. R. 1982. 'Anthropology of knowledge', *Annual Review of Anthropology* 11: 287–313.

Cullinan, K. and A. Thom (eds). 2009. *The Virus, Vitamins and Vegetables: the South African HIV/AIDS mystery*. Johannesburg: Jacana.

Daniel, J., R. Southall, and J. Lutchman. 2005. 'Introduction: President Mbeki's second term: opening the golden door?' in J. Daniel, R. Southall, and J. Lutchman (eds), *State of the Nation: South Africa 2004–2005*. Cape Town: Human Sciences Research Council Press.

Davenport, T. H. R. and C. Saunders. 2000. *South Africa: a modern history*. London: St Martin's Press.

Deacon, H. 2006. 'Towards a sustainable theory of health related stigma: lessons from the HIV/AIDS literature', *Journal of Community and Applied Social Psychology* 16: 418–25.

Deacon, H. with J. Stephney and S. Prosalendis. 2005. *Understanding HIV/AIDS Stigma: a theoretical and methodological analysis*. Cape Town: Human Sciences Research Council Press.

de Bruyn, M. 1992. 'Women and AIDS in developing countries', *Social Science and Medicine* 34 (3): 249–62.

de Gruchy, J. W. and S. de Gruchy. 2004. *The Church Struggle in South Africa*. London: Augsburg Fortress.

Delius, P. 1983. *The Land Belongs to Us: the Pedi polity, the Boers and the British in the nineteenth-century Transvaal*. Johannesburg: Ravan Press.

―――― 1990. 'Migrants, comrades and the rural revolt: Sekhukhuneland 1950–1987', *Transformation* 13: 2–26.

―――― 1996. *A Lion amongst the Cattle: reconstruction and resistance in the northern Transvaal*. Oxford: James Currey.

Delius, P. and C. Glaser. 2005. 'Sex, disease and stigma in South Africa: historical perspectives', *African Journal of AIDS Research* 4 (1): 29–36.

Delius, P. and L. Walker. 2002. 'AIDS in context', *African Studies* 61 (1): 5–13.

de Wet, D. 1995. *Moving Together, Drifting Apart: betterment planning and villagisation in a South African homeland*. Johannesburg: Witwatersrand University Press.

Dladla, N. 1997. 'African renaissance: teaching the past to find the future', *Mail and Guardian* (Johannesburg), 1 August 1997.

Drewal, M. 1991. 'The state of research on performance in Africa', *African Studies Review* 34 (3): 1–64.

Drews, A. 2000. 'Gender and *ngoma*: the power of drums in eastern Zambia' in R. van Dijk, R. Reis, and M. Spierenburg (eds), *The Quest for Fruition through* Ngoma: *political aspects of healing in Southern Africa*. Oxford: James Currey.

Eba, P. 2007. *Stigma(ta): re-exploring HIV-related stigma*. (AIDS Review) Pretoria: Centre for the Study of AIDS, University of Pretoria.

Egan, A. 2007. 'Kingdom deferred? The churches in South Africa, 1994–2006' in S. Buhlungu, J. Daniel, R. Southall, and J. Lutchman (eds), *State of the Nation 2007*. Cape Town: Human Sciences Research Council Press.

Egero, B. 1991. *South Africa's Bantustans: from dumping grounds to battlefronts*. Discussion Paper 4. Uppsala: Scandinavian Institute of African Studies.

Ellis, S. 1989. 'Tuning into pavement radio', *African Affairs* 88 (352): 321–30.

Engelke, M. 2005. 'Sticky subjects and sticky objects: the substance of African Christian healing' in D. Miller (ed.), *Materiality*. Durham NC: Duke University Press.

—— 2007. *A Problem of Presence: beyond scripture in an African church*. Berkeley CA: University of California Press.

Epstein, H. 2007. *The Invisible Cure: Africa, the West and the fight against AIDS*. London: Penguin.

Erikson, T. H. 1995. *Small Places, Large Issues*. London: Pluto Press.

Erlmann, V. 1991. *African Stars: studies in black South African performance*. Chicago IL: University of Chicago Press.

—— 1996. *Nightsong*. Chicago IL: University of Chicago Press.

Fabian, J. 1990. *Power and Performance: ethnographic explorations through proverbial wisdom and theater in Shaba, Zaire*. Madison WI: University of Wisconsin Press.

Falk Moore, S. 1999. 'Reflections on the Comaroff lecture', *American Ethnologist* 26 (2): 304–6.

Farmer, P. 1988. 'Bad blood, spoiled milk: bodily fluids and moral barometers in rural Haiti', *American Ethnologist* 15 (1): 62–83.

—— 1990. 'Sending sickness: sorcery, politics and changing concepts of AIDS in rural Haiti', *Medical Anthropology Quarterly* 4 (1): 6–27.

—— 1994. 'AIDS talk and the constitution of cultural models', *Social Science and Medicine* 38 (6): 801–9.

—— 2006 [1992]. *AIDS and Accusations: Haiti and the geography of blame*. Berkeley CA: University of California Press.

Fassin, D. 2007. *When Bodies Remember: experiences and politics of AIDS in South Africa*. Translated from French by Amy Jacobs and Gabeielle Varro. Berkeley CA and London: University of California Press.

Favret-Saada, J. 1980. *Deadly Words: witchcraft in the Bocage*. Translated from French by Catherine Cullen. Cambridge and New York NY: Cambridge University Press.

Ferguson, J. 1994. *The Anti-Politics Machine: 'development', depoliticization, and bureaucratic power in Lesotho*. Cambridge: Cambridge University Press.

—— 2006. *Global Shadows: Africa in the neoliberal world order*. Durham NC: Duke University Press.

Fernandes, M. E. L., L. A. V. D'Angelo, E. M. Vieira, and M. O'Grady (eds). 1999. *Rapid Responses: initiatives to HIV/AIDS prevention in Brazil*. Petrópolis, Brazil: Editora Vozes.

Fisher, W. 1997. 'Doing good? The politics and anti-politics of NGO practices', *Annual Review of Anthropology* 26: 439–64.

Fokwang, J. T. D. 2009. *Mediating Legitimacy: chieftaincy and democratisation in two African chiefdoms*. Bamenda, Cameroon: Langaa Research and Publishing Common Initiative Group.

Fortes, M. and E. P. Evans-Pritchard (eds). 1940 [2006]. *African Political Systems*. London: Hesperides Press.
Fraser, A. 2007. 'Land reform in South Africa and the colonial present', *Social and Cultural Geography* 8 (6): 835–51.
Freire, P. 1972. *Pedagogy of the Oppressed*. Harmondsworth: Penguin.
Fuller, C. 1997. 'Religious texts, priestly education, and ritual action in a south Indian temple', *Contributions to Indian Sociology* 31 (1): 3–26.
―――― 2003. *The Renewal of the Priesthood: modernity and traditionalism in a south Indian temple*. Princeton NJ and Oxford: Princeton University Press.
Gallant, M. and E. Maticka-Tyndale. 2004. 'School-based HIV prevention programmes for African youth', *Social Science and Medicine* 58: 1337–51.
Garner, R. C. 1998. 'Religion and economics in a South African township'. PhD thesis, University of Cambridge.
―――― 2000. 'Safe sects? Dynamic religion and AIDS in South Africa', *Journal of Modern African Studies* 38 (1): 41–69.
Gell, A. 1999. *The Art of Anthropology: essays and diagrams*. London and New Brunswick NJ: Athlone Press.
Geschiere, P. 1997. *The Modernity of Witchcraft: politics and the occult in post-colonial Africa*. Charlottesville VA: University of Virginia Press.
Gevisser, M. 2007. *Thabo Mbeki: the dream deferred*. Johannesburg: Jonathan Ball Publishers.
Giesekke, H. I. 2004. *The Berlin Mission in Venda*. Polokwane: H. I. Giesekke.
Gilbert, S. 2007. 'Singing against apartheid: ANC cultural groups and the international anti-apartheid struggle', *Journal of Southern African Studies* 33 (2): 423–41.
Gluckman, M. 1963. 'Gossip and scandal', *Current Anthropology* 4 (3): 307–16.
Gluckman, M., C. Mitchell, and J. A. Barnes. 1949. 'The village headman in British Central Africa', *Africa* 19 (2): 89–106.
Good, B. J. 1994. *Medicine, Rationality and Experience: an anthropological perspective*. Cambridge: Cambridge University Press.
Gottemoeller, M. 2000. 'Empowering women to prevent HIV: the microbicide advocacy agenda', *Agenda* 44: 32–7.
Green, E. C. 1994. *AIDS and STDs in Africa*. Boulder CO: Westview Press.
Guijt, I. and M. Shah. 1998. *The Myth of Community: gender issues in participatory development*. London: Intermediate Technology Publications.
Gumede, M. V. 1990. *Traditional Healers*. Johannesburg: Skotaville.
Gunner, L., with M. Gwala. 1991. *Musho! Zulu Popular Praises*. East Lansing MI: Michigan State University Press.
Halperin, D. T. and R. C. Bailey. 1999. 'Male circumcision and HIV infection: 10 years and counting', *Lancet* 354: 1813–15.
Hamm, C. 1987. Review of *In Township Tonight!*, *Popular Music* 6 (1): 353–5.
Hammond-Tooke, W. D. 1997. *Imperfect Interpreters: South Africa's anthropologists: 1920–1990*. Johannesburg: Witwatersrand University Press.
Harries, P. 2005. 'Consolidating democracy and building the nation: chiefs in South Africa', paper presented at conference in Neuchâtel, University of Basel, 14–16 April.
Heald, S. 1995. 'The power of sex: some reflections on the Caldwells' "African sexuality" thesis', *Africa* 65 (4): 489–505.

―――― 2006. 'Abstain or die: the development of HIV/AIDS policy in Botswana', *Journal of Biosocial Science* 38: 29–41.
Healthlink. 2007. 'What's culture got to do with HIV and AIDS?' Findings series, No. 7, <www.healthlink.org.uk> (accessed 25 February 2007).
Hebdige, D. 1979. *Subculture and the Meaning of Style*. London and New York NY: Methuen.
Hendry, J. and C. W. Watson (eds). 2001. *An Anthropology of Indirect Communication*. ASA Monographs 37. London: Routledge.
Herdt, G. 1987. 'AIDS and anthropology', *Anthropology Today* 3 (2): 1–3.
Herholdt, A. and R. J. Dombo. 1992. 'The political development of Venda: a study of a society in microcosm', *Journal for Contemporary History* 17 (1): 69–88.
Hobsbawm, E. and T. Ranger. 1983. *The Invention of Tradition*. Cambridge: Cambridge University Press.
Hope, R. 2003. 'Promoting behaviour change in Botswana: an assessment of the peer education HIV/AIDS prevention programme in the workplace', *Journal of Health and Communication* 8: 321–30.
Huges-d'Aeth, A. 2002. 'Evaluation of HIV/AIDS peer education projects in Zambia', *Evaluation and Programme Planning* 25 (4): 397–407.
Hunter, M. 2002. 'The materiality of everyday sex: thinking beyond prostitution', *African Studies* 61 (1): 99–120.
―――― 2005. 'Cultural politics and masculinities: multiple partners in historical perspective in Kwazulu-Natal' in G. Reid and L. Walker (eds), *Men Behaving Differently: South African men since 1994*. Cape Town: Double Storey.
IEC (Independent Electoral Commission). 2007. Report on the 2006 Municipal Elections, <http://www.elections.org.za/defaultPWLGEResults.asp> (accessed 2 February 2007).
Ingstad, B. 1990. 'The cultural construction of AIDS and its consequences for prevention in Botswana', *Medical Anthropology Quarterly* 4 (1): 28–40.
James, D. 1990. 'A question of ethnicity: Ndzundza Ndebele in a Lebowa village', *Journal of Southern African Studies* 16 (1): 33–54.
―――― 1997. '"Music of origin": class, social category and the performers and audience of "Kiba", a South African migrant genre', *Africa* 67 (3): 454–75.
―――― 1999. *Songs of the Women Migrants: performance and identity in South Africa*. Edinburgh: Edinburgh University Press for the International African Institute.
―――― 2001. 'Land for the landless: conflicting images of rural and urban in South Africa's land reform programme', *Journal of Contemporary African Studies* 19 (1): 93–109.
―――― 2002. '"To take the information down to the people": life skills and HIV/AIDS peer educators in the Durban area', *African Studies* 61 (1): 169–93.
―――― 2006. '"Black background": life history and migrant women's music in South Africa' in S. A. Reily (ed.), *The Musical Human: rethinking John Blacking's ethnomusicology in the twenty-first century*. Aldershot: Ashgate.
Jansen, J. M. 1992. *Ngoma: discourses of healing in Central and Southern Africa*. Berkeley CA: University of California Press.
Jeannerat, C. F. 1997. 'Invoking the female *vhusha* ceremony and the struggle for identity and security in Tshiendeulu, Venda', *Journal of Contemporary African Studies* 15 (1): 87–106.

Johnson, R. W. 2009. *South Africa's Brave New World: the beloved country since the end of apartheid*. London: Allen Lane.
Jones, S. 1993. *Assaulting Childhood: children's experiences of migrancy and hostel life in South Africa*. Johannesburg: Witwatersrand University Press.
Kaler, A. 2004. 'AIDS-talk in everyday life: the presence of HIV/AIDS in men's informal conversation in Southern Malawi', *Social Science and Medicine* 59: 285–97.
Kalipeni, E. 2000. 'Health and disease in Southern Africa: a comparative and vulnerability perspective', *Social Science and Medicine* 50 (2): 965–83.
Kalipeni, E., S. Craddock, J. Oppong, and J. Ghosh (eds). 2004. *HIV/AIDS in Africa: beyond epidemiology*. Oxford: Blackwell Publishers.
Kalipeni, E., J. Oppong, and A. Zerai. 2007. 'HIV/AIDS, gender, agency and empowerment issues in Africa', *Social Science and Medicine* 64 (5): 1015–18.
Keesing, R. and A. Strathern. 1998. *Cultural Anthropology: a contemporary perspective*. London: Harcourt Brace.
Kiernan, J. P. 1977. 'Poor and puritan: an attempt to view Zionism as a collective response to urban poverty', *African Studies* 36 (1): 31–43.
Kirkaldy, A. 2005. *Capturing the Soul: the Vhavenda and the missionaries, 1870–1900*. Pretoria: Protea House.
Koelble, T. A. and E. Lipuma. 2005. 'Traditional leaders and democracy: cultural politics in the age of globalisation' in S. Robins (ed.), *Limits to Liberation after Apartheid: citizenship, government and culture*. Oxford: James Currey.
Kopytoff, I. 1987. *The African Frontier: the reproduction of traditional African societies*. Bloomington, IN: Indiana University Press.
Kratz, C. A. 1993. '"We've always done it like this... except for a few details": "tradition" and "innovation" in Okiek ceremonies', *Comparative Studies in Society and History* 35 (1): 30–65.
Krige, E. and J. Krige. 1943. *The Realm of the Rain Queen: a study of the pattern of Lovedu society*. London: Oxford University Press.
Kruger, J. 1993. 'A Cultural Analysis of Venda Guitar Songs'. Unpublished PhD thesis, Rhodes University, South Africa.
—— 1999. '"Singing psalms with owls": a Venda twentieth-century musical history, Part 1: *Tshigombela*', *African Music* 7 (4): 122–46.
—— 1999/2000. '"Of wizards and madmen": Venda *Zwilombe* (Part 1)', *South African Journal of Musicology* 19/20: 15–29.
—— 2002. 'Playing in the land of God: musical performance and social resistance in South Africa', *British Journal of Ethnomusicology* 10 (2): 1–36.
—— 2006. '"Tracks of the Mouse": tonal reinterpretation in Venda guitar songs' in S. A. Reily (ed.), *The Musical Human: rethinking John Blacking's ethnomusicology in the twenty-first century*. Aldershot: Ashgate.
—— 2007. 'Singing psalms with owls: a Venda twentieth-century musical history, Part 2: *Tshikona*, beer songs, and personal songs', *African Music* 8 (1).
Kuper, A. 1970. 'Gluckman's village headman', *American Anthropologist* 72 (2): 355–8.
—— 1987. *South Africa and the Anthropologist*. London: Routledge and Kegan Paul.
Labour Force Survey. 2004. 'Statistics South Africa', <http://www.capegateway.gov.za/eng/publications/reports_research/L/88201> (accessed 3 February 2007).

La Fontaine, J. S. 1985. *Initiation*. London: Penguin.
Lahiff, E. 2000. *An Apartheid Oasis? Agriculture and rural livelihoods in Venda*. London: Frank Cass.
Lambek, M. 1993. *Knowledge and Practice in Mayotte: local discourses of Islam, sorcery and spirit possession*. Toronto: University of Toronto Press.
Lambert, H. and K. Wood. 2005. 'A comparative analysis of communication about sex, health and sexual health in India and South Africa: implications for HIV prevention', *Culture, Health and Sexuality* 7 (6): 527–41.
Lamptey, P. and H. Gayle. 2001. *HIV/AIDS Prevention and Care in Resource-Constrained Settings: a handbook for the design and management of programmes*. Arlington TX: Family Health International.
Lan, D. 1985. *Guns and Rain: guerrillas and spirit mediums in Zimbabwe*. London: James Currey.
Leclerc-Madlala, S. 2001. 'Virginity testing: managing sexuality in a maturing HIV/AIDS epidemic', *Medical Anthropology Quarterly* 15 (4): 533–52.
―――― 2002. 'On the virgin cleansing myth: gendered bodies, AIDS and ethnomedicine', *African Journal of AIDS Research* 1: 87–95.
―――― 2005. 'Popular responses to HIV/AIDS and policy', *Journal of Southern Africa Studies* 31 (4): 845–56.
Leonard, L., I. Ndiaye, A. Kapadia, G. Eisen, O. Diop, S. Mboup, and P. Kanki. 2000. 'HIV prevention among male clients of female sex workers in Kaolack, Senegal: results of a peer education programme', *AIDS Education and Prevention* 12: 21–37.
Le Roux, D. J. H. 1988. *Report of the Commission of Enquiry into the Causes of the Unrest in Venda during August 1988 and the Investigation of Ritual Murders*. Pretoria: Government Publisher.
Lestrade, G. P. 1930a. 'Some notes on the political organisation of the Venda tribes', *Africa* 3 (3): 306–21.
―――― 1930b. 'The *mala* system of the Venda tribes', *Bantu Studies* 4 (3): 193–204.
―――― 1932. 'Some notes on the ethnic history of the VhaVenda and their Rhodesian affinates' in N. J. van Warmelo (ed.), *Contributions Towards Venda History, Religion and Tribal Ritual*. Pretoria: Department of Native Affairs.
―――― 1949. *Some Venda Folk Tales*. Cape Town: Lovedale Press.
Leyton, R. 1997. *Introduction to Theory in Anthropology*. London: Cambridge University Press.
Liddell, C., L. Barrett, and M. Bydawell. 2005. 'Indigenous representations of illness and AIDS in sub-Saharan Africa', *Social Science and Medicine* 60: 691–700.
Lindegger, G. and J. Maxwell. 2005. 'A gender analysis of targeted AIDS interventions (TAI)'. Oxfam Australia Report, <http://www.oxfamireland.org/pdfs/longterm/johap_genderanalysis01.pdf> (accessed 20 February 2011).
Lindstrom, L. and G. M. White. 1993. 'Introduction: custom today', *Anthropological Forum* (Special Issue) 6 (4): 467–73.
Lodge, T. 2002. *Politics in South Africa: From Mandela to Mbeki*. Cape Town: David Philip.
Long, N. 1992. *Battlefields of Knowledge: the interlocking of theory and practice in social research and development*. London: Routledge.
―――― 2001. *Development Sociology: actor perspectives*. London: Routledge.

Lukhele, A. K. 1990. *Stokvels in South Africa: informal savings schemes by blacks for the black community*. Johannesburg: Amagi Books.

Luthuli, A. J. 1961. 'Nobel Peace Prize Address' in T. Karis and T. M. Gerhart (eds) (1977), *From Protest to Challenge, Volume Three: challenges and violence, 1953–1964*. Stanford: Hoover Institution Press.

Lwanda, J. 2003. 'The (in)visibility of HIV/AIDS in the Malawi public sphere', *African Journal of AIDS Research* 2 (2): 113–26.

MacDonald, D. S. 1996. 'Notes on the socio-economic and cultural factors influencing the transmission of HIV in Botswana', *Social Science and Medicine* 42 (9): 1325–33.

MacPhail, C. 2003. 'Challenging dominant norms of masculinity for HIV prevention', *African Journal of AIDS Research* 2 (2): 141–9.

MacPhail, C. and C. Campbell. 1999. 'Evaluating HIV/STD interventions in developing countries: do current indicators do justice to advances in intervention processes?', *South African Journal of Psychology* 29 (4): 149–65.

Makhulu, A. M. 2004. 'Poetic justice: Xhosa idioms and moral breach in post-aparthied South Africa' in B. Weiss (ed.), *Producing Africa Futures: ritual and reproduction in a neoliberal age*. Leiden: Brill.

Mamdani, M. 1996. *Citizen and Subject: contemporary Africa and the legacy of late colonialism*. London: James Currey.

Mare, G. and G. Hamilton. 1987. *An Appetite for Power: Buthelezi's Inkatha and the politics of 'loyal resistance'*. Johannesburg: Ravan Press.

Marks, S. 1975. 'Southern Africa and Madagascar' in R. Gray (ed.), *The Cambridge History of Africa, Volume 4*. Cambridge: Cambridge University Press.

Masanjala, W. 2007. 'The poverty-HIV/AIDS nexus in Africa: a livelihood approach', *Social Science and Medicine* 64 (5): 1932–41.

Mathews, C., K. Everett, J. Binedell, and M. Steinberg. 1995. 'Learning to listen: formative research in the development of AIDS education for secondary school students', *Social Science and Medicine* 41 (12): 1715–24.

Mavhungu, M. F. 1998. 'A changing view of death in a Venda village'. BA dissertation, Department of Anthropology, University of Venda for Science and Technology.

May, J., I. Woolard, and S. Klassen. 2000. 'The nature and measure of poverty and inequality' in J. May (ed.), *Poverty and Inequality in South Africa: meeting the challenge*. London: Zed Books.

Mayer, P. and I. Mayer. 1961. *Townsmen or Tribesmen*. Cape Town: Oxford University Press.

Mayekiso, M. 1996. *Township Politics: civic struggles for a new South Africa*. New York NY: Monthly Review Press.

Mbali, M. 2004. 'AIDS discourses and the South African state: government denialism and post-apartheid policy-making', *Transformation* 54: 104–22.

Mbeki, T. 1999. Speech at the launch of the African Renaissance Institute, <http://www.anc.org.za/ancdocs/history/mbeki/1999/tm1011.html>.

───── 2002. *Africa, Define Yourself*. Tafelberg: Mafube.

───── 2003. 'Important role for traditional leaders in development and nation building', *ANC Today* 3 (28), <http://www.anc.org.za/ancdocs/anctoday/2003/at28.htm> (accessed 14 December 2005).

Mbembe, A. 1992. 'Provisional notes on the postcolony', *Africa* 62 (1): 3–37.

McDonald, C. and E. Schatz. 2006. 'Coexisting discourses: how older women in South Africa make sense of the HIV/AIDS epidemic'. Working Paper, Institute of Behavioral Science, University of Boulder, Colorado.

McGrane, B. 1989. *Beyond Anthropology: society and the other*. New York NY: Columbia University Press.

McGregor, L. 2005. *Khabzela: the life and times of a South African*. Johannesburg: Jakana.

McNamara, J. K. 1980. 'Brothers and work mates: home friend networks in the social life of black migrant workers in a gold mine hostel' in P. Mayer (ed), *Black Villagers in an Industrial Society: anthropological perspectives on labour migration in South Africa*. Cape Town: Oxford University Press.

McNeill, F. G. 2008. '"We sing about what we cannot talk about": music as anthropological evidence in Venda, South Africa' in L. Chua, C. High, and T. Lau (eds), *How Do We Know? Evidence, ethnography and the making of anthropological knowledge*. Newcastle: Cambridge Scholars Publishing.

―――― 2009. '"Condoms cause AIDS": poison, prevention and denial in South Africa', *African Affairs* 108 (432): 353–70.

McNeill, F. G. and D. A. James. 2009. 'Singing songs of AIDS in Venda, South Africa: performance, pollution and ethnomusicology in a neo-liberal setting', *South African Music Studies* 28: 1–30.

McNeill, F. G. and I. Niehaus. 2010. *Magic!* (Aids Review 2009). Pretoria: Centre for the Study of AIDS, University of Pretoria, <http://www.csa.za.org/filemanager/fileview/157/>.

Mda, Z. 1995. *Ways of Dying*. New York NY: Picador.

Meintjes, L. 2003. *Sound of Africa! Making Music Zulu in a South African Studio*. Durham NC: Duke University Press.

―――― 2004. '"Shoot the sergeant, shatter the mountain": the production of masculinity in Zulu *ngoma* song and dance in post-apartheid South Africa', *Ethnomusicology Forum* 13 (2): 173–201.

Meyer, B. and P. Geschiere. 1999. 'Introduction' in B. Meyer and P. Geschiere (eds), *Globalization and Identity: dialectics of flow and closure*. Oxford: Blackwell.

Mills, G. 2000. *The Wired Model: South Africa, foreign policy and globalisation*. Cape Town: Tafelberg.

Moodie, T. D. 1994. *Going For Gold: men, mines and migration*. Berkeley CA: University of California Press.

Mookherjee, N. 2006. '"Remembering to forget": public secrecy and memory of sexual violence in the Bangladesh war of 1971', *Journal of the Royal Anthropological Institute* (N.S.) 12: 433–50.

Moore, H. L. and T. Sanders. 2001. 'Magical interpretations and material realities: an introduction' in H. L. Moore and T. Sanders (eds), *Magical Interpretations and Material Realities: modernity, witchcraft and the occult in postcolonial Africa*. London: Routledge.

Mosse, D. 2004. *Cultivating Development: an ethnography of aid policy and practice*. London: Pluto Press.

Msimang, S. 2000. 'African renaissance: where are the women?' *Agenda* 44: 67–84.

Mufamadi, S. 2004a. 'Announcement of Commission of Traditional Leadership Disputes and Claims', South African Ministry of Provincial and Local Government, <http://www.polity.org.za/pol/58365> (accessed 2 January 2006).

_____ 2004b. 'Press statement on the Ralushai Commission Report', South African Ministry for Provincial and Local Government.

_____ 2004c. 'Press statement on the occasion of the announcement of a Commission on Traditional Leadership Disputes and Claims', South African Ministry for Provincial and Local Government.

Muller, C. A. 1999. *Rituals of Fertility and the Sacrifice of Desire: Nazarite women's performance in South Africa*. Chicago IL: University of Chicago Press.

Murray, C. and P. Sanders. 2005. *Medicine Murder in Colonial Lesotho: the anatomy of a moral crisis*. Edinburgh: Edinburgh University Press for the International African Institute.

Myburgh, J. 2009. 'In the beginning there was Virodene' in K. Cullinan and A. Thom (eds), *The Virus, Vitamins and Vegetables: the South African HIV/AIDS mystery*. Johannesburg: Jacana.

Nattrass, N. 2004. *The Moral Economy of AIDS in South Africa*. London: Cambridge University Press.

_____ 2007. 'Disability and welfare in South Africa's era of unemployment and AIDS' in S. Buhlungu, J. Daniel, R. Southall, and J. Lutchman (eds), *State of the Nation: South Africa 2007*. Cape Town: Human Sciences Research Council Press.

_____ 2008. 'AIDS and the scientific governance of medicine in post-apartheid South Africa', *African Affairs* 107 (427): 157–76.

Naude, P. 1995. *The Zionist Christian Church in South Africa: a case study in oral theology*. Lewiston NY: Edwin Mellen Press.

Nemudzivhadi, M. 1985. *When and What: an introduction to the evolution of the history of Venda*. Thohoyandou: Office of the President.

Nettleton, A. 1992. 'Ethnic and gender identities in Venda *domba* statues', *African Studies* 51 (2): 203–30.

Ngugi, E. and D. Wilson. 1996. 'Focussed peer-mediated educational programmes among female sex workers to reduce STDs and HIV transmission in Kenya and Zimbabwe', *Journal of Infectious Diseases* 174 (Supplement 2): S240–7.

Ngwane, Z. 2004. '"Real men awaken their fathers' homesteads, the educated leave them in ruins": the politics of domestic reproduction in post-apartheid rural South Africa' in B. Weiss (ed.), *Producing African Futures: ritual and reproduction in a neoliberal age*. Leiden: Brill.

Niehaus, I. 2000. 'Towards a dubious liberation: masculinity, sexuality and power in South African lowveld schools, 1953–1999', *Journal of Southern African Studies* 26 (3): 387–407.

_____ 2001a. *Witchcraft, Power and Politics: exploring the occult in the South African lowveld*. London: Pluto Press.

_____ 2001b. 'Witchcraft in the new South Africa: from colonial superstition to postcolonial reality?' in L. H. Moore and T. Sanders (eds), *Magical Interpretations, Material Realities: modernity, witchcraft and the occult in postcolonial Africa*. London: Routledge.

_____ 2002. 'Renegotiating masculinity in the South African lowveld: narratives of male–male sex in labour compounds and in prisons', *African Studies* 61 (1): 77–99.

_____ 2007. '"Leprosy of a deadlier kind": interpretations of AIDS in the South African lowveld', paper presented at the London School of Economics Africa Series Seminar, 20 February 2005.

Niehaus, I. and G. Jonnson. 2005. 'Dr Wouter Basson, Americans and wild beasts: men's conspiracy theories of AIDS in the South African lowveld', *Medical Anthropology* 24 (2): 179–208.
Nii-Amoo, D. F., E. M. Zulu, and A. C. Ezeh. 2007. 'Urban–rural differences in the socioeconomic deprivation–sexual behaviour link in Kenya', *Social Science and Medicine* 64 (5): 1019–31.
Norman, A., M. Chopra, and S. Kadiyaki. 2005. 'HIV disclosure in South Africa: enabling the gateway to effective response', unpublished seminar paper, International Food Policy Research Institute.
Nowlin, B. 1996. *Liner notes for Radio Freedom: voice of the African National Congress and the People's Army, Umkhonto We Sizwe*. CD, Rounder Records.
O'Manique, C. 2004. *Neoliberalism and AIDS Crisis in Sub-Saharan Africa: globalization's pandemic*. Basingstoke: Palgrave Macmillan.
Oomen, B. 2000. *Tradition on the Move: chiefs, democracy and change in rural South Africa*. Leiden: Netherlands Institute for Southern Africa.
───── 2005. *Chiefs in South Africa: law, power and culture in the post-apartheid era*. Oxford: James Currey.
Oppong J. 1998. 'A vulnerability interpretation of the geography of HIV/AIDS in Ghana, 1986–1995', *The Professional Geographer* 50 (4): 437–48.
Packard, R. M. and P. Epstein. 1991. 'Epidemiologists, social scientists, and the structure of medical research on AIDS in Africa', *Social Science and Medicine* 33 (7): 771–83.
Paine, R. 1967. 'What is gossip all about? An alternative hypothesis', *Man*, n.s. 2 (2): 278–85.
Parfitt, T. 2002. *The Lost Tribes of Israel: the history of a myth*. London: Weidenfeld and Nicholson.
Parker, R. 1996. 'Empowerment, community mobilisation and social change in the face of HIV/AIDS', *AIDS* 10 (Supplement 3): S27–31.
Parker, R. and P. Aggleton. 2003. 'HIV- and AIDS-related stigma and discrimination: a conceptual framework for implications and action', *Social Science and Medicine* 57 (1): 13–24.
Philips, H. 2004. 'AIDS in the context of South Africa's epidemic history' in K. D. Kauffman and D. L. Lindauer (eds), *AIDS and South Africa: the social expression of a pandemic*. Basingstoke: Palgrave Macmillan.
Pisani, E. 2008. *The Wisdom of Whores: bureaucrats, brothels and the business of AIDS*. London: Granta.
Posel, D. 2005. 'Sex, death and the fate of the nation: reflections on the politicization of sexuality in post-apartheid South Africa', *Africa* 75 (2): 125–53.
Preston-Whyte, E. M. 2003. 'Contexts of vulnerability: sex, secrecy and HIV/AIDS', *African Journal of AIDS Research* 2 (2): 89–94.
Quinlan, T. and S. Willan. 2005. 'HIV/AIDS: finding ways to contain the pandemic' in J. Daniel, R. Southall, and J. Lutchman (eds), *State of the Nation: South Africa 2004–2005*. Cape Town: Human Sciences Research Council Press.
Ralushai, V. N. M. V. 1977. 'Conflicting Accounts of Venda History with Particular Reference to the Role of Mutupo in Social Organization'. PhD thesis, Queens University, Belfast.

Ralushai, V. N. M. V., M. G. Masingi, D. M. M. Madiba, et al. 1996. 'Report of the Commission of Enquiry into Witchcraft Violence and Ritual Murders in the Northern Province of South Africa'. Submitted to the Executive Council for Safety and Security, Northern Province.

Raman, R. 2005. 'Integrated prevention and care: including men in care'. Report, Oxfam Australia.

Rambau, V. J. 1999. 'The role of woman in the formation and operation of women's burial societies'. MA dissertation, Department of Anthropology, University of Venda for Science and Technology.

Ramushwana, M. G. 1992. 'The future of the armed forces of Transkei, Bophuthatswana, Venda and Ciskei: expectations and prospects', *Strategic Review for Southern Africa* 14 (1): 12–21.

Ranger, T. 1983. 'The invention of tradition in colonial Africa' in E. Hobsbawm and T. Ranger (eds), *The Invention of Tradition*. Cambridge: Cambridge University Press.

―――― 1993. 'The invention of tradition revisited: the case of colonial Africa' in T. Ranger and O. Vaughan (eds), *Legitimacy and the State in Twentieth-Century Africa*. London: Macmillan.

Rasing, T. 1995. *Passing on the Rites of Passage: girls' initiation rites in the context of an urban Roman Catholic community on the Zambian Copperbelt*. Avebury: African Studies Research Centre.

Reid, G. and L. Walker. 2003. 'Secrecy, stigma and HIV/AIDS: an introduction', *African Journal for AIDS Research* 2 (2): 85–8.

Reily, S. A. 1998. 'The ethnographic enterprise: Venda girls' initiation schools revisited', *British Journal of Ethnomusicology* 7: 45–68.

―――― (ed.). 2006. *The Musical Human: rethinking John Blacking's ethnomusicology in the twenty-first century*. London: Ashgate.

Rezacova, V. 'The case of the Malombo possession cult in Venda, South Africa', paper presented at the LSE Africa Seminar Series, 12 March 2007.

Richards, A. 1956. *Chisungu: a girl's initiation ceremony among the Bemba of Zambia*. London: Faber and Faber.

Robbins, J. 2001. 'Secrecy and the sense of an ending: narrative, time and everyday millennialism in Papua New Guinea and in Christian fundamentalism', *Comparative Studies in Society and History* 43: 525–51.

Robins, S. 2001. 'Whose "culture", whose "survival"? The Komani San land claim and the cultural politics of "community" and "development" in the Kalahari', *Journal of Southern African Studies* 27 (4): 833–53.

―――― 2004. '"Long live, Zakie, long live!": AIDS activism, science and citizenship after apartheid', *Journal of Southern African Studies* 30 (3): 651–72.

Rodlach, A. 2006. *Witches, Westerners and HIV: AIDS and cultures of blame in Africa*. Walnut Creek CA: Left Coast Press.

Root-Bernstein, R. 1993. *Rethinking AIDS: the tragic cost of premature consensus*. New York NY: The Free Press.

Sachs, E. S. and D. J. Sachs. 2004. 'Too poor to stay alive' in K. D. Kauffman and D. L. Lindauer (eds), *AIDS and South Africa: the social expression of a pandemic*. Basingstoke: Palgrave Macmillan.

Schapera, I. 1938. *A Handbook of Tswana Law and Custom*. London: Oxford University Press for the International Institute of African Languages and Cultures.

Schneider, H. 2002. 'On the fault line: the politics of AIDS policy in contemporary South Africa', *African Studies* 61 (1): 145–69.

Schneider, H. and J. Stein. 2001. 'Implementing AIDS policy in post-apartheid South Africa', *Social Science and Medicine* 52: 122–31.

Schutz, A. 1964. '"The well-informed citizen": an essay on the social distribution of knowledge' in A. Brodersen (ed.), *Alfred Schutz, Collected Papers, Volume 2, Studies in Social Theory*. The Hague: Martinus Nijhoff.

Scorgie, F. 2002. 'Virginity testing and the politics of sexual responsibility: implications for AIDS intervention', *African Studies* 61 (1): 55–77.

―――― 2003. 'Mobilising "Tradition" in the Post-Apartheid Era: *amasiko*, AIDS and cultural rights in KwaZulu-Natal'. PhD thesis, University of Cambridge.

Seekings, J. and N. Nattrass. 2005. *Class, Race and Inequality in South Africa*. New Haven CT: Yale University Press.

Sikwebele, A., C. Shonga, and C. Baylies. 2000. 'AIDS in Kapulanga, Mongu: poverty, neglect and gendered patterns of blame' in C. Baylies and J. Bujra (eds), *AIDS, Sexuality and Gender in Africa: collective strategies and struggles in Tanzania and Zambia*. London. Routledge.

Simmel, G. 1950. *The Sociology of Georg Simmel*. Translated by H. Wullf Kurt. New York NY: The Free Press.

Simpson, B. 2002. 'Comments', *Current Anthropology* 43 (1): 14–15.

Simpson, T. 2005. 'Sons and fathers/boys to men in the time of AIDS: learning masculinity in Zambia', *Journal of Southern African Studies* 31 (3): 569–86.

―――― 2007. 'Learning sex and gender in Zambia: masculinities and HIV/AIDS risk', *Sexualities* 10 (2): 171–86.

Sloth-Nielsen, J. 2007. 'The state of South Africa's prisons' in S. Buhlungu, J. Daniel, R. Southall, and J. Lutchman (eds), *State of the Nation: South Africa 2007*. Cape Town: Human Sciences Research Council Press.

Soler-Viñolo, M., P. Soler, M. D. Carretero, C. Martín, M. Soler-Arrebola, and J. P. A-Nacle. 1998. 'Coping strategies and psychological morbidity in asymptomatic, symptomatic and AIDS patients', *European Psychiatry* 13: 1004.

Sontag, S. 1990. *Illness as Metaphor and AIDS and Its Metaphors*. New York NY: Picador.

South African Government. 2000. 'HIV/AIDS/STI Strategic Plan for South Africa 2000–2005'. Pretoria: Government Printers, <http://www.info.gov.za/otherdocs/2000/aidsplan2000.pdf> (accessed 1 February 2007).

―――― 2005. *Government Gazette* (Regulation Gazette) Volume 476, Number 8152 (11 February 2005). Pretoria.

―――― 2006. 'National HIV and syphilis antenatal sero-prevalence survey in South Africa, 2005'. Pretoria: Department of Health.

―――― 2007. 'HIV/AIDS/STI Strategic Plan for South Africa', <http://www.doh.gov.za/docs/misc/stratplan-f.html> (accessed 3 March 2009).

―――― 2008a. 'Determination on amaZulu paramountcy'. Mimeo, <http://www.thedplg.gov.za/index.php?option=com_content&task=view&id=472&Itemid=30> (accessed 2 February 2009).

―――― 2008b. 'Determination on amaXhosa paramountcy'. Mimeo, <http://www.thedplg.gov.za/index.php?option=com_content&task=view&id=472&Itemid=30> (accessed 2 February 2009).

―――― 2008c. 'Progress report on declaration of commitment on HIV and AIDS' (Department of Health), <http://data.unaids.org/pub/Report/2008/south_africa_2008_country_progress_report_en.pdf> (accessed 9 April 2009).

―――― 2010. 'Determinations of the positions of paramount chiefs'. Mimeo, <http://www.pmg.org.za/files/docs/100729determination-chiefs.pdf> (accessed 17 November 2010).

South African Institute for Race Relations. 1980. *Survey of Race Relations in South Africa. 1979*. Johannesburg: SAIRR.

Southall, R. 2005. 'Black empowerment and present limits to a more democratic capitalism in South Africa' in S. Buhlungu, J. Daniel, R. Southall, and J. Lutchman (eds), *State of the Nation: South Africa 2005–6*. Cape Town: Human Sciences Research Council Press.

―――― 2007. 'The ANC state: more dysfunctional than developmental?' in S. Buhlungu, J. Daniel, R. Southall, and J. Lutchman (eds), *State of the Nation: South Africa 2007*. Cape Town: Human Sciences Research Council Press.

Spiegel, A. D. 2005. 'Refracting an elusive South African urban citizenship: problems with tracking *Spaza*' in S. Robins (ed.), *Limits to Liberation after Apartheid: citizenship, government and culture*. Oxford: James Currey.

Spiegel, A. D. and E. Boonzaier. 1988. 'Promoting tradition: images of the South African past' in E. Boonzaier and J. Sharp (eds), *South African Keywords: the uses and abuses of political concepts*. Cape Town: David Philip.

Stadler, J. J. 2003. 'The young, the rich, and the beautiful: secrecy, suspicion and discourses of AIDS in the South African lowveld', *African Journal for AIDS Research* 2 (2): 127–39.

Statistics South Africa. 2001.<http://mapserver2.statssa.gov.za/profiles2006/index.aspx> (accessed 9 February 2009).

―――― 2003. *Census 2001: Census in Brief*. Pretoria: SSA, <http://www.statssa.gov.za/census01/html/CInBrief/CIB2001.pdf> (accessed 2 February 2007).

Stayt, H. 1931. *The Bavenda*. London: Oxford University Press for the International Institute of African Languages and Cultures.

Stein, J. 2003. 'HIV/AIDS stigma: the latest dirty secret', *African Journal for AIDS Research* 2 (2): 95–101.

Stewart, P. J. and A. Strathern. 2004. *Witchcraft, Sorcery, Rumours and Gossip*. Cambridge: Cambridge University Press.

Tambiah, S. 1990. *Magic, Science, Religion and the Scope of Rationality*. Cambridge: Cambridge University Press.

Tawfik, L. and C. Watkins. 2007. 'Sex in Geneva, sex in Lilongwe, and sex in Balaka', *Social Science and Medicine* 64 (5): 1090–101.

Thompson, L. 1985. *The Political Mythology of Apartheid*. London: Vail-Ballou.

Thornton, R. 2008. *Unimagined Communities*. Berkeley CA: University of California Press.

Tonkinson, R. 1997. 'Anthropology and aboriginal tradition: the Hindmarsh Island Bridge affair and the politics of interpretation', *Oceania* 68 (1): 1–26.

Turner, G. and G. Shepherd. 1999. 'A method in search of a theory: peer education and health promotion', *Health Education Research* 14 (2): 235–47.

Turner, V. 1957. *Schism and Continuity in an African Society: a study of Ndembu village life*. Manchester: Manchester University Press.
———— 1967. *The Forest of Symbols*. Ithaca NY: Cornell University Press.
———— 1969a. *The Ritual Process: structure and anti-structure*. Chicago IL: Aldine Pubishing Company.
———— 1969b. 'Mukanda: the politics of a non-political ritual' in M. Swartz (ed.), *Local Level Politics*. London: University of London Press.
———— 1982. *From Ritual to Theatre: the human seriousness of play*. New York NY: PAJ Publications.
Ulin, P. 1992. 'African Women and AIDS: negotiating behavioural change', *Social Science and Medicine* 34 (1): 63–73.
UNAIDS. 2004. 'Report on the Global AIDS Epidemic'. Geneva: UNAIDS Information Centre, p. 14.
———— 2007. 'South Africa Country Profile', <http://www.unaids.org/en/Regions_Countries/Countries/south_africa.asp> (accessed 2 February 2007).
US Government. 2006. *International Religious Freedom Report*. Released by the Bureau of Democracy, Human Rights, and Labour, <http://www.state.gov/g/drl/rls/irf/2006/71325.htm> (accessed 3 March 2007).
Vail, L. 1989. *The Creation of Tribalism in Southern Africa*. Berkeley CA: University of California Press.
Vail, L. and L. White. 1983. 'Forms of resistance: songs and perceptions of power in colonial Mozambique', *American Historical Review* 88 (4): 883–919.
———— 1990. *Power and the Praise Poem*. Charlottesville VA: University of Virginia Press.
Vail, P. and S. Maseko. 'Thabo Mbeki, South Africa and the idea of an African renaissance' in S. Jacobs and R. Calland (eds.), *Thabo Mbeki's World: the politics and ideology of the South African President*. London: Zed Books.
van Dijk, R., R. Reis, and M. Spierenburg (eds). 2000. *The Quest for Fruition through Ngoma: political aspects of healing in Southern Africa*. Oxford: James Currey.
van der Vliet, V. 2004. 'South Africa divided against AIDS: a crisis of leadership' in K. D. Kauffman and D. L. Lindauer (eds), *AIDS and South Africa: the social expression of a pandemic*. Basingstoke: Palgrave Macmillan.
van Warmelo, N. J. 1932. *Contributions towards Venda History, Religion and Tribal Ritual*. Pretoria: Department of Native Affairs, Ethnological Publications, Volume 23.
———— 1948a. *Betrothal, Thaka, Wedding*. Pretoria: Department of Native Affairs, Ethnological Publications, Volume 23.
———— 1948b. *Venda Law, Part 2: Married Life*. Pretoria: Department of Native Affairs, Ethnological Publications, Volume 23.
———— 1948c. *Venda Law Part 3: Divorce*. Pretoria: Department of Native Affairs, Ethnological Publications, Volume 23.
———— 1949. *Venda Law Part 4: Inheritance*. Pretoria: Department of Native Affairs, Ethnological Publications, Volume 23.
———— 1967. *Venda Law Part 5: Property*. Pretoria: Department of Native Affairs, Ethnological Publications, Volume 50.
———— 1989. *Venda Dictionary, Tshivenda–English*. Pretoria: J. L van Schaik.

Walker, L., G. Reid, and M. Cornell. 2004. *Waiting to Happen: HIV/AIDS in South Africa*. Cape Town: Double Storey Books.

Walton, D., P. Farmer, W. Lambert, F. Leandre, S. Koenig, and J. Mukherjee. 2004. 'Integrated HIV prevention and care strengthens primary health care: lessons from rural Haiti', *Journal of Public Health Policy* 25 (2): 137–58.

Waterman, C. 1990: *Juju: a social history and ethnography of an African popular music*. Chicago IL: University of Chicago Press.

Waterston, A. 1997. 'Anthropological research and the politics of HIV prevention: towards a critique of policy and priorities in the age of AIDS', *Social Science and Medicine* 44 (9): 1381–91.

Watney, S. 1989. *Policing Desire: pornography, AIDS and the media*. London: Cassell.

Wessmann, R. 1908. *The Bawenda of the Spelonken: a contribution towards the psychology and folk-lore of African peoples*. London: The African World.

West, H. G. 2003. 'Voices twice silenced: betrayal and mourning at colonialism's end in Mozambique', *Anthropological Theory* 3 (1): 343–65.

West, H. G. and T. Luedke (eds). 2005. *Borders and Healers: brokering therapeutic resources in southeast Africa*. Bloomington, IN: Indiana University Press.

White, H. 2004. 'Ritual haunts: the timing of estrangement in a post-apartheid countryside' in B. Weiss (ed.), *Producing African Futures: ritual and reproduction in a neoliberal age*. Leiden: Brill.

White, Landeg. 1989. *Magomero: portrait of an African village*. Cambridge: Cambridge University Press.

White, Louise. 2000. *Speaking with Vampires: rumour and history in colonial Africa*. Berkeley CA: University of California Press.

Whiteside, A. and C. Sunter. 2000. *AIDS: the challenge for South Africa*. Cape Town: Human and Rousseau.

Wilson, D. 2000. 'Peer group education guidelines, volume 1'. Unpublished document, Department of Psychology, University of Zimbabwe.

Wilson, M. 1969. 'The Sotho, Venda and Tsonga' in M. Wilson and L. Thompson (eds.), *The Oxford History of South Africa, Volume 1*. Oxford: Oxford University Press.

Wojcicki, J. M. 2002. '"She drank his money": survival sex and the problem of violence in taverns in Gauteng Province, South Africa', *Medical Anthropology Quarterly* 16 (3): 267–93.

Wolf, R. C., L. A. Tawfik, and K. C. Bond. 2000. 'Peer promotion programmes and social networks in Ghana: methods for monitoring and evaluating AIDS prevention and reproductive health programmes among adolescents and young adults', *Journal of Health Communication* 5 (supplement): 61–80.

Wolpe, H. 1972. 'Capitalism and cheap labour-power in South Africa: from segregation to apartheid', *Economy and Society* 1 (4): 425–56.

Wood, K., J. Maepa, F. Maforah, and R. Jewkes. 1998. '"He forced me to love him": putting violence on adolescent sexual health agendas', *Social Science and Medicine* 47 (2): 233–43.

Wulff, W. 2006. 'Experiencing the ballet body: pleasure, pain, power' in S. A. Reily (ed.), *Rethinking John Blacking's Ethnomusicology in the Twenty-First Century*. Aldershot: Ashgate.

Yamba, C. B. 1997. 'Cosmologies in turmoil: witch finding and AIDS in Chiawa, Zambia', *Africa* 67 (2): 200–21.

Yeboah, I. E. A. 2007. 'HIV/AIDS and the construction of sub-Saharan Africa: heuristic lessons from the social sciences for policy', *Social Science and Medicine* 64 (5): 1128–50.

Young, C. (ed.) 1999. *The Accommodation of Cultural Diversity: case studies*. Basingstoke: Macmillan.

Index

abortion, as 'pollution', 190–1, 192, 196–7
African Independent Churches (AICs)
   and initiation ceremonies, 90
   and peer educators, 143–6
African National Congress (ANC)
   and African renaissance, 30, 33–4
   AIDS policy, 17
   struggle songs, 164–69
   Venda support, 13, 53–4, 55–6, 60
African renaissance
   and traditional knowledge, 198–200
   and traditional politics, 29–31, 33–4, 68–9
African Union (AU), 30, 129
Agric Rural Development Corporation (ARDC), 69
Agriven (Venda Agricultural Corporation Ltd), 52
AIDS *See* HIV/AIDS
AIDS, AIDS, AIDS, 191, 250
Amandla Cultural Ensemble, 139, 164
amaXhosa, paramountcy, 40
Amnesty International, 55
apartheid period
   resistance, 55–9
   struggle songs, 164–70, 177
   traditional leadership, 29, 47–55
AZT, 119

Bantu Authorities Act (1951), 48
Bantu Homelands Development Corporations Act (1965), 51
Bantustan system, 47–55
Bapedi ba Maroteng, paramountcy, 40
Barth, F., 193–5, 238
Barz, G., 199
beer halls, for peer education, 133–4, 137, 140–1
bepha musical expeditions, 6, 76
Biko, Steve, 30
biomedical knowledge
   and AIDS, 7, 17–18, 192, 197
   and initiation ceremonies, 97–8, 106–8
   and traditional knowledge, 74–5, 107–11, 235–41

Black Administration Act (1927), 32, 38, 47
black economic empowerment (BEE), 14
Blacking, John, 4, 5–6, 21, 43, 76, 85, 90, 158–9, 200
Bushbuckridge, 206, 208–9, 228

chieftaincy
   and initiation ceremonies, 5, 77–80. *See also Khosikhulu*; kingship; Nhlapo Commission
Christianity
   and initiation ceremonies, 89–91
   and peer educators, 142–6
circumcision. *See* male circumcision
Ciskei, paramountcy, 40
colours, symbolic, 101–2
Comaroff, J. 90–1
Commission on Disputes and Claims. *See* Nhlapo Commission
commoners, distinction from royalty, 5, 42, 44–5, 91–2
Comprehensive National HIV/AIDS and STI Strategic Plan for 2000–2005, 119
condoms
   attitudes to, 107
   as cause of AIDS, 204, 227, 231
   distribution of, 138
   use of, 201–2
Congress of the People (COPE), 13, 167
Congress of South African Trade Unions (COSATU), 120
contraception, as 'pollution', 188–90, 192
CONTRALESA (Council of Traditional Leaders in South Africa), 34, 63
Coplan, D., 157
crisis of social reproduction. *See* social reproduction

death
   attitudes to, 207–9, 230–1
   from poisoning, 211–22
democracy, and traditional leadership, 31–41

Index

development projects
  apartheid period, 50–3
  participatory approach, 129–32
  post-apartheid, 69–71
Dimbanyika, 32, 44–5
Ditike arts and crafts centre, 52
domba initiation ceremony, 1, 4, 5, 11, 70, 77–80
Dopeni, initiation ceremonies, 74, 85–101, 237, 263
Dopeni project, 80–4
Dube, Lucky, 13
Dzata, 44, 45, 54

economy, impact of AIDS, 16
employment, peer educators, 150–2
Erlmann, V., 158
ethnomusicology, medical, 201–2
Evangelical Lutheran Church of South Africa (ELCSA), 125
experience, and knowledge, 105–11, 192–7, 229–30, 237–40

Fabian, J., 157
Farisani, Simon, 13
Farmer, Paul, 206–7
farming, 9–10
Fobbe, Traugatt, 22, 80–1, 85–6
folk cosmology, HIV/AIDS, 180–202
Forum for AIDS Prevention (FAP), 3, 20, 123–6
  home-based care (HBC), 148–9, 153, 178, 225–7
  peer education, 132–41
  songs, 163–4, 178
  voluntary counselling and testing (VCT), 147, 178
  volunteers, 146–7
funerals, 16

Garvey, Marcus, 30
girls
  vhusha initiation, 87–111. *See also* women
gossip, 220–1
Growth, Employment, and Redistribution Strategy (GEAR), 14, 35, 117, 235

Ha-Matsa, peer education project, 132
Ha-Rabali, peer education project, 114, 132, 162, 175
Haiti, witchcraft and AIDS, 206–7
HIV/AIDS
  anthropological research, 19–20
  antiretroviral treatments, 119, 120, 121–3, 162
  deaths from, 207–9, 230–1, 232
  education, 3–4, 19, 74–5, 109–10
  folk cosmology, 180–202
  government policies, 116–23, 162–3
  and initiation ceremonies, 97–8, 106–11, 112–13, 235–6
  knowledge transfer, 193–8
  NGOs, 123–6
  peer educators as vectors of, 3, 204, 223–5, 231
  perception of, 15–19
  planned interventions, 126–9
  prevention of mother-to-child transmission (PMTCT), 147, 162
  silence about, 203–9, 222–31
  stigma, 207–8
  traditional knowledge, 7, 17–19, 74–5, 198–9
  traditional treatments, 111, 116–17
  women as causes of, 18–19, 180, 185, 188–91, 196–7. *See also* peer educators
hogo song, 4
home-based care (HBC), peer educators, 148–9, 153, 178, 225–7

indigenous knowledge systems (IKS), 128, 180–1
initiation ceremonies
  and AIDS education, 74–5, 97–8, 106–7
  female, 4, 11
  and knowledge transfer, 192–5, 198–9
  music, 4–7, 154
  songs, 172–6
  and traditional authority, 5, 77–80. *See also domba* initiation ceremony; *vhusha* initiation ceremony
intergenerational relations, 75, 108–9
internet generation, 10
inyanga (traditional healer), 189n7, 190–1, 211

James, D., 119, 124, 141, 151

KAP (Knowledge, Attitudes and Practice), 126–7
Khosi (chief), position of, 26n1, 37
Khosikhulu (paramount king)
  abolition of, 54–5
  battle for, 64–5
  claims, 38–41
  salary, 38
kingship, Venda, 26–73
knowledge transfer
  AIDS interventions, 126–9
  and experience, 192–7, 229–30, 237–40. *See also* biomedical knowledge; traditional knowledge

Index

KwaZulu-Natal, AIDS, 27, 28, 111

labour supply, impact of AIDS, 16
Lambek, M., 193–5, 238
Lawyers for Human Rights (LHR), 125
leadership, traditional. *See* traditional leadership
Lemba, ancestry, 5
Lemke, Harold, 123, 125, 212–13
Limpopo Province
  as 'Africa's Eden', 7–8, 27, 42–3
  paramountcy, 40–1
Love Life, 131
ludodo performance, 94–8, 105–9, 236
Lutheran Church
  and initiation ceremonies, 89–90
  peer educators, 142, 144, 159–60
Luthuli, Albert, 165
Luthuli Award ceremony, 31–2, 45, 59, 65, 68

mabepha, *see* bepha
Madzivhandila, Mmbangiseni, 184
maine (traditional healers), 189n7
male circumcision
  as AIDS prevention, 18, 27–8
  initiation ceremonies, 5
Malema, Julius, 165, 168
malende songs, 170–2, 175
malombo possession dance, 4, 143, 173–4
malwadze dza vhafumakadzi (illnesses of women), 2, 18, 188–91, 197, 201
Mandela, Nelson, 31, 53, 55, 60–1, 165
Maphanda, Edward, 191, 253
Mathase, Solomon, 22, 183–91, 195–7, 200–1, 208, 239, 244–52
Mbeki, Thabo, 15, 17, 30, 116–18, 206
medical ethnomusicology, 199–202
men
  as peer educators, 137
  zwilombe guitar songs, 22, 180–202
menstruation
  rituals, 102–5
  taboos, 188–90
Mfecane, 8, 42, 45
milayo laws, initiation ceremonies, 92–3, 101–2, 154
Modise, Joe '*Ntate*', 1, 168
Modjadji (rain queen), 43
Mokaba, Peter, 167
Motsoaledi, Aaron, 17, 121
Movement for Democracy (MDM), 55–6
Mphephu royal house
  foundation of, 45
  government of Venda, 49–50, 53–5
  removal from power, 54–5
  rivalry with Tshivhase, 26, 32–3, 40–1, 45–7, 57–9, 64–5

Mphephu, Patrick, 33, 46, 49–50, 53, 57–9
Mphephu, Toni, 33, 46, 60–1, 64
Mudau, Baldwin, 49, 55
Mufamadi, Sydney, 13, 38
mufarakano (secret lover), 107, 196, 212
Mukoma (petty headman), position of, 26n1, 37, 66
Mukwevho, Colbert, reggae band, 21, 23
Mukwevho lineage, 23
Muofhe of Tsianda, 58
murundu initiation ceremony, 4, 5
Mushasha Commission, 54, 71
mushonga/muti (medicine), 210–11
music
  initiation ceremonies, 4–7
  medical ethnomusicology, 199–202. *See also* songs
musivheto initiation ceremony, 7, 77n4, 94n17, 172
muti murders, 9, 108, 210–11

National House of Traditional Leaders, 37
ndayo dances, 93–4, 107
neoliberalism, 14
Netshitenzhe, Joel, 13
Nevirapine, 119, 162
New Partnership for Africa's Development (NEPAD), 30
ngoma (rituals of affliction), 4, 105, 174
Ngona. *See* Vhangona ethnic groups
Ngwane, Z., 108–9
Nhlapo Commission, 38–41, 54, 65, 71–2, 236
non-governmental organisations (NGOs)
  AIDS prevention, 119–20, 123–6
  health-related, 115
Nxumalo, Mpisane Eric, 39

occult economy, 221
Oomen, B. 35–6

paramountcy. *See Khosikhulu*
participatory approach, peer education, 129–32
peer educators
  activities, 115, 135–7, 180, 223
  aims, 3–4, 114–16
  attitudes to, 222–4
  biomedical knowledge, 7, 240
  employment status, 150–2
  home-based care (HBC), 148–9, 153, 179, 225–7
  male recruits, 137
  motivations, 146–52
  participatory approach, 129–32
  performances, 1–2, 137–41
  recruitment, 133–4
  religious affiliation, 141–6

peer educators (cont.)
  researching, 24
  sex workers, 133–4, 140–1, 142
  songs, 1–2, 4–5, 6–7, 24–5, 154–80, 199–200
  training, 134–5
  as vectors of AIDS, 3, 204, 223–5, 231
  Venda, 132–41
  voluntary counselling and testing (VCT), 147, 178
poisonings, 219–22
politics, traditional, 26–31
poverty reduction, 14
Project Support Group (PSG), 126, 133, 225
promiscuity, as cause of AIDS, 192
prostitution. *See* sex workers

Radio Freedom, 165–6, 167
radio jive, 166–7
Ralinala, Noriah Lowani Mbudziseni, 79–80, 85–9, 97–8, 110–11, 174n19, 236
Ralushai Commission, 40–1, 54
Ralushai, Victor, 42–3
Ramabulana, Makhado, 46
Ramabulana, Mphephu, 46
Ramaphosa, Cyril, 13
Ramushwana, Gabriel, 54–5, 64
Rathogwa, Chief, 216–18, 230
Ravele, Frank, 53–4, 57, 58n27
Reconstruction and Development Programme (RDP), 14
religion
  and initiation ceremonies, 89–92
  and peer educators, 141–6, 160
ritual knowledge. *See* traditional knowledge
royalty, distinction from commoners, 5, 42, 44–5, 91–2
rumour, 211–30

salempore girls, 89–90, 143
Sandile, Archie Velile, 40
Sapekoe, 51
Sarafina, 2, 118–19
schools, AIDS education, 103–9
secrecy, about AIDS, 204–10
Sefularo, Molefi, 121
Sekhukhune, Kgagudi Kenneth, 40
Seven Days poison, 211–22, 227–30
sex workers, 11–12, 196–7
  as peer educators, 133–4, 140–1, 142
sexual health
  and *vhusha* initiation ceremonies, 101–5, 192–3
  women, 188–91
sexually transmitted infections, 189–90.
  See also HIV/AIDS

Shaka, 8, 43
Sigcawu, Zwelidumile, 40
Simmel, G., 205
Singo clans, 44–5
Sisulu, Walter, 60, 165
social reproduction, crisis, 16, 26–7, 75, 180, 196, 232–4
songs
  adaptation of lyrics, 159–64, 168–70, 178
  anthropological analysis, 156–9
  genres, 155
  original songs, 176–8
  peer educators, 1–2, 4–5, 6–7, 24–5, 154–80, 199–200
  struggle songs, 164–70, 178
  traditional songs, 170–6
  zwilombe guitar songs, 22, 180–91. *See also* music
Sotho-Tswana, intergenerational relations, 108–9
South African Broadcasting Corporation (SABC), 166–7
South African National AIDS Council (SANAC), 119
South African Terrorism Act (1967), 55
Soutpansberg Mountains, 5, 42–3
Stadler, J. J., 110, 206, 208–9, 228
Stayt, H., 95, 103, 189, 213

tea estates, 51, 69, 221–2
Terreblanche, Eugene, 165
Tambo, Oliver, 165
Thohoyandou, 45
Thovhela (king), position of, 26n1, 37
Thulare, Thulare Victor, 40
Tomlinson Commission, 50–1
tourism, 8, 70
toyi toyi dance, 58, 166
tradition, politics of, 26–31, 75–6, 234–6
traditional healers (*inyanga*), 189n7, 190–1, 211
traditional knowledge
  and AIDS, 7, 17–19, 74–5, 198–9
  and biomedical knowledge, 74–5, 107–11, 236–41
  and experience, 193–8, 229–30, 237–8
  and initiation ceremonies, 77–80, 98–101, 105–11
traditional leadership
  apartheid period, 47–59
  post-apartheid, 31–41, 59–71
  pre-colonial, 41–7
  rivalry, 23, 26, 32–3, 40–1, 45–7, 56–9
Traditional Leadership and Governance Framework Act (2003), 36–8
traditional songs, AIDS education, 170–6

Index

transactional relationships, women, 11–12, 133–4, 196–7
Transkei
  intergenerational relations, 108–9
  paramountcy, 40
Transkei, Venda, Bophuthatswana, and Ciskei (TVBC states), 47
Treatment Action Campaign (TAC), 119, 125, 163
Tshabalala-Msimang, Manto, 116–17, 118, 120
Tshakhuma, peer education project, 132
tshifhase performance, 173–6
tshigombela songs, 7, 170, 175
Tshikombani
  leadership rivalries, 67
  peer education project, 132, 159–61
tshikona reed dance, 4, 5, 6, 67–9, 75–6
tshilombe. See zwilombe
Tshivenda language, 9
Tshivhase royal house
  foundation of, 45
  kings of, 60
  rivalry with Mphephu, 23, 26, 32–3, 40–1, 45–7, 57–9, 64–5
Tshivhase, A. A., 58
Tshivhase, John Shavhani, 59, 62
Tshivhase, Kennedy, King, 22
  consolidation of power, 65–71
  at Dopeni Project, 81–5
  and girls' initiation ceremonies, 79, 85–6, 91–2, 235–6
  paramountcy bid, 71–2, 162n6, 221n15, 234
  rise to power, 59–64
  support for, 184
  and traditional culture, 32–4, 233, 235–7
Tshivhase, Mushaisano, 23
Tshivhase, Muzila, 61
Tshivhase, Prince Thohoyandou, 59, 61
Tshivhase, Ratsimphi Frans ('Mphaya'), 31–2, 59–60, 61
Tshivhase Development Trust (TDT), 69–70, 221n15
Tshivhase Territorial Authority (TTA), 62–3, 66–7
Tshivhase Tribal Council (TTC), 62
Turner, Victor, 99, 157, 239

Uganda, AIDS education, 199
United Democratic Front (UDF), 55–6
United States, President's Emergency Plan for AIDS Relief (PEPFAR), 28, 117

van Warmelo, N. J., 103–4
Vele-la-Mbeu, 44–5

Venda
  apartheid period leadership, 47–55
  electoral support, 13–14
  kingship hierarchy, 36–7
  origin myth, 42–3
  peer education, 132–41
  post-apartheid leadership, 55–71
  pre-colonial social structure, 42–7
  socio-economic situation, 7–15
  stereotypes, 8–9
Venda Agricultural Corporation Ltd. See Agriven
Venda Development Corporation (VDC), 51–2
Venda Independence People's Party (VIPP), 49–50, 55
Venda National Party (VNP), 49, 55
Venda Sun Hotel, 52
vhakololo (royalty), distinction from commoners (*vhasiwana*), 5, 42, 44–5, 91–2
Vhamusanda/Gota (headman)
  installation of, 33–4, 65–9, 75–6
  position of, 26n1, 37
Vhangona ethnic groups, 5, 23, 43–5
vhasiwana (commoners), distinction from royalty (*vhakololo*), 5, 42, 44–5, 91–2
Vhavenda, ethnic identity, 8–9
Vhembe District Municipality, electoral support, 13
vhuhosi (installation of headmen), 33–4, 65–9, 75–6
vhusha initiation ceremonies, 4, 77, 79, 85–113
  and AIDS education, 97–8, 106–11, 112–13, 236–7
  hierarchy of authority, 98–101
  intergeneration relations, 108–9
  ludodo performance, 94–8, 105–9, 236
  milayo laws, 92–3, 101–2
  ndayo dances, 93–4, 107
  payment, 99
  and religion, 89–92
  researcher's access to, 85–7
  revival of, 88–9
  ritual knowledge, 105–11, 237–8
  for royalty or commoners, 91–2
  and sexual health, 101–5, 192–3
  songs, 172–3, 175
  stages of, 99–101
vhutungu (poison), 209–10
Virodene, 118–19
voluntary counselling and testing (VCT), 147, 178
Voluntary Services Overseas (VSO, UK), 125
Voortrekkers, 46

witchcraft, 9, 19, 206–7
women
  as causes of AIDS, 18–19, 180–1, 184, 188–91, 196–7
  'polluted', 188–91, 192
  rights, 63
  status, 12, 115
  transactional relationships, 11–12, 133–4. *See also* girls

Xhosa, circumcision, 28

Zion Christian Church (ZCC)
  and initiation ceremonies, 90–2
  peer educators, 142–4
  songs, 155, 160–1
Zulus
  circumcision, 27, 28
  kings, 39–40
Zuma, Jacob, 15, 121, 165, 168
Zwelethini, Goodwill, King, 27, 28, 39
Zwiakonda, 216, 232
'*Zwidzumbe*' (Secrets), 183–91, 200–1, 209, 244–9
zwilombe (guitar songs), 22, 181–92
zwilonda (genital sores), 188, 189, 192

TITLES IN THE SERIES

42 FRASER G. MCNEILL
    AIDS, Politics, and Music in South Africa
41 KRIJN PETERS
    War and the Crisis of Youth in Sierra Leone
40 INSA NOLTE
    Obafemi Awolowo and the Making of Remo: the local politics of a Nigerian nationalist
39 BEN JONES
    Beyond the State in Rural Uganda
38 RAMON SARRÓ
    The Politics of Religious Change on the Upper Guinea Coast: iconoclasm done and undone
37 CHARLES GORE
    Art, Performance and Ritual in Benin City
36 FERDINAND DE JONG
    Masquerades of Modernity: power and secrecy in Casamance, Senegal
35 KAI KRESSE
    Philosophising in Mombasa: knowledge, Islam and intellectual practice on the Swahili coast
34 DAVID PRATTEN
    The Man-Leopard Murders: history and society in colonial Nigeria
33 CAROLA LENTZ
    Ethnicity and the Making of History in Northern Ghana
32 BENJAMIN F. SOARES
    Islam and the Prayer Economy: history and authority in a Malian town
31 COLIN MURRAY and PETER SANDERS
    Medicine Murder in Colonial Lesotho: the anatomy of a moral crisis
30 R. M. DILLEY
    Islamic and Caste Knowledge Practices Among Haalpulaar'en in Senegal: between mosque and termite mound
29 BELINDA BOZZOLI
    Theatres of Struggle and the End of Apartheid
28 ELISHA REENE
    Population and Progress in a Yoruba Town
27 ANTHONY SIMPSON
    'Half-London' in Zambia: contested identities in a Catholic mission school
26 HARRI ENGLUND
    From War to Peace on the Mozambique–Malawi Borderland
25 T. C. MCCASKIE
    Asante Identities: history and modernity in an African village 1850–1950
24 JANET BUJRA
    Serving Class: masculinity and the feminisation of domestic service in Tanzania
23 CHRISTOPHER O. DAVID
    Death in Abeyance: illness and therapy among the Tabwa of Central Africa
22 DEBORAH JAMES
    Songs of the Women Migrants: performance and identity in South Africa
21 BIRGIT MEYER
    Translating the Devil: religion and modernity among the Ewe in Ghana

20 DAVID MAXWELL
Christians and Chiefs in Zimbabwe: a social history of the Hwesa people c. 1870s–1990s
19 A. FIONA D. MACKENZIE
Land, Ecology and Resistance in Kenya, 1880–1952
18 JANE I. GUYER
An African Niche Economy: farming to feed Ibadan, 1968–88
17 PHILIP BURNHAM
The Politics of Cultural Difference in Northern Cameroon
16 GRAHAM FURNISS
Poetry, Prose and Popular Culture in Hausa
15 C. BAWA YAMBA
Permanent Pilgrims: the role of pilgrimage in the lives of West African Muslims in Sudan
14 TOM FORREST
The Advance of African Capital: the growth of Nigerian private enterprise
13 MELISSA LEACH
Rainforest Relations: gender and resource use among the Mende of Gola, Sierra Leone
12 ISAAC NCUBE MAZONDE
Ranching and Enterprise in Eastern Botswana: a case study of black and white farmers
11 G. S. EADES
Strangers and Traders: Yoruba migrants, markets and the state in northern Ghana
10 COLIN MURRAY
Black Mountain: land, class and power in the eastern Orange Free State, 1880s to 1980s
9 RICHARD WERBNER
Tears of the Dead: the social biography of an African family
8 RICHARD FARDON
Between God, the Dead and the Wild: Chamba interpretations of religion and ritual
7 KARIN BARBER
I Could Speak Until Tomorrow: oriki, *women and the past in a Yoruba town*
6 SUZETTE HEALD
Controlling Anger: the sociology of Gisu violence
5 GUNTHER SCHLEE
Identities on the Move: clanship and pastoralism in northern Kenya
4 JOHAN POTTIER
Migrants No More: settlement and survival in Mambwe villages, Zambia
3 PAUL SPENCER
The Maasai of Matapato: a study of rituals of rebellion
2 JANE I. GUYER (ed.)
Feeding African Cities: essays in social history
1 SANDRA T. BARNES
Patrons and Power: creating a political community in metropolitan Lagos

For EU product safety concerns, contact us at Calle de José Abascal, 56–1°, 28003 Madrid, Spain or eugpsr@cambridge.org.

www.ingramcontent.com/pod-product-compliance
Lightning Source LLC
LaVergne TN
LVHW091531060526
838200LV00036B/566